NOVEL DELIVERY SYSTEMS FOR ORAL VACCINES

Edited by

Derek T. O'Hagan, Ph.D.
Director, Vaccine Formulation
United Biomedical, Inc.
Hauppauge, New York

CRC Press
Boca Raton   Ann Arbor   London   Tokyo

Library of Congress-in-Publication Data

Novel delivery systems for oral vaccines / edited by Derek T. O'Hagan.
     p.   cm.
Includes bibliographical references and index.
ISBN 0-8493-4866-8
    1. Oral vaccines--Administration.   2. Drug delivery systems.
I. O'Hagan, Derek T.
    [DNLM: 1. Drug Delivery Systems.   2. Vaccines--administration &
dosage.   3. Administraton, Oral.   QW 805 N937 1994]
RM281.N68   1994
615'.372--dc20
DNLM/DLC
for Library of Congress   93-40167
                                                         CIP

PREFACE

This book represents a timely and detailed assessment of the wide range of alternative 'antigen carriers' that are currently being investigated as prospective delivery systems for the development of new and improved oral vaccines. Oral delivery remains the "ideal" approach to vaccination, both for economic reasons and for reasons of patient acceptability. However, the oral route of immunization remains under exploited clinically, mainly because oral vaccines have traditionally proven poorly immunogenic. Nevertheless, recent developments in the formulation of nonliving antigen carrier systems, e.g., microparticles and liposomes, and in the development of live nonpathogenic carrier systems, e.g., Salmonella and Adenovirus, have given rise to real optimism that new oral vaccines will soon be developed. These new vaccines are likely to be developed both against diseases that are currently poorly controlled, e.g., diarrheal diseases, and also against diseases for which vaccines do not currently exist, e.g., many sexually transmitted diseases. It is with these new developments in antigen delivery systems that this book is concerned. Each alternative carrier system is assessed, including both its potential advantages and limitations. Furthermore, the book includes detailed considerations of "if and how" these antigen delivery systems might find applications in the development of new and improved oral vaccines for human use. This book should appeal both to clinicians and administrators involved in vaccination policy nationally and internationally and also to researchers involved in the development of antigen delivery systems and novel vaccines.

THE EDITOR

Derek T. O'Hagan, Ph.D., is Director of Vaccine Formulation at United Biomedical, Inc. in Hauppauge, New York.

Dr. O'Hagan graduated in 1983 from the Department of Pharmaceutical Sciences at the University of Nottingham, U.K., with a Bachelor of Pharmacy Degree with Honours. In 1988, he graduated again from Nottingham with a Ph.D. entitled "Pharmaceutical formulations as immunological adjuvants." He served as a Lecturer in Drug Delivery in the Department of Pharmaceutical Sciences at Nottingham from 1989 until his present position at United Biomedical in 1993.

Dr. O'Hagan is a member of the Royal Pharmaceutical Society of Great Britain (since qualification in 1984), the British Society for Immunology, the Society for General Microbiology, the European Adjuvant Group, the Society for Controlled Release and the Society for Mucosal Immunology.

Dr. O'Hagan has published over 40 research papers and has presented papers at many international meetings. His major research interests include the design, formulation, and characterization of antigen delivery systems for parenteral, oral, nasal, and vaginal immunization.

CONTRIBUTORS

Louis Alexander
Department of Microbiology
State University of New York
 at Stony Brook
Stony Brook, New York

Alan D. T. Barrett
Molecular Microbiology Group
School of Biological Sciences
University of Surrey
Guildford, Surrey, United Kingdom

Bheem M. Bhat
Biotechnology and Microbiology
 Division
Wyeth-Ayerst Research
Philadelphia, Pennsylvania

Steve N. Chatfield
Vaccine Research
Medeva Group Research
Department of Biochemistry
Imperial College of Science,
 Technology, and Medicine
London, England

Noel K. Childers
Departments of Microbiology and
 Community and Public Health Dentistry
School of Dentistry
University of Alabama at Birmingham
Birmingham, Alabama

Cecil Czerkinsky
Department of Medical Microbiology
 and Immunology
University of Göteborg
Göteborg, Sweden

Jeremy W. Dale
Molecular Microbiology Group
School of Biological Sciences
University of Surrey
Guildford, Surrey, United Kingdom

Alan R. Davis
Biotechnology and Microbiology
 Division
Wyeth-Ayerst Research
Philadelphia, Pennsylvania

Odir A. Dellagostin
Molecular Microbiology Group
School of Biological Sciences
University of Surrey
Guildford, Surrey, United Kingdom

Gordon Dougan
Department of Biochemistry
Imperial College of Science,
 Technology, and Medicine
London, England

Bruce D. Forrest
Director, Clinical Development
United Biomedical, Inc.
Hauppauge, New York

Jan Holmgren
Department of Medical Microbiology
 and Immunology
University of Göteborg
Göteborg, Sweden

Elisabeth Hörnquist
Department of Medical Microbiology
 and Immunology
University of Göteborg
Göteborg, Sweden

Paul P. Hung
Biotechnology and Microbiology
 Division
Wyeth-Ayerst Research
Philadelphia, Pennsylvania

Hui-Hua Lu
Department of Microbiology
State University of New York
 at Stony Brook
Stony Brook, New York

Michael D. Lubeck
Biotechnology and Microbiology
 Division
Wyeth-Ayerst Research
Philadelphia, Pennsylvania

Nils Lycke
Department of Medical Microbiology
 and Immunology
University of Göteborg
Göteborg, Sweden

Kevin J. Maloy
Department of Immunology
University of Glasgow
Western Infirmary
Glasgow, Scotland, United Kingdom

Johnjoe McFadden
Molecular Microbiology Group
School of Biological Sciences
University of Surrey
Guildford, Surrey, United Kingdom

Suzanne M. Michalek
Department of Microbiology
University of Alabama at Birmingham
Birmingham, Alabama

Allan McI. Mowat
Department of Immunology
University of Glasgow
Western Infirmary
Glasgow, Scotland, United Kingdom

Elizabeth Norman
Molecular Microbiology Group
School of Biological Sciences
University of Surrey
Guildford, Surrey, United Kingdom

Derek T. O'Hagan
Director, Vaccine Formulation
United Biomedical, Inc.
Hauppauge, New York

Mark Roberts
Vaccine Research
Medeva Group Research
Department of Biochemistry
Imperial College of Science,
 Technology, and Medicine
London, England

G. J. Russell-Jones
Department of Immunology
Biotech Australia Pty, Ltd.
Roseville, New South Wales, Australia

Eckard Wimmer
Department of Microbiology
State University of New York
 at Stony Brook
Stony Brook, New York

TABLE OF CONTENTS

Oral Immunization and the Common Mucosal Immune System

Derek T. O'Hagan

TABLE OF CONTENTS

I. INTRODUCTION

Oral immunization has a long-established tradition in vaccine research, and the first attempt to induce immunity more than 2000 years ago was apparently undertaken by the oral route.[1] The long history of oral immunization has been discussed in detail by Mestecky and McGhee.[2] The first book on oral immunization was published more than 60 years ago,[3] and the oral polio vaccine has been licensed for administration to humans since 1960. However, although it has been suggested that almost all vaccines could eventually be delivered by this route,[4] the oral route of immunization remains underexploited clinically.

Traditionally, vaccine research has been mainly concerned with the induction of systemic immunity through parenteral immunization, mainly involving the intramuscular or subcutaneous routes. While this approach may be appropriate against diseases caused by infectious agents which gain systemic access to the body through punctured or damaged skin, e.g., tetanus, it is widely acknowledged that the majority of pathogens naturally infect hosts through the mucosal routes, either orally, nasally, or genitally. In general, parenteral vaccines do not induce mucosal immunity, which is mediated mainly through the production of secretory immunoglobulin A (sIgA). The limited ability of parenteral vaccines to induce protective immunity against mucosally acquired pathogens

0-8493-4866-8/94/$0.00+$.50

1

may be illustrated with reference to cholera vaccines. The older parenteral vaccines offered only limited protection and showed a high incidence of adverse effects, while a new oral vaccine is effective after a single dose, with an improved safety profile.[5]

Oral vaccines are likely to be more effective at preventing or limiting mucosal infections due to their ability to induce a sIgA response. In addition, oral vaccines offer several significant advantages over parenteral vaccines. These advantages include easier administration, reduced side-effects, and the potential for almost unlimited frequency of boosting, without the need for trained personnel. Furthermore, oral vaccines will be safer than parenteral vaccines, since the protective barrier of the skin will not be breached during administration. Moreover, the avoidance of the use of needles will eliminate the possible risks of contamination and cross-infection due to reuse. In addition, the purchase cost of the needles would be eliminated. Since a product for oral administration will not be required to be manufactured under such stringent conditions as a parenteral product, oral vaccines would also be cheaper to produce. The cost of vaccines to the developing world is an important issue, and the development of less expensive vaccines would have a significant and favorable impact on the extent of vaccine coverage worldwide. Vaccines are already the most efficient and cost-effective means for disease prevention, but only 12% of the total costs for vaccination is to pay for the vaccine. The remainder is for operational costs, including trained personnel, transportation, and the maintenance of the cold chain.[6] Trained personnel would not be required to administer oral vaccines, and this is a major attraction. Clearly, oral vaccines would be particularly advantageous in the developing world, where it is often difficult for health care workers to gain access to the population to be immunized. Hence, many of the currently available vaccines would be considerably improved if they could be administered orally. Furthermore, improvements in the design of novel antigen delivery systems may allow the development of new vaccines against diseases which are currently poorly controlled, e.g., infections caused by rotavirus, influenza virus, *Escherichia coli, Shigellae, Vibrio cholerae,* and *Salmonella typhi.*

Nevertheless, despite considerable advances in recent years in understanding of the initiation, control, and maintenance of the secretory immune response, success with oral immunization has proven elusive. Degradation of antigens in the gastrointestinal tract (GIT), limited absorption, interaction with nonspecific host factors, inadequate delivery systems, and pre-existing immunity have all contrived to negatively influence the outcome following oral immunization. However, recent research has resulted in the development of several novel antigen delivery systems for oral administration. These novel delivery systems include live vectors such as salmonella, *Yersinia enterocolitica,* Bacille Calmette Guérin (BCG), adenovirus, poliovirus, and vaccinia virus, along with nonreplicating antigen carriers such as microparticles, liposomes, immune-stimulating complexes, cholera toxin, and lectins. In experimental studies, these delivery systems have been shown to induce secretory and systemic immunity to expressed, incorporated, or conjugated antigens. There are two general strategies which may be adopted for the development of improved oral vaccines. The first involves live bacterial and viral vectors which may be modified genetically to express selected antigens from unrelated microorganisms. As an alternative to this approach, microorganisms may be genetically manipulated to render them nonpathogenic but still capable of inducing protective immunity. Hence, rationally attenuated vaccines may be developed in which a known and well-defined genetic lesion has been introduced into the organism. For safety purposes, reversion of the microorganism to pathogenicity should be rendered impossible, or at least extremely unlikely. This may be achieved by selection of an appropriate site for genetic manipulation, or by the size of the genetic lesion introduced. The second approach to the development of improved oral vaccines involves the formulation of antigens into nonliving carrier systems, which are capable of protecting antigens against degradation and delivering them into the gut-associated lymphoid tissue (GALT). It is these recent developments in novel antigen delivery systems with which this book is concerned.

II. THE COMMON MUCOSAL IMMUNE SYSTEM

Prior to 1963 when sIgA was first identified, it was widely believed that serum antibody "spilled over" into the external secretions to provide mucosal antibodies. However, it is now firmly established that secretory immunity is induced and regulated by mechanisms distinct and separate from those involved in the regulation of systemic immunity. The overwhelming evidence supporting the existence of a mucosal immune system has been reviewed by Mestecky.[7] This evidence includes the observations that sIgA is predominantly locally synthesized and is transported across the epithelium into the mucosal secretions following interaction with a specific receptor produced by the epithelial cells, the secretory component (SC) (Figure 1). It has been shown that intravenously administered IgA appears in intestinal and salivary secretions at only low concentrations.[8,9] Moreover, although patients with IgA multiple myeloma show very high levels of IgA in blood, only trace amounts are found in the saliva.[10]

Accumulated experimental evidence demonstrates that the immune responses at mucosal sites are linked through the existence of a common mucosal immune system (CMIS). Consequently, oral immunization may result in the induction of secretory immune responses at all the mucosal sites. The CMIS is linked by emigrating antigen-stimulated IgA precursor cells, which are induced in the Peyer's patches (Figure 1). These IgA-committed cells are stimulated by antigens absorbed through the M cells, which are specialized "antigen-sampling" cells found in the epithelium of the Peyer's patches.[11] Thus, the Peyer's patches are the inductive sites for mucosal immunity and constitute the most important structural units of the GALT. The IgA-committed lymphoblasts leave the Peyer's patches in the mesenteric lymph and, via the thoracic duct, they enter the systemic circulation. Subsequently, they localize in mucosal tissues through interaction with specific cellular receptors on high endothelial venules.[12] Within the mucosal tissues, e.g., the lamina propria of the gut and the respiratory tract, the lymphoblasts mature into plasma cells and secrete IgA.[13] The sIgA is then transported through the epithelial cells after interaction with the SC.

The most convincing evidence for the existence of the CMIS comes from studies which have demonstrated the induction of secretory antibody responses at distant mucosal sites, e.g., tears, saliva, and genital secretions, following oral immunization.

A. IN ANIMAL MODELS

The CMIS in animals has been substantiated by lymphocyte migration studies,[12] by morphological studies,[11] and by studies showing that the Peyer's patches are an enriched source of IgA precursor cells.[14] Studies have shown migration of mesenteric lymph node lymphoblasts and T cells to the mammary glands, the salivary glands, the genital tract and the ocular system.[15] Numerous studies in mice, rats, guinea pigs, hamsters, pigs, and monkeys with a range of antigens have shown the induction of sIgA responses in saliva and the secretions of the lachrimal, bronchial, and genital tracts. Most of the studies on rodents have consistently shown the induction of a sIgA response in saliva, colostrum, and tears following oral immunization.[15]

B. IN HUMANS

Evidence for a CMIS in humans is necessarily indirect, because of the impossibility of performing studies involving adoptive transfer of lymphocytes. Nevertheless, the presence of specific antibodies in the secretions of mucosal sites which have not been directly exposed to the antigen offers compelling evidence.[15] The evidence for a CMIS in humans

4

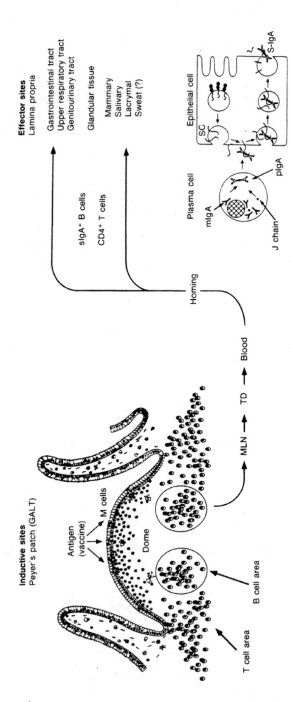

Figure 1 M cell uptake of antigens by the Peyer's patches (inductive sites) of the (GALT) sensitizes IgA-committed B cells and CD4⁺ T helper cells, which migrate via the mesenteric lymph nodes (MLN) and the thoracic duct (TD) into the blood. The cells then localize in the mucosae (effector sites), and IgA is produced by plasma cells, which have developed from the migrating B cells. Polymeric IgA (pIgA) is formed from monomeric IgA (mIgA) by the J (joining) chain and is transported through the epithelial cells after interaction with the SC to produce sIgA. (From O'Hagan, D.T., *Clin. Pharmacokin.*, 22, 1, 1992. With permission.)

is as follows: (1) oral immunization with bacteria and viruses induces a sIgA response in saliva, milk, and tears, often with little response in the serum. (2) Specific IgA antibody-secreting cells (ASC) have been detected in the peripheral blood of patients following oral immunization, and the appearance of the ASC precedes the appearance of sIgA in saliva and tears. (3) After culture *in vitro,* the IgA produced by the ASC shows the same isotype distributions and characteristics as sIgA produced in mucosal secretions.[15-17] Hence, the available evidence from humans suggests that the regulation and induction of mucosal immunity does not differ significantly from that seen in animals models.

III. MUCOSAL IMMUNITY

There are approximately (1×10^{10}) immunoglobulin-producing cells per meter of human intestine,[18] and these cells represent >75% of the total number of immunoglobulin cells in the body. Therefore, it is not surprising that sIgA accounts for approximately two thirds of the total immunoglobulins produced daily in humans.[13,19] The quantitative preeminence of IgA over alternative immunoglobulins is necessary because of the physiological role of sIgA, which is responsible for providing protection on the mucosal surfaces of the body. The GIT, respiratory, and genitourinary tracts represent a huge surface area requiring protection against many pathogens which first interact with the host at these sites. Protective mucosal immunity is mainly mediated through the local production of sIgA.

A. SECRETORY IMMUNOGLOBULIN A

Secretory IgA is a polymeric immunoglobulin, comprising two or more IgA monomers, the J chain which binds the monomers together, and the SC. The synthesis, structure, and functions of sIgA have been reviewed in detail.[13] Several of the important functions of sIgA are shown in Table 1. Since sIgA is polymeric, it has greater binding capacity than monomeric IgA and is more effective at virus neutralization.[20,21] In addition, the multivalence of sIgA allows it to more efficiently agglutinate bacteria. Secretory IgA has also been shown to neutralize bacterial toxins and enzymes.[22] Since sIgA is resistant to proteolysis, it is only slowly inactivated in the secretions.[23]

In humans, serum IgA is mainly monomeric, while IgA in the external secretions is dimeric or polymeric. Human IgA exists in two subclasses (IgA1 and IgA2), which appear in serum and secretions in different proportions.[24] In rodents, the serum IgA is polymeric and appears to have a role in clearing intestinally absorbed antigens in bile after binding to hepatocytes.[25] Thus in rodents, IgA limits antigen absorption through "immune exclusion" and also clears from the circulation small amounts of antigens that may be absorbed. The function of serum IgA in humans is unknown, but it may have a role in mediating inflammation.

Table 1 **Important biological functions of secretory IgA**

Neutralization of viruses, toxins and enzymes
Inhibition of adherence of microorganisms to mucosal surfaces; blocking of adhesins, alteration of charge and hydrophobicity of microorganisms, agglutination and entrapment in mucus
Immune exclusion of macromolecules and bacterial toxins
Suppression of antibody mediated inflammatory responses at mucosal surfaces
Synergism with innate antibacterial factors, including lactoferrin, peroxidase, and lysozyme
Clearance of absorbed antigen from the circulation
Interference with plasmid-mediated virulence determinants

1. Virus Neutralization by IgA

Although little is known about the mechanisms involved in virus neutralization,[26] neutralizing antibodies of the IgA, IgG, and IgM isotypes have been described. The ability of sIgA to neutralize the infectivity of influenza virus was demonstrated by Taylor and Dimmock.[27] It was also shown that the mechanism of neutralization for sIgA was different from that for monomeric IgA and IgG. The binding of influenza virus to a cell monolayer was prevented by sIgA, but not be monomeric IgA or IgG. Thus, it was postulated that sIgA may induce neutralization by interfering with the ability of the virus to attach to cells, or to be internalized. Monomeric IgA and IgG neutralized virus infectivity at a later stage, following internalization of the virus genome into the cell nucleus.[27]

It has recently been shown in a murine model for influenza infection that protection against virus correlated with the levels of local specific IgA.[28] This finding confirmed that of an earlier study, which showed that the presence of local IgA antibodies in the nasal cavities of mice correlated better with protection against an influenza virus challenge than the presence of serum IgG antibodies.[29] Furthermore, intranasal instillation of mouse anti-IgA has been shown to inhibit immunity to reinfection to homologous influenza virus, which is normally induced by prior infection.[30] Protection against influenza virus infection in humans has also been shown to correlate better with the presence of local antibodies in the nasal cavity than serum antibodies.[31] Nevertheless, although a positive correlation between the presence of sIgA in the nasal cavity and protection against influenza virus was described, no proof of a causal relationship was established. However, a causal relationship between local antiviral IgA antibodies and protection against infection was demonstrated in a study by Mazanec et al.[32] In this study, intranasal instillation of specific antiviral monoclonal IgA was shown to protect against Sendai virus infection in mice. It has also been demonstrated that intravenously administered polymeric IgA was transported across the nasal epithelium of mice and provided local protection against challenge with influenza virus.[33]

Monoclonal IgA has been shown to be of comparable efficacy to monoclonal IgG in providing passive protection in the respiratory tract of mice against Sendai virus infection.[34] However, IgA responses are more likely to be effective in providing clinical protection, since IgA and not IgG, is selectively transported into the airways. The unique characteristics of sIgA, including its polymeric nature, its ability to bind to mucus, and its resistance to proteolytic enzymes, all contribute to its efficiency in neutralizing viruses, including polio, echo, coxsackie, and adenovirus.[35] Recent studies have indicated that IgA may also mediate mucosal protection through intra-epithelial virus neutralization.[35a]

2. Antibacterial Activity of IgA

It is difficult to directly demonstrate the ability of sIgA to provide protection against pathogens, mainly due to the problems of obtaining sufficient quantities of well-characterized sIgA. However, a method has recently been developed to allow the production of IgA hybridomas from Peyer's patch cells.[36] Using this technique, it has been possible to demonstrate that monoclonal IgA directed against a single surface epitope of *Vibrio cholerae* can protect neonatal mice against a normally lethal dose of vibrios.[37] It has also been demonstrated in mice that monoclonal IgA can protect against infections caused by *Salmonella typhimurium*[38] and *Helicobacter felis*.[39] The latter study, involving *H. felis*, indicated for the first time that the stomach may also be part of the CMIS.[39]

The ability of sIgA to inhibit the binding of bacteria to mucosal surfaces is partly due to specific interactions with surface proteins and partly due to nonspecific interactions. Secretory IgA is particularly efficient at preventing bacterial attachment because of its multiple binding sites.[40,41] The antibacterial activity of sIgA is enhanced by its ability to potentiate the activity of innate antibacterial factors, such as lactoferrin,[42] peroxidases,[43] and lysozyme.[44] Secretory IgA has also been shown to exert antibacterial activity through an indirect mechanism, involving antibody-dependent cell-mediated cytotoxicity (ADCC). The antibacterial activity of monocytes and lymphocytes may be enhanced by sIgA, and T cells with bound IgA have been shown to effectively kill *Salmonella* and *Shigella*.[45]

3. Immune Exclusion

In association with "immune regulation" and "immune elimination", immune exclusion is thought to provide a protective barrier at mucosal surfaces to the unrestricted absorption of antigens and microorganisms (Figure 2).[46] Immune exclusion represents the "first line" of defence against pathogens and is mediated mainly through sIgA, which acts in cooperation with nonspecific defense mechanisms. It is thought that sIgA binds to microorganisms, toxins, and antigens in the lumen or the mucus, to prevent their absorption.[47] This hypothesis is supported by studies in patients with selective IgA deficiency, who have circulating immune complexes and precipitating antibodies to absorbed milk proteins.[48] In a recent clinical study in infants, recovery from cow's milk-sensitive enteropathy was shown to correlate positively with the presence of sIgA.[49] Immune exclusion is thought to cooperate with the nonspecific defense mechanisms of the mucosa and to restrict antigen absorption in several ways. In experimental animals, proteolysis of antigens has been shown to be enhanced following oral immunization,[50-52] probably because the formation of immune complexes with sIgA results in enhanced vulnerability of the antigens to digestion. Experimental evidence also suggests that the discharge of mucus from goblet cells may be immunologically mediated.[53,54] Enhanced mucus secretion will restrict the access of antigens to the enterocytes and will also limit absorption. Since immune complexes are cleared from the circulation much more readily than antigens alone,[55] immune mechanisms also restrict antigen circulation after absorption. Recent studies have suggested that IgA may be involved in the excretion of absorbed antigens from the lamina propria through the epithelium.[55a]

Nevertheless, the possibility that sIgA may in some circumstances promote viral infectivity has been raised by a study which showed the uptake of virus-antibody complexes by M cells.[56] Studies have also shown that binding of sIgA to Epstein-Barr virus (EBV) facilitates the uptake of the virus by an epithelial cell line.[57] Thus, it was

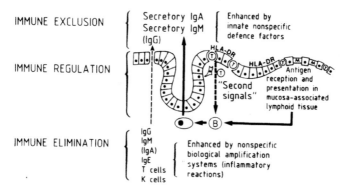

Figure 2 The three main components of mucosal defense: immune exclusion, immune regulation and immune elimination. Antigen stimulation in GALT provides "first signals" to B cells which migrate to secretory sites via the blood. "Second signals" induce local proliferation and terminal differentiation of B cells, and immunoglobulins, mainly sIgA, are transported across epithelial cells into the secretions. (From Brandtzaeg, P., *Acta Otolaryngol. (Stoch.),* 105, 172, 1988. With permission.)

postulated that IgA-mediated transport of EBV through the epithelium might promote the spread of this pathogen.[57]

4. Mediation of Inflammatory Responses by IgA

Secretory IgA may have an important role to play in restricting the development of potentially damaging inflammatory responses within the mucosa. Secretory IgA does not activate complement by either the classical or the alternative pathways, and this may be important in the maintenance of mucosal integrity. Complement activation in the mucosa due to IgG has been shown to cause local damage, which resulted in the absorption of "bystander" antigens.[58] However, the ability of IgA to inhibit complement-mediated lysis of red blood cells sensitized with IgG has been demonstrated.[59] Thus, local inflammatory reactions which could result in enhanced permeability of the mucosa to bystander antigens may be inhibited by IgA. Significantly, sIgA has been shown to be much more effective at mediating complement activation than monomeric IgA.[59] Moreover, IgA antibodies have also been shown to inhibit anaphylactic and Arthus reactions.[60] Consequently, IgA may also have a role in the suppression of hypersensitivity reactions at mucosal surfaces. Hence, a major role of IgA may be to restrict the development of inflammatory responses within the mucosa which could be initiated by alternative immunoglobulin isotypes.

B. CELL-MEDIATED IMMUNITY

Although antibody responses in the GIT are reasonably well characterized, much less is known about T cell responses. The distribution patterns and unusual phenotypes of the intraepithelial T lymphocytes (IEL) suggest that they may play a major role in the regulation of intestinal immunity. However, no role has yet been unequivocally ascribed to the IEL, and antigen specificity has not yet been demonstrated. Functional studies on the IEL are beset by isolation difficulties, which results in problems of sample purity and cell heterogeneity. These problems have all contributed to our failure to adequately define the roles of the IEL. Nevertheless, it is clear that these cells must be involved in the regulation of intestinal immunity, and their possible roles have been discussed.[61] The IEL are abundant in the small intestine and are predominantly CD8+ cells, while the lamina propria lymphocytes (LPL) are predominantly CD4+ cells. Thus, a large proportion of the LPL are of the helper T cell phenotype, and they appear to demonstrate isotype-specific help for IgA-producing plasma cells.[62] While the roles of IEL remain obscure, they may be functional suppressor cells, involved in the mediation of oral tolerance.[61]

A unique subset of T cells has been identified in mouse Peyer's patches, which induce switching of plasma cell precursors to the IgA isotype.[63] Studies in mice have shown that oral immunization preferentially induces T helper type 2 (Th2) cells in Peyer's patches.[64] Moreover, studies with the mucosal adjuvant cholera toxin have shown that oral immunization selectively induces Th2 cells in Peyer's patches and spleens.[64a] Th2 cells are thought to be the major helper cell phenotype involved in mucosal IgA responses in the GIT. Hence, the Peyer's patches may represent a major inductive site for Th2 cells, which support IgA plasma cell responses within the mucosal tissues. The roles of T cells and cytokines in the mucosal immune system has been discussed more extensively by McGhee et al.[17]

IV. FACTORS AFFECTING THE MUCOSAL IMMUNE RESPONSE

Numerous studies have demonstrated the induction of secretory immune responses following oral immunization. Nevertheless, the magnitude and the extent of the responses induced has proven very variable. While many studies have described the induction of potent sIgA responses at several mucosal sites, some have reported only limited responses

Table 2 **Factors that may affect the immune response following oral immunization**

Dose of antigen
Frequency of administration and immunization protocol
The nature of the antigen — live or killed, soluble, or particulate
Age on exposure
Immune status to specific antigen — primed or "virgin" animals
Use of adjuvants and delivery systems
Species immunized

at a single mucosal site.[15] In addition, while some have demonstrated the induction of systemic immunity following oral immunization, others have described the induction of systemic tolerance. The response to oral immunization is dependent upon a number of variables, several of which may be manipulated to increase the likelihood of the desired immune outcome (Table 2).

A. DOSE OF ANTIGEN

It has been shown in many studies that large doses of antigen are needed to induce a sIgA response following oral immunization. Michalek et al.[65] administered 10^{10} organisms of *Streptococcus mutans* daily to induce a salivary antibody response in rats. In man, oral administration with 10^{12} killed *Salmonella* was optimal for the induction of secretory immunity.[66] The dose of live typhoid vaccine (*Salmonella typhi*, Ty21a) administered to humans has been shown to exert a crucial effect on the ability of individuals to produce a secretory immune response. In previously unexposed individuals, only doses of greater than 10^{10} viable organisms were able to induce a mucosal immune response.[67,68] Children under 2 years of age living in an endemic area did not produce immune responses following a dose of 10^9 organisms,[69] and a dose of 10^9 organisms did not offer significant protection for travellers visiting an endemic area.[70] These studies also illustrated the important effect of prior immune exposure on the induction of secretory immunity. Clinical studies with a live oral cholera vaccine (CVD 103-HgR) in 5- to 9-year-old children have demonstrated a dose response relationship.[5] Clinical evidence also suggests that there may be a dose response relationship to oral polio vaccine, and reduced dosages may contribute to limited efficacy in the developing world.[71] The induction of secretory immunity to soluble protein antigens has also been shown to be dose dependent on a number of occasions. However, of more importance is the frequency of antigen exposure and the immunization protocol.

B. IMMUNIZATION PROTOCOL

Challacombe[72] investigated the salivary IgA antibody responses of mice following oral immunization with ovalbumin (OVA) and killed *S. mutans*. Single immunizations did not lead to reproducible antibody responses, nor did weekly immunizations. However, three consecutive daily immunizations induced reproducible salivary IgA antibody responses.[72] Similar findings were reported by Mowat et al.,[73] who showed that several immunizations were necessary to induce secretory IgA responses, and the frequency of exposure was much more important than the antigen dose. Nevertheless, chronic immunization with *S. mutans* resulted in the suppression of serum and salivary antibody responses.[74]

Several large-scale clinical trials have been undertaken to assess the efficacy of the oral typhoid vaccine, Ty21a.[75] Several variables were identified which affected the outcome following oral immunization. One of the most important variables was the interval between doses (Table 3).[76] Additional important variables included the frequency of immunization and the formulation of the vaccine (Table 3). One study was designed

Table 3 **The effects of vaccine formulation and immunization protocol on the protective efficacy of *Salmonella typhi* Ty21a oral vaccine in a large-scale field trial**

Vaccine and (number of doses)	Interval between doses	Number immunized	Protective efficacy (%)
Gelatin capsules with NaHCO₃ (3)	1–2 days	22,379	19
Gelatin capsules with NaHCO₃ (3)	21 days	21,541	31
Enteric-coated capsules (3)	1–2 days	22,170	67
Enteric-coated capsules (3)	21 days	21,590	49

Note: The trial was initiated in Chile in 1983 and the duration of surveillance was 3 years. All subjects enrolled in the trial were aged between 6–21 years. Adapted from Levine, M.M., Ferreccio, C., Black, R.E., Germanier, R., and Chilean Typhoid Commitee, *Lancet,* 1, 1049, 1987.

to assess the number of doses required to induce long-term protection. It was shown that 2 years after immunization, two doses of the vaccine provided 59% protection, while a single dose provided only 29% protection.[77] Another study showed that increasing the number of doses per child within an 8-day period enhanced the protective efficacy of the vaccine.[78]

C. NATURE OF THE ANTIGEN

Generally, secretory immunity is induced most effectively by living rather than killed antigens.[15] In addition, oral immunization with live organisms often results in the induction of systemic immunity.[15] Kantele et al.[79] directly compared the human immune responses to live and killed Ty21a vaccine following oral immunization. Both the live and killed vaccines induced immune responses of similar specificity, with the IgA isotype dominating. However, the response to the live vaccine was significantly more potent and longer lasting.[79] Organisms which colonize the GALT have been shown to induce potent mucosal immune responses following oral immunization.[80]

Although soluble antigens do not normally induce antibody responses following oral immunization, they may be rendered more immunogenic by presenting them to the immune system in an alternative form. Oral immunization in mice with large amounts of soluble OVA does not normally result in the induction of an immune response. However, expression of OVA in *E. coli* renders the protein strongly immunogenic by the oral route.[81] The enhanced immunogenicity may be partially due to the protection against degradation afforded the antigen by its presentation in a bacterial cell. Nevertheless, perhaps of more significance, is the inherent adjuvant activity provided by the bacterial antigen-presenting system.[82] Expression in a bacterium may also promote antigen uptake into Peyer's patches.

It is a longstanding observation that particulate antigens are more immunogenic following oral immunization than soluble antigens.[83] Cox and co-workers confirmed this observation and suggested that particulate antigens were more effective because of their ability to be taken up into the Peyer's patches.[84,85] O'Hagan et al.[86] demonstrated that biodegradable microparticles could function as effective antigen delivery systems for oral immunization. They also showed that particle size was an important factor influencing the

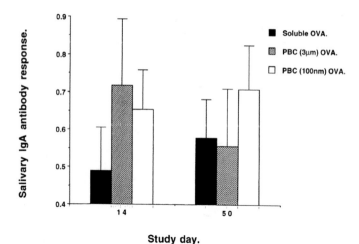

Study day.

Figure 3 Salivary IgA antibody responses in groups of 8 Wistar rats (± S.D.) following oral immunization with 1 mg ovalbumin in a soluble form, or adsorbed to poly(butyl-2-cyanoacrylate) (PBC) microparticles (3 μm and 100 nm) on 4 consecutive days. Identical booster doses of ovalbumin were administered 46 days after the primary immunizations.

outcome following oral immunization (Figure 3). The use of particulates, e.g., microparticles and liposomes, for oral immunization will be discussed in detail in Chapters 2 and 5 of Part II. The use of a liposomal antigen delivery system has allowed the anti-idiotype approach to vaccine development to be applied to the secretory immune system. Oral immunization in rats with an anti-idiotype antibody was shown to induce protection against colonization of the oral mucosa by *S. mutans*.[87]

De Aizpurua and Russell-Jones[88] investigated the ability of a range of antigens to induce antibody responses in mice following oral immunization. They showed that proteins with "lectin" or "lectin-like" binding activity to the intestinal epithelium were able to induce responses, while proteins without such activity were not (Table 4). The use of lectins as oral adjuvants will be discussed in detail in Chapter 4, Part II. Peptides from a molecule with lectin-like activity, cholera toxin B subunit (CTB), have been shown to induce serum antibody responses in mice following oral immunization.[89] This study represented the first successful use of peptides for oral immunization. The use of CTB as an oral adjuvant will be discussed in detail in Chapter 1, Part II.

D. AGE ON EXPOSURE AND PRIOR EXPOSURE

Although the levels of IgA in human serum only reach adult levels during early adolescence, adult levels of sIgA are reached only a few months after birth.[90,91] Consequently, oral vaccines could exploit this early maturation of sIgA and induce high levels of secretory immunity in newborns before systemic immunity is fully developed. The intestinal secretory immune system of humans has been shown to undergo a rapid development during the first few weeks after birth, probably in response to environmental factors.[92]

It is well established that systemic immunity is reduced with age[93] and that diseases of the respiratory tract and the GIT increase in the elderly.[94] In rats, there is strong evidence to suggest that both IgA transport across the intestinal epithelium and the numbers of plasma cells present in the lamina propria are reduced with age.[95] In addition, a study by Challacombe[96] showed that elderly mice were not able to respond to oral immunization nearly as well as younger mice (Table 5). Moreover, recent data have

Table 4 **The effect of the nature of the antigen on the serum and intestinal wash antibody responses following oral immunization**

Antigen	Serum antibodies		Intestinal wash	
	IgG	IgA	IgG	IgA
K99 pili	968 (120)	<4	3.0 (5.2)	3.2 (4.9)
987P pili	776 (64)	10.8 (8.8)	10.9 (1.7)	48.5 (1.9)
LTB	1,351 (211)	<4	<4	12.2 (4.4)
Influenza vaccine	179 (34)	<4	<4	<4
Flagella	<4	<4	<4	<4
LPS	12.1 (1)	<4	<4	<4
PS	<4	<4	<4	<4
BSA	<4	<4	<4	<4
ConA	666 (84)	<4	ND (not done)	ND

Note: Mean values from five mice (±S.D.) following oral immunization with 20 µg of antigen at days 0 and 14. The immune responses, which represent the reciprocal of the sample dilution that gave an ELISA reading of 0.5, were measured at day 21. K99 and 987P pili, flagella and heat labile enterotoxin (LTB) were isolated and purified from *Escherichia coli;* lipopolysaccharide (LPS) and polysaccharide (PS) were purified from *Salmonella typhimurium;* the lectin (Con A), bovine serum albumin (BSA), and influenza vaccine were purchased from commercial suppliers.

Adapted from De Aizpurua, H.J. and Russell-Jones, G.J., *J. Exp. Med.,* 167, 440, 1988.

demonstrated that aging compromises the intestinal immune responses in rhesus monkeys.[97] Furthermore, there is also evidence of the significant effects of old age on the mucosal immune system in humans,[98] although these findings have recently been questioned.[99] The effects of age on mucosal immunity has been reviewed by Kawanishi.[99a] Recent studies have shown that intense exercise results in a fall in the levels of IgA secretions.[99b]

It has been suggested that the efficacy of Ty21a may be dependent upon prior immune exposure to salmonellae.[68] This assertion was supported by the observation that Ty21a was only effective in individuals with evidence of prior immune priming.[100] Nevertheless, the situation is not straightforward, since Forrest[101] described limited immunogenicity of Ty21a in individuals with preexisting cross-reactive intestinal antibodies. However, a study by Dearlove et al.[102] showed that the response to an oral Ty21a-based typhoid-cholera hybrid vaccine was unaffected by prior exposure to Ty21a. Hence, the induction of immunity to Ty21a in typhoid-endemic areas appears to be dependent upon a fine balance between intestinal priming through previous exposure and the induction of blocking antibodies, which may reduce the efficacy of the vaccine. The efficacy of Ty21a will be discussed in more detail in Chapter 2, Part I.

E. MUCOSAL ADJUVANTS

The first book on oral immunization also included the first report of the use of a mucosal adjuvant. Bile was used as an adjuvant and was thought to be effective due to the removal of intestinal mucus, which resulted in enhanced intestinal permeability.[3] The bile salts are surfactants,[103] as too are the saponins, which have also been used as oral adjuvants (Table 6).[104] Acylation, the addition of fatty acid residues, has been shown to promote the

Table 5 **The effect of age on the salivary antibody response of mice to oral immunization with *Streptococcus mutans***

Age on exposure	Salivary antibody response
5 weeks	0.5 (0.2)
11 weeks	2.8 (0.3)[a]
17 weeks	5.7 (0.5)[a]
52 weeks	2.1 (0.7)

Note: Mice were orally immunized with 10^{10} *S. mutans* on 3 consecutive days, and the salivary antibody responses were determined 14 days later. The responses are mean antibody units for six mice (±S.E.).

[a] Represents a significantly different response ($p < 0.01$) in comparison to a control group of animals of the same age which were orally immunized with saline.

Adapted from Challacombe, S.J., *Mucosal Immunity IgA and Polymorphonuclear Neutrophils,* Revillard, J.P., Voisin, C., and Wierznicki, M., Eds., Fondation Franco-Allemande, Paris, 1985, 73.

Table 6 **The effect of a mucosal adjuvant (saponin) on the serum antibody responses in mice following oral immunization with inactivated rabies virus**

	Virus alone		Virus and saponin	
	Number responding	**FIMT titer**	**Number responding**	**FIMT titer**
Two doses	3/48	21	13/42	64
Three doses	2/13	28	12/14	40–2,000

Note: Mice were fed at weekly intervals, two or three doses of fixed inactivated rabies virus either alone, or in combination with *Quillaja saponaria* saponin. Blood was collected 3 days after the final dose, and the level of rabies-neutralizing antibodies in the serum was determined in a fluorescence inhibition micro test (FIMT). The number responding represents the number of seropositive animals/total tested.

Adapted from Chavali, S.R. and Campbell, J.B., *Immunobiology,* 174, 347, 1987.

immunogenicity of orally administered proteins.[105] The adjuvant effect was thought to be due to the enhanced ability of the acylated proteins to interact with macrophages and antigen-presenting cells.[105] The polycation DEAE-dextran has also been shown to exert an adjuvant effect following oral administration: enhanced numbers of antibody-secreting cells were observed in the intestinal lymph.[106] Vitamin A, which makes lysosomal membranes labile,[107] has also been shown to enhance the antibody response to an orally administered antigen.[108] Additional agents which have been shown to exert an adjuvant effect orally include lysozyme,[109] muramyl dipeptide (MDP),[110] and avridine.[111]

The majority of immunological adjuvants which have been shown to be effective orally appear to exert an effect that could best be described as "absorption enhancement".[112] The adjuvants protect antigens from intestinal degradation, or they reduce the barrier to absorption by mucolytic activity or by a direct effect on the epithelial membrane. The latter mechanism, in which epithelial membrane permeability is altered, may have potentially damaging consequences. The enhanced permeability is unlikely to be specific for the antigen of interest and enhanced absorption of unrelated bystander antigens seems likely. The potential problems associated with an impaired intestinal barrier to antigens is discussed in detail by Sanderson and Walker.[113]

The use of absorption enhancers to enhance the oral delivery of peptide and protein drugs is an area of considerable interest.[114] Several approaches to the absorption enhancement of proteins, including coadministration with enzyme inhibitors,[115] may also offer possibilities for vaccine delivery. However, the effects of the absorption enhancers on epithelial membranes and the possible implications of altered membrane permeability are a major concern.[116] Although the degree of concern may be diminished for vaccines which will only be administered on a few occasions and will not be designed for chronic administration. Nevertheless, perhaps a more acceptable approach is to deliver antigens entrapped in carrier systems such as microparticles or liposomes. These carrier systems would not exert nonspecific effects on the intestinal epithelium, but would deliver the antigens to specific sites such as the Peyer's patches. Alternatively, the antigens may be expressed and delivered in carrier organisms, including bacteria and viruses.

F. PROTECTION OF ANTIGEN AGAINST DEGRADATION

The encapsulation of antigens in delivery systems such as liposomes or microparticles may allow them to be protected from degradation in the GIT. In addition, mucosal adjuvants, e.g., bile salts, may be effective in part due to their ability to confer protection against degradation. However, alternative approaches may also be employed to ensure that antigens are protected from degradation following oral administration. In several of the large-scale clinical trials with Ty21a, the vaccine was administered in enteric-coated capsules.[75] Alternatively, the vaccine was administered with sodium bicarbonate to neutralize gastric acidity (Table 3). The second approach, involving administration of vaccine with buffer, was also employed in clinical trials with an inactivated oral cholera vaccine.[75] The use of enteric-coating polymers on the surface of microspheres has also been described.[117-120] Klipstein et al.[117] showed that entrapping *E. coli* heat-labile enterotoxin (LTB) in enteric-coated microspheres was as effective for the induction of high levels of antitoxin immunity in rats as ablation of gastric acidity by pretreatment with the drug cimetidine (Table 7). The use of enteric-coated microspheres will be discussed in detail in Chapter 2, Part II.

V. EXPLOITATION OF THE COMMON MUCOSAL IMMUNE SYSTEM

In experimental studies in man with Ty21a, convincing evidence has been obtained for the presence of a CMIS. Following oral immunization, immune responses to the vaccine were detected in serum, saliva, intestinal fluid, and in peripheral blood lymphocytes (PBL).[121] Direct measurement of the human intestinal immune response is difficult because intubation is labor-intensive, invasive, and time consuming. Therefore, indirect measurements are normally undertaken to assess the efficacy of oral vaccines. The best indicator of the intestinal IgA antibody response is the measurement of specific IgA produced by PBL.[121] The PBL represent a population of IgA-secreting cells which have been stimulated in the Peyer's patches and have subsequently migrated into the blood through the lymphatics.[122]

Studies with Ty21a in humans have shown that oral vaccines can induce antigen-specific immune responses in the lower respiratory tract.[123] In addition, a *Salmonella*-based vaccine

Table 7 **The response to oral immunization of rats with**
***Escherichia coli* heat-labile enterotoxin (LTB) in the**
presence of agents designed to protect the LTB from
degradation in the stomach

| | Antitoxin response | | % reduced secretion in immunized rats after LTB challenge |
	Serum	Mucosal	
No buffer	1	1	2 (1)
Bicarbonate	1	2	3 (1)
Cimetidine	5	6	80 (1)
Enteric-coated microspheres	5	6	97 (2)

Note: The antitoxin response is shown as the fold increase in geometric mean titers in immunized rats over control rats. Following immunization with LTB, the rats were challenged by instillation of LTB into ligated intestinal loops. Maximal fluid secretion was observed following LTB challenge in unimmunized rats. The % reduced secretions (±S.E.) induced by immunization with LTB plus the different agents is shown. An agent which completely protected LTB from degradation in the stomach might be expected to reduce secretion by 100%.
Adapted from Klipstein, F.A., Engert, R.F., and Sherman, W.T., *Infect. Immun.,* 39, 1000, 1983.

has also been shown to induce an immune response in the lungs of mice following oral immunization. The response was induced against the filamentous hemagglutinin from *Bordetella pertussis,* which was expressed by *Salmonella typhimurium.*[124] In a study in rats, Freihorst et al.[125] showed that oral immunization with *Pseudomonas aeruginosa* induced high levels of specific IgA in the intestinal and respiratory tracts. However, the immune response was not sufficient to provide protection against infection with the same bacteria.[125] Nevertheless, oral immunization with temperature-sensitive mutants of *P. aeruginosa* has been shown to enhance the lung clearance of wild-type bacteria from mice.[126]

Oral immunization with *Chlamydia trachomatis* has been shown to induce a secretory IgA antibody response in the genital tract of mice, which was protective against intravaginal challenge.[127] These findings were consistent with those from an earlier study in guinea pigs involving oral immunization with *Chlamydia psittaci.*[128] Studies in monkeys have shown that oral immunization with *C. trachomatis* can stimulate protective immunity against ocular challenge.[192] Oral immunization with herpes simplex virus type 1 (HSV-1) in mice has been shown to offer a degree of protection against subsequent genital infection with HSV-2.[130] Furthermore, oral immunization with influenza virus in mice has been shown to induce complete protection against intranasal challenge with homologous virus.[131] In addition, up to 50% cross-protection against heterologous strains was also achieved.[131]

Clancy et al.[132] provided evidence in humans that the CMIS could be exploited to modify the colonization pattern of a pathogen at a mucosal site. Oral immunization with killed *Haemophilus influenzae* provided protection against recurrent acute bronchitis in patients with smoking-related chronic lung disease (Table 8).[132] In a study in rats, it was demonstrated that the pulmonary protection against nontypeable *H. influenzae* induced by oral immunization was independent of specific antibody, but was mediated by primed T cells.[133] A vaccine prepared from the ribosomes of *Candida albicans* and adjuvanted with

Table 8 **Exploitation of the common mucosal immune
system in humans following oral immunization with killed
Haemophilus influenzae in patients prone to recurrent
acute bronchitis**

	Vaccine group (n = 20)	Placebo group (n = 20)
Number reporting infections	10	16
Number of infections	10	17
Episodes of acute bronchitis	6	16
Courses of antibiotics	5	12
Duration of symptoms in days (±S.E.)	9.4 (2.0)	12 (1.9)

Note: The study was a double-blind randomized trial conducted over a 6-month period. The vaccine group received three courses of enteric-coated tablets containing 10^{11} organisms, while the placebo group received enteric-coated tablets containing glucose.
Adapted from Clancy, R.L., Cripps, A.W., and Gebski, V., *Med. J. Aust.*, 152, 413, 1990.

membrane proteoglycan from nonencapsulated *Klebsiella pneumoniae* has shown encouraging results in a small scale clinical trial in women. Following oral immunization, the vaccine reduced the recurrence of vulvovaginal candidiasis.[134] Studies in mice have shown that oral immunization results in the induction of a secretory IgA response in the uterus.[135] In a thought-provoking study in rats, Allardyce[136] showed that oral immunization with sperm results in short- to long-term infertility, which was associated with the appearance of antisperm antibodies in genital tract secretions.

VI. CONCLUSIONS

Accumulated experimental evidence from animal models establishes the presence of a CMIS, which may be stimulated by oral immunization. Oral immunization has been shown to result in the induction of secretory IgA and T cell responses at mucosal sites, including the nasal cavity, the lungs and the genital tract. Consequently, oral immunization may be exploited for the induction of protective immunity against pathogens of the GIT and against pathogens that infect at alternative mucosal sites. Indeed, experimental evidence indicates that oral immunization can be exploited to induce protective immune responses in the nasal cavity and the genital tract. The available evidence also suggests that a CMIS is present in humans, and immune responses have been induced at several mucosal sites following oral immunization. Furthermore, there is evidence to indicate that the CMIS may be exploited to induce protective immunity in the respiratory tract of humans following oral immunization.

Nevertheless, the induction of mucosal immunity following oral immunization has been shown to depend upon a number of variables, including the dose and nature of the antigen, and the frequency of administration. However, perhaps the most crucial factor affecting the outcome of oral immunization is the selection of the antigen delivery system. A variety of antigen-delivery systems are now available, including both live and nonliving carrier systems (Table 9). These delivery systems, which may be designed to protect antigens against degradation and to deliver them into the GALT, are the subject of this book. Each chapter will deal with a prospective antigen delivery system and will discuss its relative merits and potential failings.

Table 9 **Alternative antigen delivery systems for oral immunization**

Delivery systems	Advantages	Disadvantages
Colonization of Peyer's patches with genetically engineered organisms. (e.g., *Salmonella* and poliovirus)	Potential for potent stimulation of immune response; may include several antigens	Antibodies to carrier may preclude the use of the same organism for booster immunization
Cholera toxin (B subunit)	Potent adjuvant	Probably requires whole toxin for adjuvant effect; chemical coupling may be required; immunity to carrier may restrict use
Microparticles	Promotes uptake by Peyer's patches; protects antigen; controlled release; can include adjuvants and targeting agents	Unproven efficacy in man; uptake of particles requires further study; possible denaturation of antigens during micro-encapsulation
Liposomes	May include adjuvants and targeting agents; protects antigen from degradation	Stability problems; solubilization in the gut (bile salts, lipases, etc.)
Lectins	Wide range of materials available for assessment with different specificities	Nonspecific enhancement of immune responses to gut contents possible; may require chemical coupling; toxicity?

It is highly unlikely that any one antigen delivery system will prove applicable as a universal "carrier" for a wide range of antigens. Instead, it is more likely that researchers will exploit the characteristics of one specific carrier to deliver vaccines for which it is best suited. Consequently, several or all of the vaccine delivery strategies discussed in this book may eventually be exploited for the development of more effective oral vaccines. Therefore, the alternative carrier systems may eventually be used concurrently, or even synergistically, for the delivery of a range of vaccines. For each of the novel delivery systems, there is a number of unanswered questions and concerns which must be addressed before the systems can be widely considered for the development of new and improved vaccines. This book will attempt to address at least some of the pertinent questions and wherever possible, to provide at least partial answers.

REFERENCES

1. Witebsky, E., Immunology: Views of the past and visions for the future, *Can. Med. Assoc. J.*, 97, 1371, 1967.
2. Mestecky, J. and McGhee, J.R., Oral immunization: past and present, *Curr. Top. Microbiol. Immunol.*, 146, 3, 1989.
3. Besredka, A., *Local immunization*, Williams & Wilkins, Baltimore, 1927.
4. McGhee, J.R. and Mestecky, J., In defence of mucosal surfaces: development of novel vaccines for IgA responses protective at the portals of entry of microbial pathogens, *Infect. Dis. Clin. N.A.*, 4, 315, 1990.

5. Suharyono, Simanjuntak, C., Witham, N., Punjabi, N., Heppner, D.G., Losonsky, G., Totosudirjo, H., Rifai, A.R., clemens, J., Lim, Y.L., Burr, D., Wasserman, S.S., Kaper, J., Sorenson, K., Cryz, S., and Levine, M.M., Safety and immunogenicity of single-dose oral cholera vaccine CVD 103-HgR in 5–9 year old children, *Lancet*, 340, 689, 1992.

6. Aguado, M.T. and Lambert, P.-H., Controlled release vaccines — Biodegradable polylactide/polyglycolide (PL/PG) microspheres as antigen vehicles, *Immunobiology*, 184, 113, 1992.

7. Mestecky, J., The common mucosal immune system and current strategies for induction of immune response in external secretions, *J. Clin. Immunol.*, 7, 265, 1987.

8. Delacroix, D.L., Hodgson, J.H.F., and McPherson, A., Selective transport of polymeric IgA in bile. Quantitative relationships of monomeric and polymeric IgA, IgM and other proteins in serum, bile and saliva, *J. Clin. Invest.*, 70, 230, 1982.

9. Kubagawa, H., Bertoli, L.F., and Barton, J.C., Analysis of paraprotein transport into the saliva by using anti-idiotype antibodies, *J. Immunol.*, 138, 435, 1987.

10. Tomasi, T.B., Tan, E.M., Solomon, A., and Prendergast, R.A., Characteristics of an immune system common to certain external secretions, *J. Exp. Med.*, 121, 101, 1965.

11. Owen, R.L. and Ermak, T.H., Structural specializations for antigen uptake and processing in the digestive tract, *Springer Semin. Immunopathol.*, 12, 139, 1990.

12. Stoolman, L.M., Adhesion molecules controlling lymphocyte migration, *Cell*, 56, 907, 1989.

13. Mestecky, J. and McGhee, J.R., Immunoglobulin A (IgA): Molecular and cellular interactions involved in IgA biosynthesis and immune response, *Adv. Immunol.*, 40, 153, 1987.

14. Craig, S.W. and Cebra, J.J., Peyer's patches: An enriched source of precursors for IgA-producing lymphocytes in the rabbit, *J. Exp. Med.*, 134, 188, 1971.

15. Bergmann, K.-C. and Waldman, R.H., Stimulation of secretory antibody following oral administration of antigen, *Rev. Infect. Dis.*, 10, 939, 1988.

16. Russell, M.W. and Mestecky, J., Induction of the mucosal immune response, *Rev. Infect. Dis.*, 10, S440, 1988.

17. McGhee, J.R., Mestecky, J., Dertzbaugh, M.T., Eldridge, J.H., Hirasawa, M., and Kiyono, H., The mucosal immune system: From fundamental concepts to vaccine development, *Vaccine*, 10, 75, 1992.

18. Brandtzaeg, P., Overview of the mucosal immune system, *Curr. Top. Microbiol. Immunol.*, 146, 13, 1989.

19. Conley, M.E. and Delacroix, D.L., Intravascular and mucosal immunoglobulin A: two separate but related systems of immune defence, *Ann. Intern. Med.*, 106, 892, 1987.

20. Dimmock, N.J., Mechanisms of neutralization of animal viruses, *J. Gen. Virol.*, 65, 1015, 1984.

21. Taylor, H.P. and Dimmock, N.J., Mechanisms of neutralization of influenza-virus by secretory IgA is different from that of monomeric IgA or IgG, *J. Exp. Med.*, 161, 198, 1985.

22. Kilian, M., Mestecky, J., and Rusell, M.W., Defense mechanisms involving Fc-dependent functions of immunoglobulin A and their subversion by bacterial immunoglobulin A proteases, *Microbiol. Rev.*, 52, 296, 1988.

23. Magnusson, K.-E. and Sjernstrom, I., Mucosal barrier mechanisms: Interplay between secretory IgA, IgG and mucins on the surface properties and association of salmonellae with intestine and granulocytes, *Immunobiology*, 45, 239, 1982.

24. Mestecky, J., Russell, M.W., Jackson, S., and Brown, T.A., The human IgA system, a reassessment, *Clin. Immunol. Immunopathol.*, 40, 105, 1986.

25. Brown, T.A., Russell, M.W., and Mestecky, J., Elimination of intestinally absorbed antigen into the bile by IgA, *J. Immunol.*, 132, 780, 1984.

26. Dimmock, N.J., Mechanisms of neutralization of animal viruses, *J. Gen. Virol.*, 65, 1015, 1984.

27. Taylor, H.P. and Dimmock, N.J., Mechanism of neutralization of influenza virus by secretory IgA is different from that of monomeric IgA or IgG, *J. Exp. Med.*, 161, 198, 1985.

28. Novak, M., Moldoveanu, Z., Schafer, D.P., Mestecky, J., and Compans, R.W., Murine model for evaluation of protective immunity to influenza virus, *Vaccine*, 11, 55, 1993.

29. Liew, F.Y., Russell, S.M., Appleyard, G., Brand, C.M., and Beale, T., Cross protection in mice infected with influenza A virus by the respiratory route is correlated with local IgA antibody rather than serum antibody or cytotoxic T cell reactivity, *Eur. J. Immunol.*, 14, 350, 1984.

30. Renegar, K.B. and Small, P.A., Jr., Immunoglobulin A mediation of murine nasal anti-influenza virus immunity, *J. Virol.*, 65, 2146, 1991.

31. Clements, M.L., O'Donnell, S., Levine, M.M., Chanock, R.M., and Murphy, B.R., Dose response of A/Alaska/6/77 (H3N2) cold-adapted reassortment vaccine virus in adult volunteers: Role of local antibody in resistance to infection with vaccine virus, *Infect. Immun.*, 40, 1044, 1983.

32. Manzanec, M., Nedrud, J.G., and Lamm, M.E., Immunoglobulin A monoclonal antibodies protect against Sendai virus, *J. Virol.*, 67, 2624, 1987.

33. Renegar, K.B. and Small, P.A., Passive transfer of local immunity to influenza virus infection by IgA antibody, *J. Immunol.*, 146, 1972, 1991.

34. Mazanec, M.B., Lamm, M.E., Lyn, D., Portner, A., and Nedrud, J.G., Comparison of IgA versus IgG monoclonal antibodies for passive immunization of the murine respiratory tract, *Virus. Res.*, 23, 1, 1992.

35. Cumella, J.C. and Ogra, P.L., Mucosal immune system and local immunity, in *Immunology of the Ear*, Bernstein, J. and Ogra, P.L., Eds., Raven Press, New York, 1987, 135.

35a. Mazanec, M.B., Kaetzel, C.S., Lamm, M.E., Fletcher, D., and Nedrud, J.G., *Proc. Natl. Acad. Sci. U.S.A.*, 89, 6901, 1992.

36. Weltzin, R.A., Lucia Landris, P., Michetti, P., Fields, B.N., Kraehenbuhl, J.P., and Neutra, M.R., Binding and transepithelial transport by intestinal M cells; demonstration using monoclonal IgA antibodies against enteric viral proteins, *J. Cell Biol.*, 108, 1673, 1989.

37. Winner, L.S., III, Weltzin, R.A., Mekalanos, J.J., Krahenbuhl, J.P., and Neutra, M.R., New model for analysis of mucosal immunity; intestinal secretion of monoclonal immunoglobulin A from hybridoma tumors protects against *Vibrio cholerae* infection, *Infect. Immun.*, 59, 977, 1991.

38. Michetti, P., Mahan, M.J., Slauch, J.M., Mekalanos, J.J., and Neutra, M.R., Monoclonal secretory immunoglobulin A protects mice against oral challenge with the invasive pathogen *Salmonella typhimurium*, *Infect. Immun.*, 60, 1786, 1992.

39. Czinn, S.J., Cai, A., and Nedrud, J.G., Protection of germ-free mice from infection by *Helicobacter felis* after active oral or passive IgA immunization, *Vaccine*, 11, 637, 1993.

40. Svanberg-Eden, C., Freter, C.R., and Hagbert, R., Inhibition of experimental ascending urinary tract infection by receptor analogue, *Nature*, 298, 560, 1982.

41. Freter, C.R. and Jones, G.W., Models for studying the role of bacterial attachment in virulence and pathogenesis, *Rev. Infect. Dis.*, 5, 5647, 1983.

42. Rogers, H.J. and Synge, C., Bacteriostatic effect of human milk on *Escherichia coli*, the role of IgA, *Immunology*, 34, 19, 1978.

43. Tenuovo, J., Moldoveanu, Z., Mestecky, J., Pruitt, K.M., and Rahemtulla, B.-M., Interaction of specific and innate factors of immunity: IgA enhances the antimicrobial effects of the lactoperoxidase system against *Streptococcus mutans*, *J. Immunol.*, 128, 726, 1982.

44. Adinolfi, M., Glynn, A.A., Lindsay, M., and Milne, C.M., Serological properties of A antibodies to *Escherichia coli* present in human colostrum, *Immunol.*, 10, 517, 1966.

45. Tagliabue, A., Immune response to oral *Salmonella* vaccines, *Curr. Top. Microbiol. Immunol.*, 146, 225, 1989.

46. Brandtzaeg, P., Immunobarriers of the mucosa of the upper respiratory and digestive pathways, *Acta Otolaryngol. (Stockh.)*, 105, 172, 1988.

47. Walker, W.A. and Isselbacher, K.J., Intestinal antibodies, *N. Eng. J. Med.*, 297, 767, 1977.

48. Cunningham-Rundles, C., Brandeis, W.E., Good, R.A., and Day, N.K., Bovine antigens and the formation of circulating immune complexes in selective Immunoglobulin A deficiency, *J. Clin. Invest.*, 64, 272, 1978.

49. Isolari, E., Suomalainen, H., Kaila, M., Jalonen, T., Soppi, E., Virtanen, E., and Arvilommi, H., Local immune response in patients with cow milk allergy: Follow-up of patients retaining allergy or becoming tolerant, *J. Pediatr.*, 120, 9, 1992.

50. Walker, W.A., Wu, M., Isselbacher, K.J., and Bloch, K.J., Intestinal uptake of macromolecules. III. Studies on the mechanism by which immunization interferes with antigen uptake, *J. Immunol.*, 115, 854, 1975.

51. Walker, W.A., Wu, M., Isselbacher, K.J., and Block, K.J., Intestinal uptake of macromolecules. IV. The effect of pancreatic duct ligation on the breakdown of antigen and antigen-antibody complexes on the intestinal surface, *Gastroenterology*, 69, 1223, 1975.

52. Pang, K.Y., Walker, W.A., and Bloch, K.J., Intestinal uptake of macromolecules, *Gut*, 22, 1018, 1981.

53. Lake, A.M., Bloch, K.J., Sinclair, K.J., and Walker, W.A., Anaphylactic release of intestinal goblet cell mucus, *Immunology*, 39, 173, 1980.

54. Ahlstedt, S. and Enander, I., Immune regulation of goblet cell development, *Int. Arch. Allergy Appl. Immun.*, 82, 357, 1987..

55. Walker, W.A. and Bloch, K.J., Uptake of antigen-antibody complexes prepared in antibody or antigen excess by normal rat intestine in vitro, *Gastroenterology*, 70, 948, 1976.

55a. Mazanec, M.B., Nedrud, J.G., Kaetzel, C.S., and Lamm, M.E., A three-tiered view of the role of IgA in mucosal defense, *Immunol. Today*, 14, 430, 1993.

56. Weltzin, R., Lucia-Jandris, P., Michetti, P., Fields, B.N., Kraehenbuhl, J.P., and Neutra, M.R., Binding and transepithelial transport of immunoglobulins by intestinal M cells: Demonstration using monoclonal IgA antibodies against enteric viral proteins, *J. Cell Biol.*, 108, 1673, 1989.

57. Sixby, J.W. and Yao, Q.-Y., Immunoglobulin A-induced shift of Epstein-Barr virus tissue tropism, *Science*, 255, 1578, 1992.

58. Bloch, N.J. and Walker, W.A., Effect of locally induced intestinal anaphylaxis on the uptake of a bystander antigen, *J. Allergy Clin. Immunol.*, 67, 312, 1981.

59. Russell-Jones, G.J., Ey, P.L., and Reynolds, B.L., The ability of IgA to inhibit the complement-mediated lysis of target red blood cells sensitized with IgG antibody, *Mol. Immunol.*, 17, 1173, 1980.

60. Russell-Jones, G.J., Ey, P.L., and Reynolds, B.L., Inhibition of cutaneous anaphylaxis and arthus reactions in the mouse by antigen specific IgA, *Int. Arch. Allergy Appl. Immun.*, 66, 316, 1981.

61. Trejdosiewicz, L.K., Intestinal intraepithelial lymphocytes and lymphoepithelial interactions in the human gastrointestinal mucosa, *Immunol. Lett.*, 32, 13, 1992.

62. Elson, C.O., Weiserbs, D.B., Ealding, W., and Machelski, E., T-helper cell activity in intestinal lamine propria, *Ann. N.Y. Acad. Sci.*, 409, 230, 1983.

63. Kawanishi, H., Saltzmann, L., and Strober, W., Mechanisms regulating IgA class-specific immunoglobulin production in murine gut associated lymphoid tissue. I. T cells derived from Peyer's patches that switch sIgM B cells to sIgA B cells in vitro, *J. Exp. Med.*, 157, 433, 1983.

64. Xu-Amano, J., Aicher, W.K., Taguchi, T., Kiyono, H., and McGhee, J.R., Selective induction of Th2 cells in murine Peyer's patches by oral immunization, *Int. Immunol.,* 4, 433, 1992.

64a. Xu-Amano, J., Kiyono, H., Jackson, R.J., Staats, H.F., Fujihashi, K., Burrows, P.D., Elson, C.O., Pillai, S., and McGhee, J.R., Helper T cell subsets for immunoglobulin A responses: oral immunization with tetanus toxoid and cholera toxin as adjuvant selectively induces Th2 cells in mucosa associated tissues, *J. Exp. Med.,* 178, 1309, 1993.

65. Michalek, S.M., McGhee, J.R., and Babb, J.L., Effective immunity to dental caries; dose dependent studies of secretory immunity by oral administration of *Streptococcus mutans* to rats, *Infect. Immun.,* 19, 217, 1977.

66. Dupont, H.L., Hornick, R.B., and Snyder, M.J., Studies of immunity in typhoid fever; protection induced by killed oral vaccines or by primary infection, *Bull. WHO,* 44, 667, 1971.

67. Forrest, B.D., LaBrooy, J.T., Beyer, L., Dearlove, C.E., and Shearman, D.J.C., The human humoral immune response to *Salmonella typhi* Ty21a, *J. Infect. Dis.,* 163, 336, 1991.

68. Editorial, Oral typhoid vaccine Ty21a, *Lancet,* 338, 1456, 1991.

69. Murphy, J.R., Grez, L., Schlesinger, L. et al., Immunogenicity of *Salmonella typhi* Ty 21a for young children, *Infect. Immun.,* 59, 4291, 1991.

70. Schwartz, E., Shlim, D.R., Eaton, M., Jenks, N., and Houston, R., The effect of oral and parenteral typhoid vaccination on the rate of infection with *Salmonella typhi* and *Salmonella paratyphi* A among foreigners in Nepal, *Arch. Intern. Med.,* 150, 349, 1990.

71. Patriarca, P.A., Wright, P.F., and John, T.J., Factors affecting the immunogenicity of oral poliovirus vaccine in developing countries, *Rev. Infect. Dis.,* 13, 926, 1991.

72. Challacombe, S.J., Salivary antibodies and systemic tolerance in mice after oral immunization with bacterial antigens, *Ann. N.Y. Acad. Sci.,* 409, 177, 1983.

73. Mowat, A.McI., Maloy, K.J., and Donachie, A.M., Immune stimulating complexes as adjuvants for stimulating local and systemic immunity after oral immunization with protein antigens, *Immunology,* in press.

74. Riviere, G.R., Wagoner, M.A., and Freeman, I.L., Chronic peroral immunization of conventional laboratory rats with mutans streptococci leads to stable acquired suppression of salivary antibodies, *Oral Microbiol. Immunol.,* 7, 137, 1992.

75. Gilligan, C.A. and Li Wan Po, A., Oral enteric vaccines — clinical trials, *J. Clin. Pharm. Therapeut.,* 16, 309, 1991.

76. Levine, M.M., Ferreccio, C., Black, R.E., Germanier, R., and Chilean Typhoid Commitee, Large-scale field trial of Ty21a live oral typhoid vaccine in an enteric-coated capsule formulation, *Lancet,* i, 1049, 1987.

77. Black, R.E., Levine, M.M., Ferreccio, C., Clements, M.L., Lanata, C., Rooney, J., Germanier, R., and Chilean Typhoid Commitee, Efficacy of one or two doses of Ty21a *Salmonella typhi* vaccine in enteric-coated capsules in a controlled field trial, *Vaccine,* 8, 81, 1990.

78. Ferreccio, C., Levine, M.M., Rodriguez, H., Contreras, R., and Chilean Typhoid Commitee, Comparative efficacy of two, three or four doses of Ty21a live oral typhoid vaccine in enteric-coated capsules: a filed trial in an endemic area, *J. Infect. Dis.,* 159, 766, 1989.

79. Kantele, A., Arvilommi, H., Kantele, J.M., Rintala, L., and Makela, P.H., Comparison of the human immune response to live oral, killed oral or killed parenteral *Salmonella typhi* Ty21a vaccines, *Microb. Pathogen.,* 10, 117, 1991.

80. Hohmann, A., Schmidt, G., and Rowley, D., Intestinal and serum antibody responses in mice after oral immunization with *Salmonella, Escherichia coli* and *Salmonella-Escherichia coli* hybrid strains, *Infect. Immun.,* 25, 27, 1979.

81. Dahlgren, U.I.H., Wold, A.E., Hanson, L.A., and Midtvedt, T., Expression of a dietary protein in *E. coli* renders it strongly antigenic to gut lymphoid tissue, *Immunology*, 73, 394, 1991.

82. Gustafson, G.L. and Rhodes, M.J., Bacterial cell wall products as adjuvants: early interferon gamma as a marker for adjuvants that enhance protective immunity, *Res. Immunol.*, 143, 483, 1992.

83. Strannegard, O. and Yurchison, A., Formation of agglutinating and reaginic antibodies in rabbits following oral administration of soluble and particulate antigens, *Int. Arch. Allergy Appl. Immun.*, 35, 579, 1969.

84. Cox, D.S. and Muench, D., IgA antibody produced by local presentation of antigen in orally primed rats, *Int. Arch. Allergy Appl. Immun.*, 74, 249, 1984.

85. Cox, D.S. and Taubman, M.A., Oral induction of the secretory antibody response by soluble and particulate antigens, *Int. Arch. Allergy Appl. Immun.*, 75, 126, 1984.

86. O'Hagan, D.T., Palin, K.J., and Davis, S.S., Poly (butyl-2-cyanoacrylate) particles as adjuvants for oral immunization, *Vaccine*, 7, 213, 1989.

87. Jackson, S., Mestecky, J., Childers, N.K., and Michalek, S.M., Liposomes containing anti-idiotype antibodies: an oral vaccine to induce protective secretory immune responses specific for pathogens of mucosal surfaces, *Infect. Immun.*, 58, 1932, 1990.

88. De Aizpura, H.J. and Russell-Jones, G.J., Oral vaccination; identification of classes of proteins that provoke an immune response upon oral feeding, *J. Exp. Med.*, 167, 440, 1988.

89. Guyon-Gruaz, A., Delmas, A., Pedoussat, S., Halimi, H., Milhaud, G., Raulais, D., and Rivaille, P., Oral immunization with a synthetic peptide of cholera toxin B subunit. Obtention of neutralizing antibodies, *Eur. J. Biochem.*, 159, 525, 1986.

90. Allansmith, M., McClellan, B.H., and Butterworth, M., The development of immunoglobulin levels in man, *J. Paediatr.*, 72, 276, 1968.

91. Burgio, G.R., Lanzavecchia, A., Plebani, A., Jayakar, S., and Ugazio, A.G., Ontogeny of secretory immunity: levels of secretory IgA and natural antibodies in saliva, *Pediatr. Res.*, 14, 1111, 1980.

92. Rognum, T.O., Thrane, P.S., Stoltenberg, L., Vege, A., and Brandtzaeg, P., Development of intestinal mucosal immunity in fetal life and the first postnatal months, *Pediatr. Res.*, 32, 145, 1992.

93. Makinodan, T. and Kay, M.M.B., Age influence on the immune system, *Adv. Immunol.*, 29, 287, 1980.

94. Schmucker, D.L. and Daniels, C.K., Aging, gastrointestinal infections and mucosal immunity, *J. Am. Gerontol. Soc.*, 34, 377, 1986.

95. Schmucker, D.L., Daniels, C.K., Wang, R.K., and Smith, K., Mucosal immune response to cholera toxin in aging rats. I. Antibody and antibody-containing cell response, *Immunology*, 64, 691, 1988.

96. Challacombe, S.J., Systemic tolerance and systemic antibodies after oral immunisation, in Revillard, J.P., Voisin, C., and Wierznicki, M., Eds., *Mucosal Immunity: IgA and Polymorphonuclear Neutrophils*, Fondation Franco-Allemande, Paris, 1985, 73.

97. Taylor, L.D., Daniels, C.K., and Schmucker, D.L., Aging compromises gastrointestinal mucosal immune response in the rhesus monkey, *Immunology*, 75, 614, 1992.

98. Arranz, E., O'Mahoney, S., Barton, J.R., and Ferguson, A., Immunosenescence and mucosal immunity: significant effects of old age on secretory IgA concentrations and intraepithelial lymphocyte counts, *Gut*, 33, 882, 1992.

99. Horan, M.A., Immunosenescence and mucosal immunity, *Lancet*, 341, 793, 1993.

99a. Kawanishi, H., Recent progress in senescence-associated gut mucosal immunity, *Dig. Dis. Sci.*, 11, 157, 1993.

99b. MacKinnon, L.T., Ginn, E., and Seymour, G.J., Decreased salivary immunoglobin A secretion rate after intense interval exercise in elite kayakers, *Eur. J. Appl. Physiol.*, 67, 180, 1993.

100. Ferguson, A. and Sallam, J., Mucosal immunity to oral vaccines, *Lancet,* 339, 179, 1992.
101. Forrest, B.D., Impairment of immunogenicity of *Salmonella typhi* Ty21a due to pre-existing cross-reacting intestinal antibodies, *J. Infect. Dis.,* 166, 210, 1992.
102. Dearlove, C.E., Forrest, B.D., van den Bosch, L., and La Brooy, J.T., The antibody response to an oral Ty21a-based typhoid-cholera hybrid is unaffected by prior oral vaccination with Ty21a, *J. Infect. Dis.,* 165, 182, 1992.
103. Helenius, A. and Simons, K., Solubilization of membranes by detergents, *Biochem. Biophys. Acta,* 415, 29, 1975.
104. Chavali, S.R. and Campbell, J.B., Adjuvant effects of orally administered saponins on humoral and cellular immune responses in mice, *Immunobiology,* 174, 347, 1987.
105. Heatley, R.V. and Stark, J.M., Immunogenicity of lipid conjugated protein in the intestine, *Immunology,* 29, 143, 1975.
106. Beh, K.J., Antibody containing cell response in lymph of sheep after intra intestinal infusion of ovalbumin with and without DEAE-dextran, *Immunology,* 37, 229, 1979.
107. Dingle, J.T., Studies on the mode of action of excess vitamin A. Release of bound protease by the action of vitamin A, *Biochem. J.,* 79, 509, 1961.
108. Falchuk, K.R., Walker, W.A., Perrotto, J.L., and Isselbacher, I., Effect of vitamin A on the systemic and local antibody responses to intragastrically administered bovine serum albumin, *Infect. Immun.,* 17, 361, 1977.
109. Lodinova, R. and Jouja, V., Influence of oral lysozyme administration on serum immunoglobulin and intestinal secretory IgA levels, *Acta Paediat. Scand.,* 66, 709, 1977.
110. Taubman, M.A., Ebersole, J.L., Smith, D.J., and Stack, W., Adjuvants for secretory immune responses, *Ann. N.Y. Acad. Sci.,* 409, 637, 1983.
111. Jensen, K.E., Synthetic adjuvants: Avridine and other interferon inducers, in *Advances in Carriers and Adjuvants for Veterinary Biologics,* Nervig, R.M., Gough, P.M., Kaeberle, M.L., and Whetstone, C.A., Eds., Iowa State University Press, Ames, 1986, 79.
112. O'Hagan, D.T. and Illum, L., Absorption of proteins and peptides from the respiratory tract and the potential for development of locally administered vaccine, *Crit. Rev. Ther. Drug Carr. Sys.,* 7, 35, 1990.
113. Sanderson, I.R. and Walker, W.A., Uptake and transport of macromolecules by the intestine: Possible role in clinical disorders (an update), *Gastroenterology,* in press.
114. Smith, P.L., Wall, D.A., Gochoco, C.H., and Wilson, G.W., Oral absorption of peptides and proteins, *Adv. Drug. Deliv. Rev.,* 8, 253, 1992.
115. Saffran, M., Franco-Saenz, R., Kong, A., and Szoka, F., A model for the oral administration of peptide hormones, *Can. J. Biochem.,* 57, 548, 1979.
116. Ennis, R.D., Borden, L., and Lee, W.a., The effects of permeation enhancers on the surface morphology of the rat nasal mucosa: a scanning electron microscope study, *Pharm. Res.,* 7, 468, 1990.
117. Klipstein, F.A., Engert, R.F., and Sherman, W.T., Peroral immunization with *Escherichia coli* heat-labile enterotoxin delivered by microspheres, *Infect. Immun.,* 39, 1000, 1983.
118. Maharah, I., Nairn, J.G., and Campbell, J.B., Simple rapid method for the preparation of enteric-coated microspheres, *J. Pharm. Sci.,* 73, 39, 1984.
119. Lin, S.Y., Tzan, Y.L., Lee, C.J., and Weng, C.N., Preparation of enteric-coated microspheres of *Mycoplasma hyopneumoniae* vaccine with cellulose acetate phthalate. I. Formation condition and micromeritic properties, *J. Microencap.,* 8, 317, 1991.
120. Lin, S.Y., Tzan, Y.L., Lee, C.J., and Weng, C.N., Preparation of enteric-coated microspheres of *Mycoplasma hyopneumoniae* vaccine with cellulose acetate phthalate. II. Effect of temperature and pH on the stability and release behaviour of microspheres, *J. Microencap.,* 8, 537, 1991.

121. Forrest, B.D., Indirect measurement of intestinal immune responses to an orally administered bacterial vaccine, *Infect. Immun.*, 60, 2023, 1992.

122. Forrest, B.D., The identification of an intestinal immune response using peripheral blood lymphocytes, *Lancet*, i, 81, 1988.

123. Forrest, B.D., LaBrooy, J.T., Robinson, P., Dearlove, C.E., and Shearman, D.J.C., Specific immune response in the human respiratory tract following oral immunization with live typhoid vaccine, *Infect. Immun.*, 59, 1206, 1991.

124. Guzman, C.A., Brownlie, R.M., Kadurugamuwa, J., Walker, M.J., and Timmis, K.N., Antibody response in the lungs of mice following oral immunization with *Salmonella typhimurium* aroA and invasive *Escherichia coli* strains expressing the filamentous hemagglutinin of *Bordetella pertussis*, *Infect. Immun.*, 59, 4391, 1991.

125. Freihorst, J., Merrick, J.M., and Ogra, P.l., Effect of oral immunization with *Pseudomonas aeruginosa* on the development of specific antibacterial immunity in the lungs, *Infect. Immun.*, 57, 235, 1989.

126. Hooke, A.M., Cerquetti, M.C., Wan, K.S., Wang, Z., Sordelli, D.O., and Bellanti, J.A., Oral immunization of mice with temperature-sensitive *Pseudomonas aeruginosa* enhances pulmonary clearance of the wild-type, *Vaccine*, 9, 294, 1991.

127. Cui, Z.-D., Tristram, D., La Scolea, L.J., Kwiatokowski, T., Jr., Kopti, S., and Ogra, P.L., Induction of antibody response to *Chlamydia trachomatis* in the genital tract by oral immunization, *Infect. Immun.*, 59, 1465, 1991.

128. Nichols, R.L., Murray, E.S., and Nisson, P.E., Use of enteric vaccines in protection against chlamydial infections of the genital tract and the eye of guinea pigs, *J. Infect. Dis.*, 138, 742, 1978.

129. Taylor, H.R., Young, E., MacDonald, A.B., Schachter, J., and Prendergast, R.A., Oral immunization against chlamydial eye infection, *Opthalmol. Vis. Sci.*, 28, 249, 1987.

130. Sturn, B. and Schneweis, K.-E., Protective effect of an oral infection with Herpes simplex virus type 1 against subsequent genital infection with Herpes simplex virus type 2, *Med. Microbiol. Immunol.*, 165, 119, 1978.

131. Chen, K.-S. and Quinnan, G.V., Jr., Efficacy of inactivated influenza vaccine delivered by oral administration, *Curr. Top. Microbiol. Immunol.*, 146, 101, 1989.

132. Clancy, R.L., Cripps, A.W., and Gebski, V., Protection against recurrent acute bronchitis after oral immunization with killed *Haemophilus influenzae*, *Med. J. Aust.*, 152, 413, 1990.

133. Wallace, F.J., Cripps, A.W., Clancy, R.L., Husband, A.J., and Witt, C.S., A role for intestinal T lymphocytes in bronchus mucosal immunity, *Immunology*, 74, 68, 1991.

134. Levy, D.A., Bohbot, J.M., Catalan, F., Normier, G., Pinel, A.M., and Dussourd d'Hinterland, L., Phase II study of D.651, an oral vaccine designed to prevent recurrences of vulvovaginal candidiasis, *Vaccine*, 7, 337, 1989.

135. Parr, E.L. and Parr, M.B., A comparison of antibody titres in mouse uterine fluid after immunization by several routes and the effect of the uterus on antibody titres in vaginal fluid, *J. Reproduct. Fertil.*, 89, 619, 1990.

136. Allardyce, R.A., Effect of ingested sperm on fecundity in the rat, *J. Exp. Med.*, 159, 1548, 1984.

Part I: Live Antigen Delivery Systems

Chapter 1

Salmonella as Carriers of Heterologous Antigens

Mark Roberts, Steve N. Chatfield, and Gordon Dougan

I. INTRODUCTION

Immune responses to live vaccines are generally of greater magnitude and of longer duration than those produced by nonreplicating immunogens.[1,2] A single dose of a live attenuated organism can provide solid protection against infection with wild-type organisms. Live vaccines are particularly efficacious at eliciting cell-mediated immune responses

(CMI).[1,3] The reasons for this are unknown, but might be connected with the ability of some live vaccines to replicate in antigen presenting cells such as macrophages.[3] Live vaccines also have advantages over nonreplicating immunogens when given mucosally. Most infections are acquired by contact of a pathogen with a mucosal surface. The specific and nonspecific defenses of mucous membranes therefore provide a first line defense against infectious disease. Thus it is desirable to be able to prime the mucosal-associated lymphoid tissue (MALT) by vaccination. Parenteral vaccination alone is inefficient at inducing mucosal immune responses; stimulation of the MALT usually requires direct contact between the immunogen and the mucosal surface.[4-6] Unfortunately most nonreplicating antigens are poorly immunogenic when given orally, stimulating weak (if any) secretory antibody response and undetectable serum responses.[4-6] The goal of oral immunization is not only to stimulate the MALT but also to induce good systemic immune responses because this may be necessary for a complete immunity to certain infection.

Attenuated strains of enteric pathogens such as *Salmonella* can be administered by the natural route of infection (peroral) and so are able to interact with the MALT. *Salmonella* can translocate from the lumen of the gut to the submucosa, where, depending on the species and the host, they may disseminate systemically. *Salmonella* can achieve this by either directly invading enterocytes or by entering the M cells overlying Peyer's patches.[7-9] Salmonellae are able to persist and replicate in Peyer's patches, thus presenting and retaining antigens at the inductive sites of the secretory immune system.[7,10] Salmonellae have a predilection for macrophages and take up residence in the fixed macrophages of the mononuclear phagocytic system in such organs as liver, spleen, and regional lymph nodes.[1,9,11-13] Because of its particular life style, infection with *Salmonella* or immunization with avirulent *Salmonella* strains can elicit humoral, secretory, and CMI responses.[14-19] The poor oral immunogenicity of purified immunogens can be overcome by expressing the genes for these antigens in attenuated *Salmonella* that can be used to deliver the foreign antigens to the local and systemic lymphoid tissue. Early experiments using attenuated *Salmonella* expressing the model antigen *E. coli* β-galactosidase showed that following oral immunization mice developed serum and secretory antibodies and delayed type hypersensitivity (DTH) to β-galactosidase.[14] Therefore it is feasible that multicomponent oral vaccines can be developed using *Salmonella* as a carrier. The capacity of *Salmonella* to deliver heterologous antigens is dependent on the viability of the carrier strain and is not merely because particular antigens are taken up more readily by M cells. Killed *Salmonella* are not effective at delivering heterologous antigens orally.[17,20]

Other advantages of live vaccines are that they are relatively easy and cheap to manufacture. They do not require purification of antigens or formulation with adjuvants. They can be used to developed vaccines against organisms that are difficult or impossible to culture, or which yield minute quantities of antigen, by expressing the genes for the critical immunogen in the live carrier. The close genetic relationship between *E. coli* and *Salmonella* means that expression systems developed for use in *E. coli* function well in *Salmonella* (we and others have found that in many cases foreign genes are expressed to higher levels in *Salmonella* than in *E. coli*). Also, systems for introducing genetic material into *Salmonella* are advanced and efficient.

The main drawbacks to the use of live vaccines in the past have been their propensity to cause severe infections in immunocompromised individuals and also their potential to revert to full virulence because the lesion(s) causing attenuation are not characterized. This is because vaccine strains were selected by empirical means such as multiple passage *in vitro* or using immunogenically related animal isolates that did not (usually) cause disease in humans.[21] However, it is possible with modern molecular genetic techniques to introduce precise nonreverting (deletions) mutations in specific genes in order to attenuate bacteria. These techniques are now being used to construct stable, attenuated strains of *Salmonella typhi* that can be used as safe nonreactogenic single-dose oral typhoid vaccines. Development of such strains is a prerequisite for using *S. typhi* as an antigen delivery system in humans.

II. DEVELOPMENT OF LIVE *SALMONELLA* VACCINES

The ideal live vaccine should have the following properties: it should give solid, long-lasting immunity with a single dose; be well tolerated; possess well-characterized mutations in specific genes; be stable and should therefore carry deletions in at least two genes; grow to high densities in fermenters and recover well from lyophilization. At present, strains that have all these characteristics are not commercially available.

Initial attempts to produce live typhoid vaccines relied on empirical methods to isolate attenuated strains, either mutants were spontaneously arising or induced by chemical or U.V. mutagenesis.[15,18,22,23] The search for attenuated *S. typhi* strains has also been hampered by the lack of a good small animal model. *S. typhi* is not virulent for mice perorally.[1,24] The test for virulence in this animal requires *S. typhi* to be administered intraperitoneally (I/P) with or without hog gastric mucin.[24,25] Other strains of *Salmonella* such as *S. typhimurium*, *S. dublin*, or *S. enteritidis* will cause typhoid-like disease in susceptible mice following oral or parenteral challenge and will cause death if sufficient bacteria are administered.[1,26,27] The murine typhoid model has proved very useful in elucidating components of *Salmonella* that are essential for virulence and also for studying the anti-*Salmonella* immune response. However, it has not proved possible to extrapolate totally from results obtained using mice to the behavior of *S. typhi* in humans (see below). A full history of the development of live typhoid vaccines is beyond the scope of this review; those interested can find fuller details elsewhere.[15,22,23,28,29]

A. *S. TYPHI* TY21A

The first generation licenced oral typhoid vaccine, Ty21a, was developed by Germanier and colleagues. They showed that *S. typhimurium* strains with rough LPS due to mutations in *gal*E gene are avirulent in mice and make good vaccines.[30,31] Several rounds of chemical mutagenesis (nitrosoguanidine) of *S. typhi* Ty2 were used to produce the *gal*E mutant (Ty21a). This strain was shown to be attenuated and very well tolerated in volunteers, even doses at 10^{11} colony forming units (CFU).[32] Details of clinical trials with Ty21a are presented in the next chapter, but in summary, the findings of a number of studies were that multiple doses of the vaccine (>3) are necessary to give acceptable levels of protection. Reported efficacy varies between 60 and 80%, comparable to heat-killed parenteral vaccine but with much lower reactogenicity. The presentation of the vaccine is important; liquid suspensions are superior to enteric-coated capsules, which in turn are superior to gelatin-encapsulated bacteria. Immunization with Ty21a has been shown to stimulate humoral, cellular, and mucosal immune responses.[11,23]

The *gal*E mutation was believed, until recently, to be the attenuating lesion in Ty21a. The product of *gal*E, the enzyme uridine 5′-diphosphate (UDP) glucose-4-epimerase, catalyzes the formation of UDP-galactose from glucose which is essential for the synthesis of smooth LPS. In the absence of exogenous galactose, *gal*E mutants are rough. However, in the presence of galactose, *gal*E mutants undergo lysis after a number of generations due to the accumulation of a toxic intermediate of galactose metabolism.[32] The role of a *gal*E mutation in attenuating *S. typhi* is now in doubt. When a Ty2 derivative with a site-directed mutation in *gal*E was tested in human volunteers, it retained virulence.[33] The strain also possessed a deletion in the *via* locus which abolished ability to make the Vi capsular antigen, a defect shared with Ty21a, which demonstrates that this capsule is not an essential virulence factor for *S. typhi*, as it was at one time thought.[33] Also, GalE⁺ revertants of Ty21a are still avirulent.[34] Ty21a is known to possess numerous mutations, a consequence of the method used to mutagenize the strain, and those lesions that are important for reducing virulence remain unknown.[22] Interestingly, a *S. typhimurium* strain with a deletion in *gal*E is avirulent for mice.[35] This reinforces the view that caution must be taken when extrapolating from data obtained in the mouse to other animal hosts.

Ty21a does not have all the properties of an ideal live typhoid vaccine, but in terms of reactogenicity it is a huge improvement over the parenteral vaccine and has proved to be stable (in terms of attenuation) after being administered to many thousands of individuals without virulent revertants being isolated.[22,23] Ty21a has therefore provided confidence that the development of a single dose of oral typhoid vaccine is a realistically achievable goal. Modern molecular techniques coupled with the identification of genes involved in *Salmonella* virulence has enabled the construction of defined mutants that can be evaluated as vaccine candidates.

B. THE USE OF MOLECULAR GENETICS TO RATIONALLY ATTENUATE *SALMONELLAE*

Pathogenic bacteria can be attenuated by mutating genes falling into one of three main groups: first, genes whose products are classical virulence factors, such as toxins or invasins, for example, a strain of *Vibrio cholerae* which possesses deletions in the genes encoding cholera toxin has reduced virulence;[36] second, regulatory genes which control the expression of a number of other genes, including these essential for survival *in vivo*. The *bvg* locus of *Bordetella* sp. positively regulates the transcription of virulence genes, while Bvg– strains are avirulent;[37,38] third, particular housekeeping genes, such as those encoding enzymes whose products cannot be supplied or assimilated from the host, for example, those involved in LPS biosynthesis.[30,31,35,39] Until very recently, genes encoding classical virulence factors have not been well characterized in *Salmonella,* and so attenuation has been achieved by mutating genes belonging to the latter two groups. It should be stressed that attenuating a strain may not render it useful as a live vaccine. It is possible that the mutant may be over-attenuated, so that it no longer stimulates a sufficiently powerful or appropriate immune response (see *purA* mutants below). This possibly may be because the mutant does not survive for long enough in the host, or because expression of a critical immunogen has been abolished. Alternatively, a strain, although it has reduced virulence and may no longer cause lethal infection, may still be too reactogenic to be considered for clinical or veterinary use.

It is desirable that future vaccine strains harbor mutations in at least two loci preferably separated by some distance on the chromosome so as to reduce the chance of reversion to virulence in the field due to transfer of DNA from wild-type organisms (by transfection, transformation, or conjugation). It is also important to select the combination of mutations carefully because again over-attenuation may result (see below). Mutations that cannot be suppressed by additional mutations at secondary sites or that can be overcome by factors supplied by the host should be selected. It is also important to avoid introducing mutations that induce a hyper mutable state that could lead to secondary mutations.

Genes that are important for virulence can be identified by a variety of techniques. Commonly this is done by insertional inactivation using transposons such as Tn*10*. Strains harboring Tn*10* are identified using the selectable antibiotic-resistance gene (tetracyclin) they carry. Isolates can then be characterized *in vivo* and *in vitro*. However, it is not desirable for vaccine strains to carry antibiotic resistance. Also, transposons are not totally stable; they can excise from the chromosome leaving a functional gene. This property can be exploited when using Tn*10* which can excise imprecisely from host DNA, leaving a deletion at the site of insertion and at the same time curing the strain of tetracycline resistance (this rare event can be selected for, using fusaric acid).[40] The development of hybrid transposons that allow the identification of insertions into secreted proteins such as Tn*pho*A can aid in the identification of virulence gene products which are believed to reside at the surface of the bacteria where they are in a position to interact with the host.[41-43] Alternatively, virulence genes can be identified by preparing a genomic library of a virulent strain, introducing these clones into an appropriate avirulent host and characterizing recombinants to see if they have phenotypes that are associated with virulence, such as the increased ability to adhere to, invade, or survive in eukaryotic cells or the ability to produce a virulence-associated product like toxins or capsules.

There are now more sophisticated ways of introducing defined deletions into the genome to produce candidate vaccine strains that do not harbor antibiotic resistance. The gene of interest is cloned on a suicide vector and mutagenized by removing an internal fragment of the gene.[44,45] The mutated construct can be introduced into the virulent strain of choice by conjugation, transformation, transfection, or electroporation. Homologous recombination at a single site between the target gene on the host genome and the mutated gene on the suicide vector leads to integration of the suicide plasmid and mutated gene into the chromosome. Recombinants can be selected using the antibiotic resistance marker on the vector. A second recombination event between host sequences carried by the suicide vector and the host chromosome can result in the mutated allele being left on the chromosome and the wild-type allele being lost from the cell along with the suicide vector upon replication. Isolating such double recombinants requires screening colonies for loss of antibiotic resistance by replica plating. The genotype of antibiotic-sensitive isolates needs to be determined by Southern blotting or PCR. The LPS phenotype of the strain should be examined because rough strains take up DNA more readily. New suicide vectors which allow for positive selection of the second recombination event should make this task easier.[45] The process can be repeated to introduce mutations into additional genes. The use of these techniques has led to the construction of candidate oral typhoid strains that harbor completely defined mutations. These are now being evaluated in human volunteers (see below).

III. RECOMBINANT *SALMONELLA* MUTANTS AS LIVE VACCINES

A. AUXOTROPHIC MUTANTS

Mutants of *S. typhi* that require *p*-aminobenzoic acid (PABA) for growth *in vitro* were found by Bacon et al. to have reduced virulence in mice.[46] PABA is synthesized from chorismate, a starting compound for the biosynthesis of a number of aromatic compounds in the cell, such as aromatic amino acids, dihydroxybenzoate, certain vitamins, and PABA.[47] Chorismate is formed via a number of intermediates by enzymes encoded by *aro* genes. This pathway is known as the prechorismate or aromatic pathway.[47] Stocker and colleagues constructed a PABA auxotroph of *S. typhimurium* by introducing a mutation into the *aro*A gene (encoding 5-enolpyruvylshikimate-3-phosphate synthetase) using the Tn*10* excision method.[48] This strain was highly attenuated in mice by the oral and intravenous (IV) routes.[26,48] *Aro*A mutants of *S. typhimurium* do not have measurable oral LD_{50}s and the IV LD_{50}s are about 10^6 higher than that of wild-type strains.[26,48] Auxotrophs requiring purine for growth were also shown by Bacon et al. to have reduced virulence.[46] This observation was exploited by Stocker et al. to construct *S. typhi* strains with two attenuating lesions: they introduced deletions in *aro*A and the *pur*A genes rendering the strains dependent on aromatic compounds and adenine (or adenosine) for growth.[49] A nonattenuated mutation in the *his* operon was also introduced to act as a marker for the strains. Two strains were constructed from *S. typhi* CDC10-80, 541Ty and 543Ty, the latter being a Vi-derivative of 541Ty that was selected by resistance to Vi-specific phage.[49] In adult volunteers, the two strains were tolerated well when administered orally in bicarbonate at doses of 1×10^8 to 2×10^{10} CFU. Volunteers mounted T cell responses to both vaccines. Unfortunately, 90% of vaccinees failed to mount a significant serum or enteric antibody response to any of the O, H, Vi antigens or *S. typhi* lysates.[50] The poor antibody responses in vaccinees were disappointing. It suggested that the strains were too attenuated and may not provide adequate protection against *S. typhi* challenge, although this was not investigated and indicates that the strains may not be useful as carriers, particularly if a strong humoral response to the foreign antigen is desired.

Subsequent work has indicated that attenuation caused by inactivation of the *purA* gene is too severe, producing strains that can no longer stimulate effective immunity.[51,52] Table 1 compares the properties of *aroA, purA*, and *aroA purA* mutants. Therefore, other mutations were necessary to combine with single *aro* mutants in order to produce stable effective vaccine strains. Interestingly, a mutation in a different gene coding for an enzyme within the purine pathway, *purE*, reduced virulence to a much lesser extent than either *purA* or *aroA* mutations.[51,55] *purA purE* strains were considered too "hot" for vaccine strains.

We investigated the possibility of combining mutations into *aro* genes in order to produce a strain with a low chance of reversion. The *aro* genes are attractive in this regard because they are widely spaced on the *Salmonella* chromosome.[47] *Salmonella typhimurium* strains harboring deletions in *aroC* or *aroD*, as well as different combinations with *aroA* (including *aroA aroD aroC* mutants) were all shown to be attenuated to similar levels and make excellent single-dose oral *Salmonella* vaccines in mice.[56-58] *Aro* mutants of various *Salmonella* strains have also been found to be efficacious single-dose oral vaccines in domestic animals including chickens, calves, and sheep.[59-65]

Aro mutants are believed to be attenuated because they are unable to obtain essential metabolites *in vivo*. Vertebrates do not possess the pre-chorismate pathway and the products of this pathway are believed not to be present in mammalian tissues or fluids or to exist at levels that do not permit sustained bacterial replication. Starvation for PABA is thought to be the major cause of attenuation, since strains with mutations in the *pabB* gene are as attenuated as *aro* mutants.[66] PABA is an intermediate in the synthesis of folate, which is a co-factor in pyrimidine biosynthesis. Bacteria cannot assimilate folate from their host. *Aro* mutants also appear to have a defect in their ability to synthesize fmet-tRNA, which is necessary to initiate translation and may contribute to attenuation.[67] Because the reduced virulence of *aro* mutants results from starvation for essential nutrients and not an inability to deal with the onslaught of the hosts' nonspecific and specific immune system, *aro* mutants should remain attenuated in immunocompromised individuals. As mentioned previously, the propensity of some traditional live vaccines to cause serious infections in this group has been a problem. The LD_{50} of *aro* mutants is not increased in mice sublethally irradiated, in mice treated with anti-TNF-α, in mice treated with antimacrophage agents, or in mice with genetically determined immunodeficiencies.[53,54,66,68-70] *Aro* mutants may therefore be safe to use in areas of the world where lowered immunocompetence is common or in individuals that are immunodeficient, such as those infected with HIV. Strains of *S. typhi* with precise deletions in *aroC* and *aroD* have now been constructed and are being evaluated in human volunteers.[71,72]

B. REGULATORY MUTANTS

Strains of *Salmonella* with deletions in the adenylate cyclase *(cya)* and the cAMP receptor protein *(crp)* genes do not cause disease in mice and induce immunity against wild-type *S. typhimurium* challenge.[17,73,74] Mutations in these two genes affect the activity of a large number of other genes, particularly those involved in carbohydrate and amino acid metabolism.[17] Curing *cya crp* double mutants of their large virulence plasmid, required for the full virulence of murine *Salmonella* strains but not present in *S. typhi*, does not affect their immunogenicity but introduces an additional level of safety.[73] The *in vitro* growth rate of *cya crp* strains is half that of their wild-type parent, which may account for their attenuation.[73]

Table 1 Comparison of the properties of *aroA*, *purA*, and *aroA purA* mutants of *S. typhimurium*

Mutation	LD$_{50}$ Oral	IV	Multiplication in liver and spleen[b]	Persistance in liver and spleen (d)[b]	Splenomegally	Specific protection against *Salmonella*[c] Oral	IV	Dose needed to induce non-sp. protection (log CFU)[d]	Immune response to *Salmonella*[e] Serum Ab	T cell prolif.
aroA	>10	7.4	+	<35	+	+++	+++	5	+++	+++
purA	>10	8.6	–	>70	–	–	+	7	++	+++
aroA purA	ND	8.9	–	>70	–	–	–	ND	ND	ND

[a] Mutants derived from *S. typhimurium* HWSH.
[b] Following IV inoculation.
[c] Against challenge with SL1344.
[d] Protection against IV challenge with *Listeria monocytogenes*.
[e] Responses measured using heat-killed *S. typhimurium* as antigen.
Data compiled from References 51 and 52.

The *omp*R gene forms a two-gene operon with *env*Z.[75,76] These two genes are members of a family of two component regulatory genes that consist of a cytoplasmic membrane protein (EnvZ) that senses the external environment and transmits signals to a cytoplasmic regulator protein (OmpR).[75,76] EnvZ transmits information on the external osmolarity to OmpR, which modulates transcription of various genes including those encoding the major porin proteins OmpC and OmpF.[76] We have shown that *S. typhimurium* SL1344 harboring a mutation in *omp*R is attenuated both orally and parenterally in mice.[77] Orally immunized mice are also well protected against challenge with the virulent parent strain.[77] Further studies revealed that an *omp*C *omp*F double mutant does not mimic the behavior of an *omp*R mutant.[10] Although attenuated to a similar level orally, it exhibited little attenuation when given intravenously. This suggests that other *omp*R-regulated genes play a role in the early stages of the natural infectious process.[10]

Another two-component regulatory system has also proved to be a fruitful target for attenuation in *Salmonella*. The *phoP/phoQ* regulatory genes are responsive to phosphate levels and also other environmental conditions, such as those expected to be experienced by *Salmonella* residing intracellularly within macrophages, for example low pH.[78-82] The *phoP/phoQ* affects, positively or negatively, the expression of a number of other genes. One of the positively regulated genes, *pagC*, is an outer membrane protein that appears to be essential for survival in macrophages.[81] Interestingly, mutants in *phoP* that allow constitutive expression of *pagC (phoP^c)* are attenuated and are superior to *phoP^-* strains as live oral vaccines.[83,84] The *phoP^-* and *phoP^c* mutations have been combined successfully with *aroA* mutations in *S. typhimurium* to make live oral vaccines.[84]

C. OTHER MUTATIONS

Tn*phoA* mutagenesis identified the *htrA* gene as important for survival of *Salmonella in vivo* but not *in vitro*.[85] The product of this gene is a stress-induced protein, DegP, that is responsible for removing erroneously folded proteins in the periplasm. Although the equivalent gene in *E. coli* is necessary for survival at elevated growth temperatures, this is not the case in *Salmonella;* rather the mutants appear to be more sensitive to oxidizing agents and so are thought to be less able to survive in the phagolysosome of macrophages.[85] Like *purA* mutants, *S. typhimurium htrA* mutants do not exhibit replication *in vivo* and persist at lower levels in tissues than *aro* mutants.[86] However, *S. typhimurium htrA* and *S. typhimurium htrA aroA* strains are good single dose oral vaccines.[86] This was somewhat surprising, because we had previously believed that the initial period of replication exhibited by *aro* mutants was essential for inducing protective immunity.

D. EVALUATION OF DEFINED *S. TYPHI* DOUBLE MUTANTS IN HUMANS

A human volunteer study was carried out using double mutants of two *S. typhi* strains, Ty2 and ISP1820 (a recent Chilean isolate). Strains were constructed to harbor deletions in either the *aroC* and *aroD* genes (CVD906, ISP1820 Δ*aroC* Δ*aroD;* CVD908, Ty2 Δ*aroC* Δ*aroD*) or *cya* and *crp* (χ3927, Ty2 Δ*crp* Δ*cya*).[25,71] The virulence of the strains was assessed in mice by injection IP with hog gastric mucin. The ISP1820 strain was at least 100-fold less virulent than Ty2 in this model, and consequently CVD906 was the least virulent strain, followed by CVD908 and χ3927.[25] A double-blind study was performed to assess the behavior of the strains in humans. Small groups of volunteers received a single oral dose of one of the three strains, suspended in PBS. Two dose levels were used, 5×10^4 and 5×10^5 CFU. In contrast to the results in mice, the ISP1820 background appeared more virulent because two individuals that received CVD906 (one from each of the two different dose groups) developed a fever ($\geq 38.2°C$) and malaise.[25] CVD906 was also recovered from the blood of the individual with fever who received the higher doses. CVD908 did not produce clinical symptoms in any recipient nor was it isolated from the blood. χ3927 was isolated from the blood of one individual from each of the two dose groups (they did not exhibit any clinical symptoms), and a third individual developed fever.[25] Although the numbers were small, it would appear that in humans as in mice the *cya crp* mutants retains more virulence than the *aro* mutants. However, despite its apparent lack of reactogenicity, the immunogenicity of CVD908 was comparable to the other strains, all of which induce serum IgG antibodies against *S. typhi* LPS in ca. 50% of recipients. Evidence of stimulation of the MALT was demonstrated by detecting circulating IgA antibody-secreting cells (ASC) specific for LPS and flagellin in over half of the recipients.[25] Because of the absence of adverse reactions, CVD908 has been selected for further volunteer studies. Subsequently the vaccine was given at higher doses (5×10^7 CFU or three doses of 5×10^5 CFU). In this study, the vaccine strain was isolated from the blood of two of the six people receiving 5×10^7 CFU and one of seven individuals given 5×10^5 CFU. In no case was this associated with clinical symptoms.[87]

The immunogenicity of CVD908 was compared with the reported responses generated by other oral typhoid vaccine strains[87] (Table 2). Although only small numbers of individuals were involved, a greater percentage of CVD908 vaccinees responded compared to volunteers given other vaccines, even when 100 to 100,000 fewer organisms were administered[87] (Table 2). Phase II studies are now planned to extend the safety and immunogenicity data on this strain prior to planning a phase III field trial. If these studies are successful, CVD908 will be an attractive candidate for a live oral carrier. Many foreign antigens have already been expressed successfully in *aro* mutants of mouse virulent strains of *Salmonella* (Table 1).

IV. *SALMONELLA* AS A LIVE CARRIER OF HETEROLOGOUS ANTIGENS

Because of the spectrum of immune responses they induce and the availability of good genetic manipulation techniques, attenuated *Salmonella* strains are ideal candidates for use as vectors in delivering heterologous antigens. A number of different genes from bacteria, viruses, parasites, and mammals have been successfully expressed in attenuated *Salmonella* (Table 5), and the recombinant strains have been used to immunize small and domestic animals. Importantly, several investigators have shown that immunization of humans orally with Ty21a (considered a poor carrier) expressing LPS antigens from other enteric bacteria can induce circulating and secretory antibody responses towards the

Table 2 **Comparison of the immunogenicity of different live oral typhoid vaccine strains**

Vaccine strain	Dose (CFU)	No. dose	IgG anti-LPS[a] (%)
Ty21a	10^9	1	5/36 (14)
Ty21a Vi+	10^7	1	2/6 (33)
	10^9	1	1/6 (17)
	10^9	3	6/9 (67)
541 Ty/543Ty	10^8	1	1/19 (11)
	10^9	1	1/10 (10)
	10^{10}	1	1/4 (25)
CVD908	10^4	1	4/7 (57)
	10^5	1	2/5 (40)
	10^7	1	5/6 (83)

[a] No. of individuals responding/No. of individuals.

From Tacket, C. O., Hone, D. M., Losonsky, G. A., Guers, L., Edelman, R., and Levine, M. M., *Vaccine,* 10, 443, 1992. With permission.

foreign LPS,[88-94] thus proving that using *Salmonella* as an oral delivery system is feasible in man.

A. STABILITY OF FOREIGN GENES

The major obstacle to overcome with using *Salmonella* as an oral carrier is to obtain stable expression of the foreign gene at sufficient levels to provoke the required immune response and to ensure that the expression is controlled in such a way that it is not deleterious to the carrier strain. Conventional expression vectors, which may exist at high copy number, allow for high level expression of the antigen of interest. However, these vectors are often very unstable *in vitro* and *in vivo* without antibiotic selection (unacceptable for veterinary and human use), and even if stable *in vitro,* they may not be so *in vivo.* Several approaches have been devised to try to overcome this problem. Integration of the foreign gene(s) into the chromosome should stabilize the genes. This can be achieved by cloning a fragment of the *Salmonella* chromosome that carries particular genes (e.g., *aro* genes) into an appropriate suicide vector that cannot be maintained in *Salmonella.* A multiple cloning site can be introduced into the coding sequence of the cloned gene to allow foreign genes to be inserted along with appropriate promoter sequences. The constructs are then introduced into *Salmonella* and the foreign gene is integrated into the chromosome by homologous recombination between sequences flanking the foreign gene and homologous sequences on the chromosome. Recombinants can be selected positively, if the integrated DNA contains an antibiotic resistance gene as well as the foreign DNA, or negatively, if the integration causes an auxotrophic mutation by replica plating. Vectors that allow integration into the *his*[95] locus or the *aroC*[96] gene have been devised, the latter system having the advantage that integration creates an additional attenuating lesion in the carrier strain. The drawback to this approach is that only a single copy of the gene is present in the host strain. The level of expression will consequently be lower than if the gene was present on a multicopy plasmid and the antigen concentration in the *Salmonella* may be subimmunogenic (see below). A possible solution to this problem is to integrate several copies of the gene of interest into the genome either at several different sites or using multiple copies at a single site.

An alternative approach is to utilize plasmids carrying determinants that are essential to the survival of *Salmonella* in the host. One such system uses plasmids that harbor the *asd* gene, which codes for the protein aspartate β-semialdehyde dehydrogenase, an enzyme common to the biosynthesis of several amino acids as well as diaminopymelic acid (DAP), is an essential component of the bacterial peptidoglycan. DAP cannot be supplied by the host, and *asd* mutants of *S. typhimurium* are avirulent.[17,97] Plasmids carrying *asd* can be utilized in strains with deletions in several attenuating genes such as *cya* and *crp* as well as *asd.*[97] In *asd* mutants, plasmids carrying the *asd* gene are very stable *in vitro* in the absence of DAP.[97] In animals, loss of the plasmid by the *asd Salmonella* mutant would be lethal. This selection does not prevent segregation; rather, plasmidless bacteria die. However, selective pressure may be such that the plasmid may be retained by enough of the population to engender an immune response. Similar systems based around the *purA* and *thyA* gene have been developed.[18,98]

Unregulated high level expression of foreign proteins, particularly secreted products such as toxins and outer membrane proteins, may be toxic to *Salmonella* and will lead to selection of plasmid "cured" strains. A way around this is to control the expression of the foreign gene using promoters that are only active at a certain phase of the life cycle of *Salmonella* or when the *Salmonella* occupies a particular cellular compartment. There is now a greater understanding of which genes are regulated by host environmental signals. For example, certain genes may be controlled by direct contact with eukaryotic cells, osmolarity, oxygen tension of the environment, or by the concentration of certain nutrients such as iron[99,100] (see below).

B. OTHER FACTORS AFFECTING THE EFFICACY OF *SALMONELLA* AS A DELIVERY SYSTEM

As well as instability of the foreign genes, there are a number of other factors that may have an influence on *Salmonella*-based carrier systems but for which we as yet do not have any systematic rules:

1. What Level of Antigen Expression is Necessary to Elicit the Desired Immune Response?

This almost certainly depends on the individual antigen and the type of response required. We have found that integrating the gene for the C terminal 50-kDa portion of tetanus toxin (fragment C), which is nontoxic and carries protective epitopes,[101] into the *aroC* gene of *S. typhimurium aroA* (SL3261) increases stability of the gene, but the quantity of fragment C produced was subimmunogenic.[96] (See below and Table 3)

The same *aroC* integration system was used to express the gene for the P.69 outer membrane protein of *Bordetella pertussis* from the chromosome of an *aroA aroD S. typhimurium* mutant.[58] Serum and mucosal antibodies against the carried antigen were not detected following two oral or IV doses. However, the recombinant strain did induce protective immunity (enhanced clearance of *B. pertussis* from the lungs of aerosol-challenged mice).[58] Upon further analysis of the immune response, it was found that splenic T cells from immunized mice proliferated vigorously *in vitro* in the presence of P.69[58] and produced large amounts of γ-interferon (γ-IFN) but not interleukin (IL) 5[102] (Table 4).

Murine helper T cells can be divided into two groups on the pattern of the cytokines they secrete.[103] Th1 cells produce IL-2, γ-IFN, and lymphotoxin and Th2 cells produce IL-4, IL-5, IL-6, and IL-10.[103,104] Th1 helper T cells are primarily responsible for promoting cellular immunity (CMI), including activating macrophages, and cytotoxic T lymphocytes (CTL), and Th2 cells provide help for antibody production.[103,104] There is some evidence that immunization with low amounts of an antigen promotes primarily CMI whereas large doses of an antigen induces antibody responses, at least in rodents, and the two types of responses are mutually exclusive.[99] This can now be explained by the reciprocal antagonism of Th1 and Th2 helper T cells.[103,104] We are examining if the concentration of antigen in the *Salmonella* carrier determines the type of immune response by expressing model antigens at different levels. It may be possible to produce the required response by coexpressing immunomodulating agents such as particular cytokines along with the foreign antigens; for example, Th1 responses might be generated by using *Salmonella* expressing cytokines such as IL-2, γ-IFN, and Th2 responses by expressing IL-4 and IL-10. We have recently demonstrated the feasibility of this approach by showing that *Salmonella* can produce functional IL-1 *in vivo*.[105]

2. How Does the Location or Form of the Foreign Antigen in *Salmonella* Affect the Resulting Immune Response?

Again this will probably vary according to the individual antigen. Early studies with *aroA S. typhimurium* expressing β-galactosidase, a cytoplasmically located antigen, demonstrated that CMI, humoral, and secretory antibodies can be elicited.[14] It is possible, however, that if the conformation of the antigen is critical to the formation of certain epitopes, then the folding of the protein could be altered if it resides in a foreign environment. This needs to be tested using conformation-dependent monoclonal antibodies or appropriate protection models. Tetanus toxin is normally a secreted protein. However the critical epitopes of fragment C are maintained when the protein is located in the cytoplasm of *Salmonella*.[20,106]

If correct folding does not occur in the cytoplasm, then translocation of the protein through the cytoplasmic membrane can be attempted. If the gene or the antigen includes

Table 3 Heterologous Antigens Expressed in Attenuated *Salmonella*

Antigen	Organism	*Salmonella* strain	Immune response[a]				Ref.
			Ab	CMI	CTL	Protection[b]	
Bacterial							
C-fragment	*C. tetani*	*S. typhimurium aroA, aroA aroD aroA aroC*	+	ND[c]	ND	+	20, 96, 106
P.69	*B. pertussis*	*S. typhimurium aroA aroC aroD*	−	+	ND	+	58
FHA	*B. pertussis*	*S. typhimurium aroA*	+	ND	ND	ND	140, 141
PTX-S1	*B. pertussis*	*S. typhimurium aroA*	+	ND	ND	ND	142
M protein	*S. pyogenes*	*S. typhimurium aroA*	+	ND	ND	+	123
LTB	*E. coli*	*S.typhimurium aroA, S. enteridis aroA, S. dublin aroA, S. typhi Ty21a*	+	ND	ND	+	19, 26, 113, 143–145
K1 capsule	*E. coli*	*S. typhimurium aroA*	−	ND	ND	+	114
K88	*E. coli*	*S. typhimurium aroA, galE*	+	ND	ND	+	145–147
β-Galactosidase	*E. coli*	*S. typhimurium aroA, galE*	+	+	ND	ND	14
Hemagglutinin	*P. gingivalis*	*S. typhimurium aroA*	+	+	ND	ND	149
28-kD OMP	*N. meningitidis*	*S. typhimurium aroA*	+	ND	ND	ND	150
Lipoprotein	*P. aeruginosa*	*S. dublin aroA*	+	ND	ND	ND	19
Various	*T. pallidum*	*S. typhimurium aroA, aroA aroC*	±	ND	ND	−[d]	96, 151
31 kDa	*B. abortis*	*S. cholerasuis cya crp cdt, S. typhimurium cya crp*	+	−	−	ND	152–154
17 kDa	*F. tularensis*	*S. typhimurium cya crp asd*	+	ND	ND	+	154, 155
O antigen	*S. sonnei*	*S. typhi Ty21a*	+	ND	ND	±	88, 92, 157–160
O antigen	*S. flexneri*	*S. typhi Ty21a*	+	ND	ND	+	115
O antigen	*V. cholerae*	*S. typhi Ty21a*	+	ND	ND	±	89–91, 93, 94, 161–163
SpaA	*S. mutans*	*S. typhimurium cya crp*	ND	ND	ND	ND	163–165

Antigen	Source	Salmonella strain					Ref.
SpaA	*S. sobrinus*	*S. typhimurium cya crp, cya crp asd*	+	ND	ND	ND	74, 97
Viral							
Nucleoprotein	Influenza A	*S. typhimurium aroA*	+	+	+[e]	+[f]	113
Core protein	Hepatitis B	*S. typhimurium aroA, aroA aroD, cya crp, S.dublin aroA*	+	+	ND	ND	19, 167, 168 (P. Londono unpub.)
gpD	Herpes simplex	*S. typhimurium aroA*	ND	ND	ND	+	169
Envelope antigen	Dengue 4	*S. typhimurium aroA*	ND	ND	ND	ND	170
Parasites							
Core protein	Wood chuck	*S. typhimurium cya crp*	+	ND	ND	ND	19
VP7	Rotavirus SA11	*S. typhimurium cya crp*	−	ND	ND	ND	171
CSP	*P. berghei*	*S. typhimurium WR4017, WR4024*	−	+	+	+	127, 128
CSP	*P. falciparum*	*S. typhimurium WR4024*	−	+	+	ND	128
CSP	*P. yoleii*	*S. typhimurium aroA*	−	+	+	−	129
gp63	*L. major*	*S. typhimurium aroA*	−	+	ND	+	133
Species specific Ag	*E. multilocularis*	*S. typhimurium galE*	+	+	ND	+	172
Cytokines							
IL-1β	Human	*S. typhimurium aroA*	+	ND	ND	+[g]	105
Epitopes							
LTB-HBsAg	Hepatitis B	*S. dublin aroA*	−	+	ND	ND	145
LTB-HBsAg	Hepatitis B	*S. typhimurium cya crp asd*	−	+	−	ND	145
LTB-SpA	*S. sobrinus*	*S. typhimurium cya crp asd*	ND	ND	ND	ND	173
LTB-Dextranase	*S. sobrinus*	*S. typhimurium cya crp asd*	ND	ND	ND	ND	173
Core-preS2	Hepatitis B	*S.dublin aroA, S. typhimurium aroA*	+	ND	ND	ND	168
Flagellin-M	*S. pyogenes*	*S. dublin aroA*	+	ND	ND	+	124

Table 3 (continued) **Heterologous Antigens Expressed in Attenuated *Salmonella***

Antigen	Organism	*Salmonella* strain	Immune response[a]			Protection[b]	Ref.
			Ab	CMI	CTL		
Flagellin-CTB	*V. cholerae*	*S. dublin aroA*	+	ND	ND	ND	112
Flagellin-HBsAg	Hepatitis B	*S. dublin aroA*	+	–	–	ND	174
Flagellin-HA	Influenza A	*S. dublin aroA*	+	ND	ND	–	175
OmpA-HA	Influenza A	*S. typhimurium cya crp asd*	–	ND	ND	±	176
OmpA-HRPII	*P. falciparum*	*S. typhimurium cya crp asd*	+	–	–	ND	111
OmpA-SERP	*P. falciparum*	*S. typhimurium cya crp asd*	+	–	–	ND	111
LamB-Shiga toxin B-subunit	*S. dysenteriae*	*S. typhimurium aroA* +	–	–	–	ND	110

[a] Ab, antibody response; CMI, cell-mediated response, i.e., macrophage activation, T cell proliferation, production of particular cytokines or delayed-type hypersensitivity; CTL, generation of cytotoxic T cells.

[b] Protection in an animal model or in human volunteers or neutralisation *in vivo*.

[c] ND, not determined.

[d] Immunization enhanced the development of syphilitic lesions in rabbits.

[e] CD4+ class II-restricted CTL.

[f] Protection requires intranasal boosting with purified nucleoprotein.

[g] Radio protection.

Table 4   Effect of fragment C gene copy number, stability, and expression on the immunogenicity of *Salmonella*-delivered fragment C

Promoter	Expression	Gene location[a]	Copies of gene	Solubility[b]	Stability[c]	Immunization[d]	Dose	Protection[e]	Ref.
trpE	Constitutive	P	Multiple	−	Low	O, IV	2	None	(N. Fairweather, personal communication)
tac	Constitutive	P	Multiple	+	Low	O O IV	1 2 1	Partial Partial to full Full	20, 106 20, 106 20
tac	Constitutive	C	Single	+	High	O, IV	2	None	96 (N. Fairweather, personal communication)
nirB	Inducible	P	Multiple	+	High	O, IV	1	Full	106

Note: The *Salmonella* strains used were either *S. typhimurium* SL3261 (*aroA*) or *S. typhimurium* BRD509 (*aroA aroC*)

[a] P, Plasmid; C, chromosomal.
[b] −, insoluble; +, soluble.
[c] Stability in tissues in vivo.
[d] O, Oral; IV, intravenous.
[e] Protection against 50 LD_{50}s of tetanus toxin.
[f] Induced by anaerobiosis.

them, then the natural secretion sequence for the protein (signal sequence) can be used or, if not, the secretion signals from well-characterized proteins such as OmpA or MalE can be utilized.[107] Alternatively, if the critical epitope(s) have been identified, the DNA sequences encoding the epitope can be cloned internally in the gene that encodes a surface located protein such as PhoE, LamB, OmpA, or flagellin.[107-112] Sites within the carrier protein are selected on the basis of being surface located and that can allow insertions without disrupting the overall structure of the protein (permissive sites).[107] Recently, quite large foreign polypeptides have been expressed on the surface of *Salmonella* using OmpA.[111]

3. How Does Prior Exposure (Immunity) to the Carrier Strain Affect the Response to the Foreign Antigen?

This is a question that is often asked, but surprisingly little work has been carried out in this area. It is possible that a preexisting immune response to the *Salmonella* carrier would clear the carrier strain more quickly following immunization than in a naive individual, thereby reducing the response to the carried antigen. Alternatively, the vigorous anamnestic immune response to the carrier may potentiate the response to a foreign antigen. In the single reported investigation into this area using the murine *Salmonella* model, the latter appeared to be the case. Exposure to the carrier strain *(S. dublin aroA)* led to an enhanced response to the carried antigen (LTB) when the mice were subsequently given *S. dublin* expressing LTB.[113] Interestingly, priming the mice with a heterologous serotype *(S. typhimurium aroA)* also boosted the serum response to LTB, but only priming with the homologous strain augmented the secretory antibody response.[113] In humans, immunization with Ty21a did not impede the immune response to *Vibrio cholerae* LPS when individuals were subsequently given Ty21a expressing this antigen.[93] However, high preexisting anti-*V. cholerae* LPS antibodies did appear to reduce the subsequent development of vibrocidal antibodies following immunization with Ty21a expressing cholera LPS.[94]

4. Does the Foreign Gene or Antigens Affect the Behavior of the Carrier?

For multivalent vaccines where immunity against *Salmonella* is also desired, it is important to test that the foreign antigen does not interfere with development of anti-*Salmonella* immunity. In many reported studies of *Salmonella* carrying heterologous antigens this has not been explored. We have so far not found any foreign antigen which interferes with *Salmonella* immunity in mice. The presence of the K1 polysaccharide capsule of virulent *E. coli* on the surface of *S. typhimurium aroA* did alter its behavior *in vivo*, however.[114] The K1+ positive strain was cleared more slowly from the livers and more rapidly from the spleens than the isogenic K1− strain. Mice immunized with the K1+ strain did not exhibit splenomegaly, but they were immune to challenge with *S. typhimurium*.[114]

Ty21a engineered to express the LPS antigens of *S. flexneri* 2a no longer immunized mice against *S. typhi* challenge (immunization and challenge IP), but the animals were immune to *S. flexneri* challenge.[115] It will be interesting to determine if similar problems are encountered using *Salmonella* carrier strains that do not have defects in their ability to produce complete LPS.

V. SPECIFIC EXAMPLES OF USING *SALMONELLA* AS A CARRIER OF HETEROLOGOUS ANTIGENS

As can be seen from Table 3, a large number of different heterologous antigens have been expressed in attenuated *Salmonella*. However in very few instances, even in mice, has the "gold standard" of this approach to immunization been achieved, namely, solid protection against challenge with a heterologous pathogen or toxin following a single oral immunization. In many instances, the efficacy of the *Salmonella* delivery system cannot be assessed because the mouse is not an appropriate host for certain pathogens (such as hepatitis B virus). The following are notable examples of the use of *Salmonella* delivery systems to immunize against heterologous challenge.

A. IMMUNIZATION AGAINST BACTERIAL DISEASES
1. Oral Tetanus Vaccine

We have for some time been trying to develop an oral tetanus vaccine. This would be invaluable in the third world, where the majority of the 1 million deaths per year attributable to tetanus occur.[116] The problems with the current vaccine are the need for a cold chain for storage, the use of needles for administration, and the requirement of multiple doses for full protection. When given orally, 600 to 1000-fold more tetanus toxoid is necessary to induce the level of protection that can be achieved by parenteral immunization[126] (P. Knight, personal communication) and so this is not a practical means of vaccination. These problems may be overcome by using *Salmonella* to deliver the nontoxic forms of tetanus toxin. The prospect for success with this approach is improved by the fact that a serum immune response to a single invariant immunogen (tetanus toxin) mediates protection. Fragment C is a 50-kDa C-terminal fragment of tetanus toxin that can be generated by proteolytic cleavage of tetanus toxin or by expressing defined DNA fragments of *Clostridium tetani* DNA that specify this region of tetanus toxin.[101] Fragment C is nontoxic and can immunize mice against tetanus.[101,118]

Initial fragment C expression plasmids produced fragment C as fusion proteins to either a portion of the B fragment of tetanus toxin or the TrpE protein.[118] These recombinant proteins were insoluble in *E. coli* but were capable of inducing protection against tetanus toxin challenge.[118] These plasmids were introduced into *S. typhimurium* SL3261; they did not confer the ability to immunize mice against challenge, or to induce antitetanus antibodies, probably because they were very unstable (N. Fairweather, personal communication). The problem of insolubility was overcome by expressing only the DNA sequences encoding the fragment C polypeptide presumably because it allowed correct folding of the protein.[20] Two pAT153-based plasmids expressing fragment C from *Ptac* were constructed, pTETtac2 and pTETtac4. The latter was derived from pTETtac2 by removal of a restriction enzyme fragment containing the *lacI* gene.[20] Both constructs were introduced into SL3261. Fragment C is produced from pTETtac4 constitutively in *Salmonella*, whereas pTETtac2 requires induction with IPTG and therefore should not be expressed *in vivo*.[20] Two oral or a single IV inoculation of SL3261 pTETtac4 induced complete protection against challenge with up to 500 LD_{50}s of tetanus toxin.[20] A single oral dose gave incomplete protection (ca. 74%). There were no survivors among mice receiving SL3261 or SL3261pTETtac2.[20]

Subsequent studies were aimed at improving the immunogenicity of the *Salmonella* fragment C strains to produce a single-dose oral vaccine. To overcome the instability of pTETtac4, the fragment C gene was introduced into the chromosome of SL3261, using the *aroC* integration vector.[96] Although this stabilized the fragment C gene in *Salmonella*, the level of fragment C synthesized was very low[96] (only detectable in total cell lysates by Western blotting), and immunization of mice by the oral or IV routes did not induce antitetanus toxin antibodies or protection against tetanus toxin challenge (N. Fairweather, personal communication), so alternative means of augmenting the immune response to *Salmonella* fragment C were sought. The level of fragment C produced by *E. coli* was increased (from 3 to 4% to 11 to 14% total cell protein) by substituting codons in the *C. tetani* DNA sequence that are rarely used in *Enterobacteriacae* with codons more commonly utilized.[119]

We also experimented with using different promoters to express fragment C. High level of expression of fragment C from the constitutive *Ptac* promoter probably contributes to the instability of plasmids carrying this gene. We found that the *nirB* promoter was useful for expressing proteins with vaccine potential in *E. coli* grown in fermenters.[120] This promoter controls the expression of the NADH-dependent nitrite reductase gene and is regulated by the oxygen and nitrite concentration in the media. it is optimally active under anaerobic conditions.[121] To determine the utility of expressing foreign antigens using the *nirB* promoter, the *tac* promoter from the plasmid encoding the codon-optimized fragment C (pTETtac85) was replaced with an oligonucleotide containing the *nirB* promoter.[106] The plasmids pTETtac85 and pTETnir15 (the P*nirB* fragment C plasmid) were introduced into *S. typhimurium* BRD509 *(aroA aroD)*. Fragment C was produced constitutively in BRD753 (BRD509 pTETtac85), whereas in BRD847 (BRD509 pTET*nir*15) fragment C was inducible under anaerobic conditions.[106] BRD847 induced solid protection in BALB/c mice against tetanus toxin challenge after a single oral dose.[106] In contrast, only partial protection was provided by two oral doses of BRD753.[106] The degree of protection induced by the two strains correlated with the serum anti-fragment C response. Plasmid pTETnir15 was much more stable *in vivo* than pTETtac85, and this may be the reason for the greater immunogenicity of BRD847.[106] We are currently investigating at what stage during colonization of the host the *nirB* promoter is active. It has been found that controlling expression of other foreign antigen using P*nirB* enhances the humoral immune response to *Salmonella*-delivered antigens (C. Hormaeche, personal communication). The effect of copy number, stability, solubility, and promoters on the immune response to *Salmonella*-delivered fragment C is summarized in Table 4. Other workers have shown that different environmentally regulated promoters can be used to improve the host response to foreign antigens expressed by *Salmonella*.[110]

2. Immunization against *Streptococcus pyogenes*

The M protein of *S. pyogenes* and other streptococci is the major virulence factor and immunogen. Type-specific antibodies against the M protein neutralizes its antiphagocytic properties and allow elimination of the organism.[122] Poirier et al. expressed the entire type 5 M protein (pepM5) of *S. pyogenes* from a plasmid (pMK207) in SL3261.[123] M protein was confined to the cytoplasmic compartment in *Salmonella*. Mice immunized twice orally, (6 days apart) developed serum type-specific antibody against pepM5 that peaked around week 9. Boosting of mice 1 day prior to bleeding with purified pepM5 greatly enhanced the titer (10-16 fold).[123] IgA anti-pepM5 was also demonstrated in the saliva from immunized mice.[132] Oral immunization with two doses of SL3261 pMK207 ($\geq 2 \times 10^5$ CFU) provided protection against intraperitoneal and intranasal challenge with M type 5 *S. pyogenes* (but not M type 24 streptococci), and also protection against wild type *S. typhimurium*.[123]

The problem with developing anti-*S. pyogenes* vaccines based on M protein is twofold. First, M proteins can induce antibodies that cross-react with human cardiac antigens. Second, immunity is type specific. Therefore, a successful vaccine should elicit antibodies against the protective epitopes of numerous M proteins without stimulating antibodies that cross-react with the host. Expressing only those regions of M protein responsible for inducing protective antibodies will overcome the problem of auto antibodies. It is theoretically possible to express multiple protective epitopes from different M proteins in *Salmonella*.

Stocker and colleagues used their flagellin foreign epitope expression system to construct an *aroA S. dublin* strain producing a protective epitope of pepM5 (the N terminal 15-amino acid residues).[124] An oligonucleotide specifying the M5 peptide was introduced into the EcoRV site of the flagellin gene *(fliC)*. The oligo was designed so that functional flagellin would only be produced by constructs with the correct orientation. The resultant plasmid restored the motility of a flagellin-negative strain of *aroA S. dublin*.[124] The flagella produced by this strain was reactive with antibodies raised against pepM5.[124] Multiple intraperitoneal immunizations (6 doses of 1×10^6 to 2×10^6 CFU) induced type-specific opsonic antibodies and partial (four out of five mice) protection against intraperitoneal challenge with *S. pyogenes*.[124]

3. Oral Whooping Cough Vaccine

The P.69 outer membrane protein (also known as pertactin) is a virulence factor believed to be involved in the attachment of *B. pertussis* to eukaryotic cells.[38,125] It is also a protective immunogen and a candidate for inclusion in future acellular pertussis vaccines. To investigate the possibility of developing an oral whooping cough vaccine based on *Salmonella*, we expressed the gene for P.69 *(prn)* in *S. typhimurium* vaccine strain BRD509.[58] P.69 is made as a precursor of 93 kDa that is processed prior to its appearance on the surface of the cell by removal of an N-terminal signal sequence and a large (ca. 30 kDa) region from the C terminus.[126] *E. coli* harboring a plasmid (pAYL1) encoding *prn* under the control of *Ptrc* synthesized and correctly processed the 93-kDa precursor to produce P.69 on their surface.[58] However, high-level expression was lethal, and the plasmid was very unstable in the absence of antibiotics.

To ensure stable expression in *Salmonella*, the plasmid was integrated into the chromosome of BRD509 using the *aroC* integration vector.[58] *Salmonella* produced P.69 to levels comparable to *B. pertussis*, and P.69 was processed normally and located at the surface of *Salmonella* in correct conformation as determined by immunoelectron microscopy or agglutination.[58] The presence of P.69 did not affect the tissue tropism or persistence of *S. typhimurium* in mice. The response of mice immunized with P.69 expressing *S. typhimurium* is summarized in Table 5.

B. IMMUNIZATION AGAINST PARASITES
1. *Plasmodium*

Plasmodium species cause malaria in a variety of mammals. Rodent *Plasmodium* strains are often used as models of human malaria. *Plasmodium* exists in several different forms during its life cycle and expresses numerous antigens. At present no consensus exists as to which parasite antigens are important for protection. The major surface antigen of the infective sporozoite form, the circumsporozoite protein (CSP) has received much attention. Two groups have used *Salmonella* to deliver CSP from different *Plasmodium* strains. Although the carrier strains and expression systems were different, the resulting immune responses were almost identical. Sadoff and co-workers expressed the CSP gene from *P. berghei* from the λ P_L promoter on a plasmid (pMGB2) in *S. typhimurium* WR4017 or WR4204 (strains impaired in macrophage replication).[127,128] Orally immunized mice did not develop serum anti-CSP antibodies although such antibodies were detected transiently in subcutaneously immunized mice.[127] Mice were challenged intravenously with *P. berghei* salivary gland sporozoites, and protection was assessed by determining the number of mice infected with *P. berghei*. A single oral dose of WR4017pMGB2 induced protection in 60 to 70% of animals. Subcutaneous immunization was poorly protective (30 to 44%).[127] Complete protection against infection was achieved by IV immunization of mice with irradiated sporozoites.[127]

It was subsequently demonstrated that the protective effects of immunization could be abolished by treatment with anti-CD8 antibodies.[128] Interestingly, immunity arising from vaccination with irradiated sporozoites was not affected by anti-CD8 treatment. *In vitro* cytotoxicity assays revealed that class I-restricted CD8+ CTLs were induced by immunization with *S. typhimurium* expressing CSP of *P. berghei* or *P. falciparum*.[128]

Flynn et al. induced CD8+ CTLs against *P. yoelii* CSP by multiple (3×) oral immunization with *S. typhimurium aroA* (SL3235) expressing *P. yoelii* CSP from the bacterial chromosome.[129] The CSP gene under the control of the *lac*UV5P promoter was inserted randomly into the chromosome of *Salmonella* using a modified mini-transposon,

Table 5 Cellular, humoral, and protective immune response in mice immunized orally with *Salmonella* expressing the *B. pertussis* P.69 protein

Strain[a]	Dose[b]	Protection against Salmonella[c]	B. pertussis in lungs (CFU)[d]	Antibody response[e]		Cellular response[f]		
				Serum	Mucosal	Proliferation	IFN	IL-5
BRD640 (aroA aroC aroD, P69+)	1	+	1.5×10^4	−	−	+	+	−
	2	+	3.2×10^3	±	−	+	+	−
BRD509 (aroA aroD)	2	+	9.5×10^5	−	−	−	−	−

[a] Both strains derived from *S. typhimurium* SL1344.

[b] Mice received 3 to 5 × 109 CFU/dose. The second dose was administered 28 d after the first.

[c] Protection against oral challenge with wild-type *S. typhimurium*.

[d] Levels of *B. pertussis* in the lungs of immunized mice 10 d after aerosol challenge.

[e] Serum anti-P.69 response measured by ELISA and the presence of P.69-specific B cells in the respiratory tract by ELISPOT.

[f] P.69-specific cellular responses: proliferation of splenic T cells determined by 3H-thymidine: secretion of γ-IFN or IL-5 by splenic lymphocytes *in vivo* in the presence of P.69 measured by ELISA.

mini-Tn*10*-kan.[129] As with *Salmonella* expressing CSP from other *Plasmodium* species, oral immunization with SL3235 expressing *P. yoelii* CSP did not induce a CSP serum response.[129] In contrast to the results with *Salmonella* expressing *P. berghei* CSP, immunization did not reduce parasitemia.[129]

There is an interesting example of *Salmonella* enhancement of protective immune response to *Plasmodium* species, by co-administration of the *Salmonella* strain and the *Plasmodium* antigens. *P. vinckei* causes lethal infection in mice. Immunization of BALB/c mice with combinations of live *S. typhimurium aroA* (SL3235 BV) and killed *P. vinckei,* but not either component alone, protected mice against *P. vinckei* challenge.[129] The protection was active even when *Salmonella* and *P. vinckei* antigens were administered by different routes.[129] Protection was attributed to nonspecific activation of the splenic defenses by the *Salmonella* and specific CD4+ T cell-dependent responses to *P. vinckei* antigens. The protection seen was dependent on a functional spleen, and the role played by *Salmonella* cannot be substituted by adjuvants such as complete Freunds adjuvant or *B. pertussis*.[129] It will be interesting to see if the response is the same if the *Salmonella* strain expresses the *P. vinckei* antigen(s).

2. Leishmania

Immunity to *Leishmania* sp. in susceptible mice can be achieved by immunization with killed *Leishmania* or certain purified antigens such as the gp63 protein or lipophosphoglycan.[131,132] Protection is associated with induction of a Th1 response to the *Leishmania* antigens. Th2 responses to *Leishmania* exacerbate the course of infection.[131,132] The route of immunization is critical to the type of immune response elicited and hence protection. Th1 responses to *Leishmania* in mice result from IV or IP immunization, Th2 follow subcutaneous immunization.[131,132] The IV and IP routes are unacceptable in humans. Yang et al. investigated the oral route of immunization using *S. typhimurium* SL3261 expressing the *L. major* gp63 from a plasmid (pKK-Imm63-67, p63).[133] The plasmid was relatively unstable *in vivo* in CBA mice; nevertheless splenic T cells from SL3261 p63 immunized mice (2 × oral) proliferated and produced γ-IFN and IL-2 but not IL-4 (a Th1 response) in the presence of *L. major* antigens.[133] Low levels of serum anti-gp63 antibodies were detected, but delayed type hypersensitivity did not develop in response to challenge with parasite antigens.[133] Mice immunized orally with SL3261 p.63 also controlled *Leishmania* infections better than control mice in terms of size of the lesions produced following subcutaneous challenge with *L. major* promastogotes.[133]

C. IMMUNIZATION AGAINST VIRAL INFECTIONS
1. Influenza

A plasmid (pNP-2) specifying the nucleoprotein (NP) of influenza A virus was introduced into SL3261. NP was produced at high levels in the cytoplasm of SL3261pNP-2 (BRD350). Mice immunized with BRD350 did not develop class I-restricted NP-specific CTLs, although oral immunization with BRD350 did induce activation of NP-specific helper T cells (proliferation) and a serum antibody response to NP.[134] Influenza virus A/PR8 was cleared more rapidly from the lungs of mice receiving two oral doses of BRD350 and boosted IN with purified NP compared to SL3261 immunized controls (500-fold lower virus titre in lung homogenates 6 days following IN challenge).[134] Because NP is an internal antigen and CD8+ CTLs were not elicited, it is not readily apparent how immunization with BRD350 enhances clearance of influenza from the respiratory tract. It is possible that the cytokines produced by CD4+ T cells promote antiviral activity of other cells.

VI. FUTURE CONSIDERATIONS

The planned extended safety and immunogenicity studies with CVD908 should establish if this strain is safe and sufficiently immunogenic to continue development as a second generation oral typhoid vaccine. If CVD908 does fulfill its potential, then studies in humans using this strain or closely related strains expressing foreign antigens should follow rapidly. This should establish if using double *aro* mutants of *S. typhi* as a live carrier for foreign antigens is practical in humans. We have already constructed such strains expressing fragment C from both the chromosome and on plasmids under the control of different promoters[72] (S. Chatfield, unpublished).

If it proves that plasmids are the most effective and convenient vehicles for carrying and expressing foreign genes in *Salmonella,* then alternatives to antibiotic resistant markers will need to be sought, such as mercury resistance or auxotrophic markers described above. If prior immunity to *S. typhi* is detrimental to development of immunity to foreign antigens delivered by *S. typhi,* then attenuated strains of other serotypes of human *Salmonella* such as *S. paratyphi* or enteritis-causing strains could be used as carriers to overcome this problem. It is possible that strains attenuated by different means may differ in their effectiveness as carriers. For instance, *htrA* mutants which do not produce the DegP protease[85] may degrade foreign antigens less readily and therefore may be capable of presenting higher levels of antigen to the immune system.

Although this review has focused on *Salmonella,* attenuated mutants of other bacteria could also be exploited as live mucosal carriers for heterologous antigens, and in certain instances may offer advantages over *Salmonella*-based systems. For example, because of the common mucosal immune systems, stimulation of the gut MALT can lead to secretory IgA responses at distant sites.[5,135-138] However, the immune response is usually greatest at the site of induction,[5] i.e., the gut in the case of *Salmonella.* Therefore, if strong secretory responses are desired at nonenteric sites, such as the respiratory tract, then attenuated respiratory pathogens may be more effective as carriers. *B. pertussis aroA* mutants are attenuated and immunogenic when given by aerosol to mice, and these may have potential to deliver foreign antigen to the human respiratory tract MALT.[138] Also, live carriers based on bacteria such as *Listeria* which can induce strong CD8+ CTLs may be more effective at inducing cytotoxic T cell responses if this is required.[139] BCG has recently been used successfully as a live carrier of foreign antigens in mice (see Chapter 3, Part I).

As well as being used to construct practical vaccines, *Salmonella* expressing foreign antigens can be used as probes to study the immune response to particular immunogens of different pathogens in isolation, for instance, studies with the BRD640, which expresses the *B. pertussis* P.69 protein, revealed that a CMI response to this pertussis antigen in the absence of an antibody response can contribute to protection against pertussis infection.[58]

REFERENCES

1. Collins, F. M., Vaccines and cell-mediated immunity, *Bact. Rev.,* 38, 371, 1974.
2. Hormaeche, C. E., Joysey, H. S., DeSilva, L., Izhar, M., and Stocker, B. A., Immunity induced by live attenuated *Salmonella* vaccines, *Res. Microbiol.,* 141, 757, 1990.
3. Mackaness, G. B., Resistance to intracellular infection, *J. Infect. Dis.,* 123, 439, 1971.
4. Waldman, R. H. and Ganguly, R., Immunity to infections on secretory surfaces, *J. Infect. Dis.,* 130, 419, 1974.
5. McGhee, J. R., Mestecky, J., Dertzbaugh, M. T., Eldridge, J. H., Hirasawa, M., and Kiyono, H., The mucosal immune system: from fundamental concepts to vaccine development, *Vaccine,* 10, 75, 1992.

6. Holmgren, J. and Czerkinsky, C., Cholera as a model for research on mucosal immunity and development of oral vaccines, *Curr. Opin. Immunol.*, 4, 387, 1992.
7. Carter, P. B. and Collins, F. M., The route of enteric infection in normal mice, *J. Exp. Med.*, 139, 1189, 1974.
8. Takeuchi, A., *Electron Microscope Studies of Experimental* Salmonella *Infection. I. Penetration into the Intestinal Epithelium by* Salmonella typhimurium, American Society for Microbiology, Los Angeles, CA, 1966, 109.
9. Finlay, B. B. and Falkow, S., *Salmonella* as an intracellular parasite, *Mol. Microbiol.*, 3, 1833, 1989.
10. Chatfield, S. N., Dorman, C. J., Hayward, C., and Dougan, G., Role of *ompR*-dependent genes in *Salmonella typhimurium* virulence: mutants deficient in both *ompC* and *ompF* are attenuated *in vivo, Infect. Immun.*, 59, 449, 1991.
11. Buchmeier, N. and Heffron, F., Induction of *Salmonella* stress proteins upon infection of macrophages, *Science*, 248, 730, 1990.
12. Buchmeier, N. A. and Heffron, F., Inhibition of macrophage phagosome-lysosome fusion by *Salmonella typhimurium, Infect. Immun.*, 59, 2232, 1991.
13. Nnalue, N. A., Shnyra, A., Hultenby, J., and Lindberg, A. A., *Salmonella choleraesuis* and *Salmonella typhimurium* associated with liver cells after intravenous inoculation of rats are localised mainly in Kupffer cells and multiply intracellularly, *Infect. Immun.*, 60, 2758, 1992.
14. Brown, A., Hormaeche, C. E., DeMarco de Hormaeche, R., Winther, M., Dougan, G., Maskell, D. J., and Stocker, B. A. D., An attenuated *aroA Salmonella typhimurium* vaccine elicits humoral and cellular immunity to cloned β-galactosidase in mice, *J. Infect. Dis.*, 155, 86, 1987.
15. Dougan, G., Smith, L., and Heffron, F., Live bacterial vaccines and their application as carriers for foreign antigens, in *Advances in Veterinary Science and Comparative Medicine*, Vol. 33, Bittle, J. L., Ed., Academic Press, Orlando, FL, 1989, 271.
16. Chatfield, S. N., Strugnell, R. A., and Dougan, G., Live *Salmonella* as vaccines and carriers of foreign antigenic determinants, *Vaccine*, 7, 495, 1989.
17. Curtiss, R. I., Kelly, S. M., Gulig, P. A., and Nakayama, K., Selective delivery of antigens by recombinant bacteria, *Curr. Top. Microbiol. Immunol.*, 146, 35, 1989.
18. Hackett, J., *Salmonella*-based vaccines, *Vaccine*, 8, 5, 1990.
19. Schodel, F., Prospects for oral vaccination using recombinant bacteria expressing viral epitopes, *Adv. Virus Res.*, 41, 409, 1992.
20. Fairweather, N. F., Chatfield, S. N., Makoff, A. J., Strugnell, R. A., Bester, J., Maskell, D. J., and Dougan, G., Oral vaccination of mice against tetanus by use of a live attenuated *Salmonella* carrier, *Infect. Immun.*, 10, 1323, 1990.
21. Bittle, J. L. and Muir, S., Vaccines produced by conventional means to control major infectious diseases of man and animals, *Advances in Veterinary Science and Comparative Medicine*, 33, 1989.
22. Hone, D. and Hackett, J., Vaccine against enteric bacterial diseases, *J. Infect. Dis.*, 11, 853, 1989.
23. Levine, M. M. and Hone, D. M., New and improved vaccines against typhoid fever, in *New Generation Vaccines*, Woodrow, G. C. and Levine, M. M., Eds., Marcel Dekker, New York, 269, 1990.
24. Dougan, G., Maskell, D., Pickard, D., and Hormaeche, C. E., Isolation of stable *aroA* mutants of *Salmonella typhi* Ty2: properties and preliminary characterization in mice, *Mol. Gen. Genet.*, 207, 402, 1987.
25. Tacket, C. O., Hone, D. M., Curtiss, R., III, Kelly, S. M., Losonsky, G., Guers, L., Harris, A. M., Edelman, R., and Levine, M. M., Comparison of the safety and immunogenicity of delta *aroC* delta *aroD* and delta *cya* delta *crp Salmonella typhi* strains in adult volunteers, *Infect. Immun.*, 60, 536, 1992.

26. Maskell, D. J., Sweeney, K. J., O'Callaghan, D., Hormaeche, C. E., Liew, F. Y., and Dougan, G., *Salmonella typhimurium aro*A mutants as carriers of the *Escherichia coli* heat-labile enterotoxin B subunit to the murine secretory and systemic immune systems, *Microb. Pathogen.*, 2, 211, 1987.

27. Hsu, H. S., Pathogenesis and immunity in murine salmonellosis, *Microbiol. Rev.*, 53, 390, 1989.

28. Levine, M. M., Ferreccio, C., Black, R. E., Tacket, C. O., and Germanier, R., Progress in vaccines against typhoid fever, *Rev. Infect. Dis.*, 11, S552, 1989.

29. Levine, M. M. and Edelman, R., Future vaccines against enteric pathogens, *Infect. Dis. Clin. N. Am.*, 4, 105, 1990.

30. Germanier, R., Immunity in experimental salmonellosis. I. Protection induced by rough mutants of *Salmonella typhimurium*, *Infect. Immun.*, 2, 309, 1970.

31. Germanier, R. and Furer, E., Immunity in experimental salmonellosis. II. Basis for the avirulence and protective capacity of galE mutants of *Salmonella typhimurium*, *Infect. Immun.*, 4, 663, 1971.

32. Gilman, R. H., Hornick, R. B., Woodward, W. E., DuPont, H. L., Snyder, M. J., Levine, M. M., and Libonati, J. P., Evaluation of a UDP-glucose-4-epimeraseless mutant of *Salmonella typhi* as a live oral vaccine, *J. Infect. Dis.*, 136, 717, 1977.

33. Hone, D. M., Attridge, S. R., Forest, B., Morona, R., Daniels, D., LaBrooy, J. T., Bartholomeusz, R. C. A., Shearman, D. J. C., and Hackett, J., A galE via (Vi antigen-negative) mutant of *Salmonella typhi* Ty2 retains virulence in humans, *Infect. Immun.*, 56, 1326, 1988.

34. Silva-Salinas, B. A., Rodriguez-Aguayo, L., Maldonado-Ballesteros, A., Valenzuela-Montero, M. E., and Seoane-Montecinos, M., Properties of two gal+ derivatives from vaccine strain *S. typhi* mutant Ty21a, *Bol. Hosp. Infant. Mex.*, 42, 234, 1985.

35. Hone, D., Morona, R., Attridge, S., and Hackett, J., Construction of defined galE mutants of *Salmonella* for use as vaccines, *J. Infect. Dis.*, 156, 167, 1987.

36. Levine, M. M., Kaper, J. B., Herrington, D., Losonsky, G., Morris, J. G., Clements, M. L., Black, R. E., Tall, B., and Hall, R., Volunteer studies of deletion mutants of *Vibrio cholerae* O1 prepared by recombinant techniques, *Infect. Immun.*, 56, 161, 1988.

37. Weiss, A. A., Hewlett, E. L., Myers, G. A., and Falkow, S., Pertussis toxin and extracytoplasmid adenylate cyclase as virulence factors of *Bordetella pertussis*, *J. Infect. Dis.*, 150, 219, 1984.

38. Roberts, M., Fairweather, N. F., Leininger, E., Pickard, D., Hewlett, E. L., Robinson, A., Hayward, C., Dougan, G., and Charles, I. G., Construction and characterization of *Bordetella pertussis* mutants lacking the *vir*-regulated P.69 outer membrane protein, *Mol. Microbiol.*, 5, 1393, 1991.

39. Collins, L. V., Attridge, S., and Hackett, J., Mutations are rfc or pmi attenuate *Salmonella typhimurium* virulence for mice, *Infect. Immun.*, 59, 1079, 1991.

40. Bochner, B. R., Huang, H. C., Schieven, G. L., and Ames, B. N., Positive selection for loss of tetracycline resistance, *J. Bacteriol.*, 170, 108, 1980.

41. Manoil, C. and Beckwith, J., TnphoA: a transposon probe for protein export signals, *Proc. Natl. Acad. Sci. U.S.A.*, 82, 8129, 1985.

42. Miller, I., Maskell, D., Hormaeche, C., Pickard, D., and Dougan, G., The isolation of orally attenuated *Salmonella typhimurium* following TnphoA mutagenesis, *Infect. Immun.*, 57, 2758, 1989.

43. Finlay, B. B., Starnbach, M. N., Francis, C. L., Stocker, B. A. D., Chatfield, S., Dougan, G., and Falkow, S., Identification and characterisation of TnphoA mutants of *Salmonella* that are unable to pass through a polarized MDCK epithelial cell monolayer, *Mol. Microbiol.*, 2, 757, 1988.

44. Miller, V. L. and Mekalanos, J. J., A novel suicide vector and its use in construction of insertion mutations: Osmoregulation of outer membrane proteins and virulence determinants in *Vibrio cholerae* requires *tox*R, *J. Bacteriol.*, 170, 2575, 1988.

45. Donnenberg, M. S. and Kaper, J. B., Construction of an *eae* deletion mutant of enteropathogenic *Escherichia coli* by using a positive selection suicide vector, *Infect. Immun.*, 59, 4310, 1991.

46. Bacon, G. A., Burrows, T. W., and Yates, M., The effects of biochemical mutation on the virulence of *Bacterium typhosum:* the loss of virulence of certain mutants, *Br. J. Exp. Pathol.*, 32, 85, 1951.

47. Pittard, A. J., Biosynthesis of the aromatic amino acids, in Escherichia coli *and* Salmonella typhimurium: *Cellular and Molecular Biology*, Vol. 1, Neidhardt, F. C., Ingraham, J. L., Magasanik, B., Low, K. B., Schaechter, M., and Umbarger, H. E., Eds., American Society for Microbiology, Washington, D.C., 368, 1987.

48. Hoiseth, S. K. and Stocker, B. A. D., Aromatic-dependent *Salmonella typhimurium* are non-virulent and effective as live vaccines, *Nature*, 291, 238, 1981.

49. Edwards, M. F. and Stocker, B. A. D., Construction of *aro*A his *pur* strains of *Salmonella typhi*, *J. Bacteriol.*, 170, 3991, 1988.

50. Levine, M. M., Herrington, D., Murphy, J. R., Morris, J. G., Losonsky, G., Tall, B., Lindberg, A. A., Svenson, S., Baqar, S., Edwards, M. F., and Stocker, B., Safety, infectivity, immunogenicity, and *in vivo* stability of two attenuate auxotrophic mutant strains of *Salmonella typhi*, 541Ty and 543Ty, as live oral vaccines in humans, *J. Clin. Invest.*, 79, 888, 1987.

51. O'Callaghan, D., Maskell, D., Liew, F. Y., Easmon, C. S. F., and Dougan, G., Characterisation of aromatic- and purine-dependent *Salmonella typhimurium:* attenuation, persistence, and ability to induce protective immunity in BALB/c mice, *Infect. Immun.*, 56, 419, 1988.

52. O'Callaghan, D., Maskell, D., Tite, J., and Dougan, G., Immune responses in BALB/c mice following immunization with aromatic compound or purine-dependent *Salmonella typhimurium* strains, *Immunology*, 69, 184, 1990.

53. Tite, J. P., Dougan, G., and Chatfield, S. N., The involvement of tumor necrosis factor in immunity to *Salmonella* infection, *J. Immunol.*, 147, 3161, 1991.

54. Mastroeni, P., Arena, A., Costa, G. B., Liberto, M. C., Bonina, L., and Hormaeche, C. E., Serum TNFα in mouse typhoid and enhancement of the infection by anti-TNFα antibodies, *Microb. Pathogen.*, 11, 33, 1991.

55. McFarland, W. C. and Stocker, B. A. D., Effect of different purine auxotrophic mutations on mouse virulence of a Vi-positive strain of *Salmonella dublin* and of two strains of *Salmonella typhimurium*, *Microb. Pathogen.*, 3, 129, 1987.

56. Dougan, G., Chatfield, S., Pickard, D., Bester, J., O'Callaghan, D., and Maskell, D., Construction and characterisation of vaccine strains of salmonella harbouring mutations in two different *aro* genes, *J. Infect. Dis.*, 158, 1329, 1988.

57. Miller, I. A., Chatfield, S., Dougan, G., DeSilva, L., Joysey, H. S., and Hormaeche, C., Bacteriophage P22 as a vehicle for transducing cosmid gene banks between smooth strains of *Salmonella typhimurium:* use in identifying a role for *aro*D in attenuating virulent *Salmonella* strains, *Mol. Gen. Genet.*, 215, 312, 1989.

58. Strugnell, R., Dougan, G., Chatfield, S., Charles, I., Fairweather, N., Tite, J., Li, J. L., Beesley, J., and Roberts, M., Characterization of a *Salmonella typhimurium aro* vaccine strain expressing the P.69 antigen of *Bordetella pertussis*, *Infect. Immun.*, 60, 3994, 1992.

59. Smith, B. P., Reina-Guerra, M., and Hoiseth, S. K., Aromatic-dependent *Salmonella typhimurium* as modified live vaccines for calves, *Am. J. Vet. Res.*, 45, 59, 1984.

60. Mukkur, T. K. S., McDowell, G. N., Stocker, B. A. D., and Lascelles, A. K., Protection against salmonellosis in mice and sheep by immunisation with aromatic-dependent *Salmonella typhimurium, J. Med. Microbiol.,* 24, 11, 1987.

61. Cooper, G. L., Nicholas, R. A., Cullen, G. A., and Hormaeche, C. E., Vaccination of chickens with a *Salmonella enteritidis aro*A live oral *Salmonella* vaccine, *Microb. Pathogen.,* 9, 255, 1990.

62. Cooper, G. L., Venables, L. M., Nicholas, R. A., Cullen, G. A., and Hormaeche, C. E., Vaccination of chickens with chicken-derived *Salmonella enteritidis* phage type 4 *aro*A live oral *Salmonella* vaccines, *Vaccine,* 10, 247, 1992.

63. Jones, P. W., Dougan, G., Hayward, C., Mackensie, N., Collins, P., and Chatfield, S. N., Oral vaccination of calves against experimental salmonellosis using a double *aro* mutant of *Salmonella typhimurium, Vaccine,* 9, 29, 1990.

64. Barrow, P. A., Hassan, J. O., Lovell, M. A., and Berchieri, A., Vaccination of chickens with *aro*A and other mutants of *Salmonella typhimurium* and *S. enteritidis, Res. Microbiol.,* 141, 851, 1990.

65. Segall, T. and Lindberg, A. A., *Salmonella dublin* experimental infection in calves: protection after oral immunization with an auxotrophic *aro*A live vaccine, *Zentralbl. Veterinaermed.,* 38, 142, 1991.

66. Stocker, B. A., Aromatic-dependent *Salmonella* as live vaccine presenters of foreign epitopes as inserts in flagellin, *Res. Microbiol.,* 1990, 787, 1990.

67. Hagarvall, T. G., Jonsson, Y. H., Edmonds, C. G., McCloskey, J. A., and Bjork, G. R., Chorismic acid, a key metabolite in modification on tRNA, *J. Bacteriol.,* 172, 252, 1990.

68. Izhar, M., DeSilva, L., Joysey, H. S., and Hormaeche, C. E., Moderate immunodeficiency does not increase susceptibility to *Salmonella typhimurium aro*A live vaccines in mice, *Infect. Immun.,* 58, 2258, 1990.

69. Killar, L. M. and Eisenstein, T. K., Immunity to *Salmonella typhimurium* infection in C3H/HeJ and C3H/HeNCr1BR mice: studies with an aromatic-dependent live *S. typhimurium* as a vaccine, *Infect. Immun.,* 47, 605, 1985.

70. Izhar, M., Desilva, L., Joysey, H. O., and Hormaeche, C. E., Moderate immune suppression does not increase susceptibility to *aro*A salmonella vaccine strains, *Infect. Immun.,* 58, 2258, 1990.

71. Hone, D. M., Harris, A. M., Chatfield, S., Dougan, G. and Levine, M. M. Construction of genetically defined double *aro* mutants of *Salmonella typhi, Vaccine,* 9, 810, 1991.

72. Chatfield, S. N., Fairweather, N. F., Charles, I., Pickard, D., Levine, M., Hone, D., Posada, M., Strugnell, R. A., and Dougan, G., Construction of a genetically defined *Salmonella typhi* Ty2 *aro*A, *aro*C mutant for the engineering of a candidate oral typhoid-tetanus vaccine, *Infect. Immun.,* 10, 53, 1992.

73. Curtiss, R., III and Kelly, S. M., *Salmonella typhimurium* deletion mutants lacking adenylate cyclase and cyclic AMP receptor protein are avirulent and immunogenic, *Infect. Immun.,* 55, 3035, 1987.

74. Curtiss, R. I., Goldschmidt, R. M., Fletchall, N. B., and Kelly, S. M., Avirulent *Salmonella typhimurium cya crp* oral vaccine strains expressing a streptococcal colonization and virulence antigen, *Vaccine,* 6, 155, 1988.

75. Forst, S., Conneau, D., Noroika, S., and Inouye, M., Localization and membrane topology of EnvZ, a protein involved in osmoregulation of OmpF and OmpC in *Escherichia coli, J. Biol. Chem.,* 262, 16433, 1987.

76. Dorman, C. J. and Bhriain, N. N., Global regulation of gene expression during environmental adaptation: implications for bacterial pathogens, in *Molecular Biology of Bacterial Infection: Current Status and Future Perspectives,* Hormaeche, C. E., Penn, C. W., and Smyth, C. J., Eds., University of Dublin, Trinity College: Cambridge University Press, 1992, 193.

77. Dorman, C. J., Chatfield, S., Higgins, C. F., Hayward, C., and Dougan, G., Characterisation of porin and *omp*R mutants of a virulent strain of *Salmonella typhimurium: omp*R mutants are attenuated *in vivo, Infect. Immun.*, 57, 2136, 1989.

78. Fields, P. I., Groisman, E. A., and Heffron, F., A *Salmonella* locus that controls resistance to microbicidal proteins from phagocytic cells, *Science*, 243, 1059, 1989.

79. Foster, J. W. and Hall, H. K., Adaptive acidification tolerance response of *Salmonella typhimurium, J. Bacteriol.*, 172, 771, 1990.

80. Groisman, E. A., Chiao, E., Lipps, C. J., and Heffron, F., *Salmonella typhimurium phoP* virulence gene is a transcriptional regulator, *Proc. Natl. Acad. Sci. U.S.A.*, 86, 7077, 1989.

81. Miller, S. I., Kukral, E. A., and Mekalanos, J. J., A two component regulatory system (*phoP/phoQ*) controls virulence of *Salmonella typhimurium, Proc. Natl. Acad. Sci.*, 86, 5054, 1989.

82. Galan, J. E. and Curtiss, R. I., Virulence and vaccine potential of *phoP* mutants of *Salmonella typhimurium, Microb. Pathogen.*, 6, 433, 1989.

83. Miller, S. I. and Mekalanos, J. J., Constitutive expression of the PhoP regulon attenuates *Salmonella* virulence and survival within macrophages, *J. Bacteriol.*, 172, 2485, 1990.

84. Miller, S. I., Mekalanos, J. J., and Pulkkinen, W. S., *Salmonella* vaccines with mutations in the *phoP* virulence regulon, *Res. Microbiol.*, 141, 817, 1990.

85. Johnson, K., Charles, I., Dougan, G., Pickard, D., O'Gaora, P., Costa, G., Ali, T., Miller, I., and Hormaeche, C., The role of a stress-response protein in *Salmonella typhimurium* virulence, *Mol. Microbiol.*, 5, 401, 1991.

86. Chatfield, S. N., Strahan, K., Pickard, D., Charles, I. G., Hormaeche, C. E., and Dougan, G., Evaluation of *Salmonella typhimurium* strains harbouring defined mutations in *htr*A and *aro*A in the murine salmonellosis model, *Microb. Pathogen.*, 12, 145, 1992.

87. Tacket, C. O., Hone, D. M., Losonsky, G. A., Guers, L., Edelman, R., and Levine, M. M., Clinical acceptability and immunogenicity of CVD908 *Salmonella typhi* vaccine strain, *Vaccine*, 10, 443, 1992.

88. Black, R. E., Levine, M. M., Clements, M. L., Losonsky, G., Herrington, D., Berman, S., and Formal, S. B., Prevention of shigellosis by a *Salmonella typhi-Shigella sonnei* bivalent vaccine, *J. Infect. Dis.*, 155, 1260, 1987.

89. Tacket, C. O., Forrest, B., Morona, R., Attridge, S. R., LaBrooy, J., Tall, B. D., Reymann, M., Rowley, D., and Levine, M. M., Safety, immunogenicity, and efficacy against cholera challenge in humans of a typhoid-cholera hybrid vaccine derived from *Salmonella typhi* Ty21a, *Infect. Immun.*, 58, 1620, 1990.

90. Forrest, B. D., LaBrooy, J. T., Attridge, S. R., Boehm, G., Beyer, L., Morona, R., Shearman, D. J., and Rowley, D., Immunogenicity of a candidate live oral typhoid/cholera hybrid vaccine in humans (letter), *J. Infect. Dis.*, 159, 145, 1989.

91. Forrest, B. D. and LaBrooy, J. T., *In vivo* evidence of immunological masking of the *Vibrio cholerae* O-antigen of a hybrid *Salmonella typhi* Ty21a-*Vibrio cholerae* oral vaccine in humans, *Vaccine*, 9, 515, 1991.

92. Van de Verg, L., Herrington, D. A., Murphy, J. R., Wasserman, S. S., Formal, S. B., and Levine, M. M., Specific immunoglobulin A-secreting cells in peripheral blood of humans following oral immunization with a bivalent *Salmonella typhi-Shigella sonnei* vaccine or infection by pathogenic *S. sonnei, Infect. Immun.*, 58, 2002, 1990.

93. Dearlove, C. E., Forrest, B. D., van den Bosch, L., and LaBrooy, J. T., The antibody response to an oral Ty21a-based typhoid-cholera hybrid is unaffected by prior oral vaccination with Ty21a (letter), *J. Infect. Dis.*, 165, 182, 1992.

94. Attridge, S., Oral immunization with *Salmonella typhi* Ty21a-based clones expressing *Vibrio cholerae* O-antigen: serum bactericidal antibody responses in man in relation to pre-immunization antibody levels, *Vaccine*, 9, 877, 1991.

95. Hone, D., Attridge, S., Van den Bosch, L., and Hackett, J., A chromosomal integration system for stabilisation of heterologous genes in *Salmonella* based vaccine strains, *Microb. Pathogen.*, 5, 407, 1988.

96. Strugnell, R. A., Maskell, D., Fairweather, N., Pickard, D., Cockayne, A., Penn, C., and Dougan, G., Stable expression of foreign antigens from the chromosome of *Salmonella typhimurium* vaccine strains, *Gene*, 88, 57, 1990.

97. Nakayama, K., Kelly, S. M., and Curtiss, R., Construction of an Asd expression-cloning vector: stable maintenance and high level expression of cloned genes in a *Salmonella* vaccine strain, *Bio/Technology*, 6, 693, 1988.

98. Morona, R., Yeadon, J., Considine, A., Morona, J. K., and Manning, P. A., Construction of plasmid vectors with a non-antibiotic selection system based on the *Escherichia coli* thyA+ gene: application to cholera vaccine development, *Gene*, 107, 139, 1991.

99. Griffiths, E., Environmental regulation of bacterial virulence — implications for vaccine design and production, *Tibtech*, 9, 309, 1991.

100. Mekalanos, J. J., Environmental signals controlling expression of virulence determinants in bacteria, *J. Bacteriol.*, 174, 1, 1991.

101. Heltvig, T. B. and Nau, H. H., Analysis of the immune response to papain digestion products of tetanus toxin, *Acta Pathol. Microbiol. Scand. Sect.*, 92, 59, 1984.

102. Roberts, M., Dougan, G., Li, J. L., Chatfield, S., and Strugnell, R., Immunisation against *Bordetella pertussis* infection of mice using a *Salmonella typhimurium aro* vaccine strain expressing the *Bordetella pertussis* P.69 antigen, *Biologicals*, 21, 4, 1993.

103. Mosmann, T. R., Cherwinski, H., Bond, M. W., Giedin, M. A., and Coffman, R. L., Two types of murine helper T cell clone I Definition according to profiles of lymphokine activities and secreted proteins, *J. Immunol.*, 136, 2348, 1986.

104. Mosman, T. R. and Moore, K. W. The role of IL-10 in crossregulation of Th1 and Th2 responses, *Immunology Today*, 12, 49, 1991.

105. Carrier, M. J., Chatfield, S. N., Dougan, G., Nowicka, U. T., O'Callaghan, D., Beesley, J. E., Milano, S., Cillari, E., and Liew, F. Y., Expression of human IL-1 beta in *Salmonella typhimurium*: a model system for the delivery of recombinant therapeutic proteins *in vivo*, *J. Immunol.*, 148, 1176, 1992.

106. Chatfield, S. N., Charles, I. G., Makoff, A. J., Oxer, M. D., Dougan, G., Pickard, D., Slater, D., and Fairweather, N. F., Use of the *nir*B promoter to direct the stable expression of heterologous antigens in *Salmonella* oral vaccine strains: development of a single-dose oral tetanus vaccine, *BioTechnology*, 10, 888, 1992.

107. O'Callaghan, D., Charbit, A., Martineau, P., Leclerc, C., van der Werf, S., Nauciel, C., and Hofnung, M., Immunogenicity of foreign peptide epitopes expressed in bacterial envelope proteins, *Res. Microbiol.*, 141, 963, 1990.

108. Agteberg, M., Adriaanse, H., Lankhof, H., Meloen, R., and Tommassen, J., Outer membrane protein PhoE protein of *Escherichia coli* as a carrier for foreign antigenic determinants: immunogenicity of epitopes of food-and-mouth disease virus, *Vaccine*, 8, 85, 1990.

109. Leclerc, C., Charbit, A., Molla, A., and Hofnung, M., Antibody response to a foreign epitope expressed at the surface of recombinant bacteria: importance of the route of immunization, *Vaccine*, 7, 242, 1989.

110. Su, G. F., Brahmbhatt, H. N., Wehland, J., Rohde, M., and Timmis, K. N., Construction of stable LamB-Shiga toxin B subunit hybrids: analysis of expression in *Salmonella typhimurium aro*A strains and stimulation of B subunit-specific mucosal and serum antibody responses, *Infect. Immun.*, 60, 3345, 1992.

111. Schorr, J., Knapp, B., Hundt, E., Kupper, H. A., and Amann, E., Surface expression of malarial antigens in *Salmonella typhimurium*: induction of serum antibody response upon oral vaccination of mice, *Vaccine*, 9, 675, 1991.

112. Newton, S. M. C., Jacob, C. O., and Stocker, B. A. D., Immune response to cholera toxin epitope inserted in *Salmonella* flagellin, *Science*, 244, 70, 1989.

113. Bao, J. X. and Clements, J. D., Prior immunologic experience potentiates the subsequent antibody response when *Salmonella* strains are used as vaccine carriers, *Infect. Immun.*, 59, 3841, 1991.

114. O'Callaghan, D., Maskell, D. J., Beesley, J. E., Lifely, M. R., Roberts, M., Boulnois, G., and Dougan, G., Characterisation and *in vivo* behaviour of a *Salmonella typhimurium aroA* strain expressing *Escherichia coli* K1 polysaccharide, *FEMS Microbiol. Lett.*, 52, 269, 1988.

115. Baron, L. S., Kopecko, D. J., Formal, S. J., Seid, R., Guerry, P., and Powell, C., Introduction of *Shigella flexneri* 2a type and group antigens genes into oral typhoid vaccine strain *Salmonella typhi* Ty21a, *Infect. Immun.*, 55, 2797, 1987.

116. Stanfield, J. P. and Galazka, A., Neonatal tetanus in the third world today, *WHO Bull.*, 62, 647, 1984.

117. Baljer, G., Oral immunization against tetanus, in 14th Congr. Int. Assoc. Biol. Standardization, Karker, S., Ed., Douglas, Isle of Man, 1975, 63.

118. Fairweather, N. F., Lyness, V. A., and Maskell, D. J., Immunization of mice against tetanus with fragment of tetanus toxin synthesized in *Escherichia coli*, *Infect. Immun.*, 55, 2541, 1987.

119. Makoff, A. J., Oxer, M. D., Romanos, M. A., Fairweather, N. F., and Ballantine, S., Expression of tetanus toxin fragment C in *E. coli*: high level expression by removing rare codons, *Nucleic Acids Res.*, 17, 10191, 1989.

120. Oxer, M. D., Bently, C. M., Doyle, J. G., Peakman, T. C., Charles, I. G., and Makoff, A. J., High level heterologous expression in *E. coli* using the anaerobically-activated *nir*B promoter, *Nucleic Acids Res.*, 19, 1889, 1991.

121. Peakman, T., Crouzet, J., Jayaux, J. F., Busby, S., Mohan, S., Harborne, N., Wooton, J., Nicholson, R., and Cole, J., Nucleotide sequence, organisation and structural analysis of the products of genes in the *nir*B-*cys*B region of the *Escherichia coli* K-12 chromosome, *Eur. J. Biochem.*, 191, 315, 1990.

122. Robinson, J. H. and Kehoe, M. A., Group A streptococcal M proteins: virulence factors and protective antigens, *Immunol. Today*, 13, 362, 1992.

123. Poirier, T. P., Kehoe, M. A., and Beachey, E. H., Protective immunity evoked by oral administration of attenuated *aroA Salmonella typhimurium* expressing cloned streptococcal M protein, *J. Exp. Med.*, 168, 25, 1988.

124. Newton, S. M., Kotb, M., Poirier, T. P., Stocker, B. A., and Beachey, E. M., Expression and immunogenicity of a streptococcal M protein epitope inserted in *Salmonella flagellin*, *Infect. Immun.*, 59, 2158, 1991.

125. Leininger, E., Roberts, M., Kenimer, J. G., Charles, I. G., Fairweather, N. F., Novotny, P., and Brennan, M. J., Pertactin, an Arg-Gly-Asp-containing *Bordetella pertussis* surface protein that promotes adherence of mammalian cells, *Proc. Natl. Acad. Sci. U.S.A.*, 88, 345, 1991.

126. Charles, I. G., Dougan, G., Pickard, D., Chatfield, S., Smith, M., Novotny, P., Morrissey, P., and Fairweather, N. F., Molecular cloning and characterisation of protective outer membrane protein P.69 from *Bordetella pertussis*, *Proc. Natl. Acad. Sci. U.S.A.*, 86, 3554, 1989.

127. Sadoff, J. C., Ballou, W. R., Baron, L. S., Majarian, W. R., Brey, R. N., Hockmeyer, W. T., Young, J. F., Cryz, J. J., Ou, J., Lowell, G. H., and Chulay, J. D., Oral *Salmonella typhimurium* vaccine expressing circumsporozoite protein protects against malaria, *Science*, 240, 236, 1988.

128. Aggarwal, A., Kumar, S., Jaffe, R., Hone, D., Gross, M., and Sadoff, J., Oral *Salmonella*: malaria circumsporozoite recombinants induce specific CD8+ cytotoxic T cells, *J. Exp. Med.*, 172, 1083, 1990.

129. Flynn, J. L., Weiss, W. R., Norris, K. A., Seifert, H. S., Kumar, S., and So, M., Generation of cytotoxin T-lymphocyte response using a *Salmonella* antigen-delivery system, *Mol. Microbiol.*, 4, 2111, 1990.

130. Kumar, S., Gorden, J., Flynn, J. L., Berzofsky, J. A., and Miller, L. H., Immunization of mice against *Plasmodium vinckei* with a combination of attenuated *Salmonella typhimurium* and malarial antigen, *Infect. Immun.*, 58, 3425, 1990.

131. Liew, F. Y., Functional heterogeneity of CD4+ T-cells in leishmaniasis, *Immunol. Today*, 10, 40, 1989.

132. Locksley, R. M. and Scott, P., Helper T-cell subsets in mouse leishmaniasis: induction, expansion and effector function, *Immunol. Today*, 12, 58, 1991.

133. Yang, D. M., Fairweather, N., Button, L. L., McMaster, W. R., Kahl, L. P., and Liew, F. Y., Oral *Salmonella typhimurium* (AroA-) vaccine expressing a major leishmanial surface protein (gp63) preferentially induces T helper 1 cells and protective immunity against leishmaniasis, *J. Immunol.*, 145, 2281, 1990.

134. Tite, J. P., Gao, X. M., Jenkins, M., Lipscombe, M., O'Callaghan, D., Dougan, G., and Liew, F. Y., Anti-viral immunity induced by recombinant nucleoprotein of Influenza A virus. III. Delivery of recombinant nucleoprotein to the immune system using attenuated *Salmonella typhimurium* as a live carrier, *Immunology*, 70, 540, 1990.

135. Bienenstock, J., McDermott, M., Befus, D., and O'Neil, L. M., A common mucosal immunologic system involving the bronchus, breast and bowel, *Adv. Exp. Med. Biol.*, 107, 53, 1978.

136. McDermott, M. R. and Bienenstock, J., Evidence for a common mucosal immunologic system. 1. Migration of B immunoblasts into intestinal, respiratory, and genital tissues, *J. Immunol.*, 122, 1892, 1979.

137. Mestesky, J., McGhee, J. R., Russell, M. W., Michalek, S. M., Kutteh, W. H., Gregory, R. L., Scholler-Guinard, M., Brown, T. A., and Crago, S. S., Evidence for a common mucosal immune system in humans, *Prot. Biol. Fluids*, 32, 25, 1985.

138. Roberts, M., Maskell, D., Novotny, P., and Dougan, G., Construction and characterisation *in vivo* of *Bordetella pertussis aro*A mutants, *Infect. Immun.*, 58, 732, 1990.

139. Schafer, R., Portnoy, D. A., Brassell, S. A., and Paterson, Y., Induction of a cellular immune response to a foreign antigen by a recombinant *Listeria monocytogenes* vaccine, *J. Immunol.*, 149, 53, 1992.

140. Molina, N. C. and Parker, C. D., Murine antibody response to oral infection with live *aro*A recombinant *Salmonella dublin* vaccine strains expressing filamentous hemagglutinin antigen from *Bordetella pertussis*, *Infect. Immun.*, 58, 2523, 1990.

141. Guzman, C. A., Brownlie, R. M., Kadurugamuwa, J., Walker, M. J., and Timmis, K. N., Antibody responses in the lungs of mice following oral immunization with *Salmonella typhimurium aro*A and invasive *Escherichia coli* strains expressing the filamentous hemagglutinin of *Bordetella pertussis*, *Infect. Immun.*, 59, 4391, 1991.

142. Walker, M. J., Rohde, M., Timmis, K. N., and Guzman, C. A., Specific lung mucosal and systemic immune responses after oral immunization of mice with *Salmonella typhimurium aro*A, *Salmonella typhi* Ty21a, and invasive *Escherichia coli* expressing recombinant pertussis toxin S1 subunit, *Infect. Immun.*, 60, 4260, 1992.

143. Clements, J. D. and El-Morshidy, S., Construction of a potential live oral bivalent vaccine for typhoid fever and cholera-*Escherichia coli*-related diarrhoeas, *Infect. Immun.*, 46, 564, 1984.

144. Clements, J. D., Lyon, F. L., Lowe, K. L., Farrand, A. L., and El-Morshidy, S., Oral immunization of mice with attenuated *Salmonella enteritidis* containing a recombinant plasmid which codes for production of the B subunit of heat-labile *Escherichia coli* enterotoxin, *Infect. Immun.*, 53, 685, 1986.

145. Schodel, F., Enders, G., Jung, M. C., and Will, H., Recognition of a hepatitis B virus nucleocapsid T-cell epitope expressed as a fusion protein with the subunit B of *Escherichia coli* heat labile enterotoxin in attenuated salmonellae, *Vaccine*, 8, 569, 1990.

146. Stevenson, G. and Manning, P. A., Galactose epimeraseless (*galE*) mutant G30 of *Salmonella typhimurium* is a good potential live oral vaccine carrier for fimbrial antigens, *FEMS Microbiol. Lett.*, 28, 317, 1985.

147. Dougan, G., Sellwood, R., Maskell, D., Sweeney, K., Liew, F. Y., Beesley, J., and Hormaeche, C., *In vivo* properties of a cloned K88 adherence antigen determinant, *Infect. Immun.*, 52, 344, 1986.

148. Attridge, S., Hackett, J., Morona, R., and Whyte, P., Towards a live oral vaccine against enterotoxigenic *Escherichia coli*, *Vaccine*, 6, 387, 1988.

149. Dusek, D. M., Produlske-Fox, A., Whitlock, J., and Brown, T. A., Isolation and characterization of a cloned *Porphyromonas gingivalis* hemagglutinin from an avirulent strain of *Salmonella typhimurium*, *Infection and Immunity*, 61, 940, 1993.

150. Tarkka, E., Muotiala, A., Karvonen, M., Saukkonen Laitinen, K., and Sarvas, M., Antibody production to a meningococcal outer membrane protein cloned into live *Salmonella typhimurium aroA* vaccine strain, *Microb. Pathogen.*, 6, 327, 1989.

151. Strugnell, R., Schouls, L., Cockayne, A., Bailey, M., van Embdon, J., and Penn, C., Experimental syphilis vaccines: use of *aroA Salmonella typhimurium* to deliver recombinant *Treponema pallidum* antigens, in *Vaccines for Sexually Transmitted Diseases*, Meheus, A. and Spier, R. E., Eds., Butterworths, Oxford, U.K., 1989, 107.

152. Stabel, T. J., Mayfield, J. E., Tabatabai, L. B., and Wannemuehler, M. J., Oral immunization of mice with attenuated *Salmonella typhimurium* containing a recombinant plasmid which codes for production of a 31-kilodalton protein of *Brucella abortus*, *Infect. Immun.*, 58, 2048, 1990.

153. Stabel, T. J., Mayfield, J. E., Tabatabai, L. B., and Wannemuehler, M. J., Swine immunity to an attenuated *Salmonella typhimurium* mutant containing a recombinant plasmid which codes for production of a 31 kilodalton protein of *Brucella abortus*, *Infect. Immun.*, 59, 2941, 1991.

154. Stabel, T. J., Mayfield, J. E., Morfitt, D. C., and Wannemuehler, M. J., Oral immunization of mice and swine with an attenuated *Salmonella choleraesuis* [*cya*-12 (*crp-cdt*)19] mutant containing a recombinant plasmid, *Infect. Immun.*, 61, 610, 1993.

155. Sjostedt, A., Sandstrom, G., and Tarnvik, A., Immunization of mice with an attenuated *Salmonella typhimurium* strain expressing a membrane protein of *Francisella tularensis*. A model for identification of bacterial determinants relevant to the host defence against tularemia, *Res. Microbiol.*, 141, 887, 1990.

156. Sjostedt, A., Sandstrom, G., and Tarnvik, A., Humoral and cell-mediated immunity in mice to a 17-kilodalton lipoprotein of *Francisella tularensis* expressed by *Salmonella typhimurium*, *Infect. Immun.*, 60, 2855, 1992.

157. Formal, S. B., Baron, L. S., Kopecko, D. J., Powell, C., and Life, C. A., Construction of a potential bivalent vaccine strain: Introduction of *S. sonnei* form 1 antigen genes into the *galE Salmonella typhi* Ty21a typhoid vaccine strain, *Infect. Immun.*, 34, 746, 1981.

158. Tramont, E. C., Chung, R., Berman, S., Keren, D., Kapfer, C., and Formal, S. B., Safety and antigenicity of typhoid-*Shigella sonnei* vaccine (strain 5076-1C), *J. Infect. Dis.*, 149, 133, 1984.

159. Hartman, A. B., Ruiz, M. M., and Shultz, C. L., Molecular analysis of variant plasmid forms of a bivalent *Salmonella typhi-Shigella sonnei* vaccine strain, *J. Clin. Microbiol.*, 29, 27, 1991.

160. Seid, R. C. J., Kopecko, D. J., Sadoff, J. C., Schneider, H., Baron, L. S., and Formal, S. B., Unusual lipopolysaccharide antigens of a *Salmonella typhi* oral vaccine strain expressing the *Shigella sonnei* form I antigen, *J. Biol. Chem.*, 259, 9028, 1984.

161. Attridge, S., Forrest, B., Hackett, J., LaBrooy, J., Levine, M. M., Morona, R., et al., Construction and efficacy of a live oral baterial cholera-typhoid vaccine, *Proc. 8th Australian Biotech. Conf.*, Sydney, 25, 1989.

162. Attridge, S. R., Daniels, D., Morona, J. K., and Morona, R., Surface co-expression of *Vibrio cholerae* and *Salmonella typhi* O-antigens on Ty21a clone EX210, *Microb. Pathogen.*, 8, 177, 1990.

163. Attridge, S. R., Dearlove, C., Beyer, L., van den Bosch, L., Howles, A., Hackett, J., Morona, R., LaBrooy, J., and Rowley, D., Characterization and immunogenicity of EX880, a *Salmonella typhi* Ty21a based clone which produces *Vibrio cholerae* O antigen, *Infect. Immun.*, 59, 2279, 1991.

164. Curtiss, R. I., Genetic analysis of *Streptococcus mutans* virulence and prospects for an anticaries vaccine, *J. Dent. Res.*, 65, 1034, 1986.

165. Katz, J., Michalek, S. M., Curtiss, R. I., Harmon, C., Richardson, G., and Mestecky, J., Novel oral vaccines: the effectiveness of cloned gene products on inducing secretory immune responses, *Adv. Exp. Med. Biol.*, 216B, 1741, 1987.

166. Michalek, S. M., Childers, N. K., Katz, J., Denys, F. R., Berry, A. K., Eldridge, J. H., McGhee, J. R., and Curtiss, R. I., Liposomes as oral adjuvants, *Curr. Top. Microbiol. Immunol.*, 146, 1989.

167. Schodel, F. and Will, H., Expression of hepatitis B virus antigens in attenuated salmonellae for oral immunisation, *Res. Microbiol.*, 141, 831, 1990.

168. Schodel, F., Milich, D. R., and Will, H., Hepatitis B virus nucleocapsid/pre-S2 fusion proteins expressed in attenuated *Salmonella* for oral vaccination, *J. Immunol.*, 145, 4317, 1990.

169. Bowen, J. C., Alpar, O., Phillpotts, R., Roberts, I. S., and Brown, M. R., Preliminary studies on infection by attenuated *Salmonella* in guinea pig and on expression on herpes simplex virus, *Res. Microbiol.*, 141, 873, 1990.

170. Cohen, S., Powell, C. J., Dubois, D. R., Hartman, A., Summers, P. L., and Eckels, K. H., Expression of the envelope antigen of dengue virus in vaccine strains of *Salmonella, Res. Microbiol.*, 141, 855, 1990.

171. Salas, V. E., Plebanski, M., Castro, S., Perales, G., Mata, E., Lopez, S., and Arias, C. F., Synthesis of the surface glycoprotein of rotavirus SAL1 in the *aro*A strain of *Salmonella typhimurium* SL3261, *Res. Microbiol.*, 141, 883, 1990.

172. Gottstein, B., Muller, N., Cryz, S. J. J., Vogel, M., Tanner, I., and Seebeck, T., Humoral and cellular immune response in mice and dogs induced by a recombinant *Echinococcus multilocularis* antigen produced by a *Salmonella typhimurium* vaccine strain, *Parasite Immunol.*, 12, 163, 1990.

173. Jagusztyn-Krynicka, E., Clark-Curtiss, J. E., and Curtiss, R. I., *Escherichia coli* heat labile toxin subunit B fusions with *Streptococcus sobrinus* antigens expressed by *Salmonella typhimurium* oral vaccine strains: importance of the linker for antigenicity and biological activities of the hybrid proteins, *Infect. Immun.*, 61, 1004, 1993.

174. Wu, J. Y., Newton, S., Judd, A., Stocker, B., and Robinson, W. S., Expression of immunogenic epitopes of hepatitis B surface antigen with hybrid flagellin proteins by a vaccine strain of *Salmonella, Proc. Natl. Acad. Sci. U.S.A.*, 86, 4726, 1989.

175. McEwen, J., Levi, R., Horwitz, R. J., and Arnon, R., Synthetic recombinant vaccine expressing influenza haemagglutinin epitope in *Salmonella* flagellin leads to partial protection in mice, *Vaccine*, 10, 405, 1992.

176. Pistor, S. and Hobom, G., OmpA-Haemagglutinin fusion proteins for oral immunization with live attenuated *Salmonella, Res. Microbiol.*, 141, 879, 1990.

Chapter 2

Clinical Evaluation of Attenuated *Salmonella typhi* Vaccines in Human Subjects

Bruce D. Forrest

TABLE OF CONTENTS

I. CLINICAL EVALUATION OF ATTENUATED LIVE ORALLY ADMINISTERED TYPHOID VACCINES

Typhoid fever remains a disease of serious consequences, associated with world-wide incidence rate of 560/100,000, and with significant morbidity and substantial mortality.[1]

0-8493-4866-8/94/$0.00+$.50
© 1994 by CRC Press Inc.

The mainstay typhoid vaccine remains the parenterally administered heat-inactivated whole *Salmonella typhi* vaccine, despite many attempts to replace it. A variety of approaches have been utilized in vaccine development which have been associated with varying degrees of success. One of these approaches has been the development of specifically attenuated bacterial vaccines, where a pathogenic organism is rendered avirulent losing all potential to cause disease, while retaining its immunogenicity and ability to grow. Attenuated live whole organism vaccines are possibly best suited for protecting against pathogens which access the body through the mucosal surfaces, and so much of the development has focused on enteric and respiratory pathogens, where strong local immune responses have been shown to be responsible for long-term protection against reinfection. This approach has been used to develop the live oral typhoid vaccine *S. typhi* Ty21a ("Vivotif", Swiss Serum and Vaccine Institute, Berne, Switzerland), and a promising monovalent attenuated orally administrable single-dose cholera vaccine.[2]

Therefore, the objectives for the rational design of an effective vaccine must include the ability to block those processes essential for the establishment of infection; to neutralize those substances produced by the infective agent that mediate the pathological effects; and to enhance the specific immune defenses of the host. It is generally accepted that an orally administered live attenuated vaccine will provide the most convenient and effective means of vaccinating against enteric disease. The success of the live attenuated (Sabin) poliovirus vaccines provides support for this approach, which is most likely to be effective when utilized in cooperation with other primary health care interventions.[3] The basis for the use of attenuated live orally administrable *S. typhi* organisms as vaccines against typhoid fever is dependent on the assertion that the ideal vaccine is one that retains the protective antigens of the pathogenic bacterial cell and mimics the behavior of the pathogenic form, but to a far lesser extent, through retaining the ability to penetrate intestinal mucus, adhere to the intestinal epithelium, and invade or penetrate the epithelium, and colonize and proliferate in the epithelial layer.

II. EVALUATIONS OF EARLY ATTENUATED VACCINES

A. STREPTOMYCIN-DEPENDENT LIVE TYPHOID VACCINE

The early methods of attenuation such as those of Pasteur are considered as being largely unsuitable for the modern era due to questionable safety resulting from the absence of understanding of the mechanisms of attenuation in those processes, and so without guarantees of inability to retain or regain virulence. The first method of rational vaccine development was the creation of auxotrophic strains of the pathogen. This was first proposed in 1948 by Iverson and Waksman, using streptomycin dependence as a means of developing a rationally attenuated vaccine.[4]

In 1967, Reitman reported the immunogenicity and antigenicity of a streptomycin-dependent (Sm-D) *S. typhi* in animals.[5] This strain, known as *S. typhi* 27V, exhibited several desirable traits as a viable vaccine: stability, antigenicity, lack of degradation, and safety in animals. Subsequently another Sm-D *S. typhi*, a Vi-negative variant *S. typhi* 20SD candidate vaccine, was derived from the streptomycin-sensitive parent of the *S. typhi* 27V strain, *S. typhi* 19V. This vaccine strain was made Vi negative because of the then prevailing belief that Vi antigen played little or no role in the protective immunity in typhoid fever.[6] However, orally administered *S. typhi* 20SD failed to provide adequate protection in chimpanzees against virulent challenge with *S. typhi* Ty2.

In 1969, DuPont et al.[7] administered the Sm-D *S. typhi* 27V vaccine strain to adult volunteers in doses of $\approx 10^8$ or $\approx 10^9$ viable bacteria with or without streptomycin. Some of these volunteers were challenged with virulent *S. typhi* and not protected against disease. However, other studies demonstrated the effectiveness of the Sm-D *Shigella* vaccines using greater doses ($>10^{10}$ viable organisms) and pretreating vaccine recipients with oral sodium hydrogen carbonate solution,[8] and resulted in the Sm-D *S. typhi* 27V strain being reevaluated.

DuPont et al.[9] reevaluated the vaccine strain in a study comprising 30 men who received six weekly doses of between 3×10^{10} and 1×10^{11} live *S. typhi* 27V organisms either with or without sodium hydrogen carbonate pretreatment and either with or without oral streptomycin. These men, along with 26 unvaccinated control subjects, were subsequently challenged with virulent *S. typhi*. The overall protective efficacy of this vaccine preparation against clinical disease was reported to be 67%. No breakdown of the differing groups and their respective protection was provided. When the serum antityphoid antibody responses were evaluated postvaccination, 9% of subjects were reported as having four-fold or greater rise in serum anti-O antigen antibody responses, 54% having a similar rise in anti-H antibody responses, and 12% in Vi haemagglutination responses. The investigators' conclusion was the same as that drawn by other investigators using the parenterally administered heat-inactivated preparations some 40 years earlier, in that the humoral antibody response was not predictable after oral vaccination.

In a series of subsequent studies using the 27V strain to further evaluate its protective efficacy, Levine et al.[10] consistently demonstrated that the protective efficacy of this strain was in the range of 66%-78%. However, the lyophilized preparation of the 27V strain only provided a nonsignificant protective efficacy of 29%. More subjects receiving the fresh preparation of the *S. typhi* 27V vaccine strain demonstrated an anti-H antibody response than those receiving the lyophilized preparation (58% vs. 33%). No correlation was found to exist between the serum anti-Vi and anti-O antibody responses and protection. Similarly, no difference in the attack rate was observed between the vaccinated subjects with (21%) and those without (26%) anti-H antibody at the time of challenge.

Following their success with a streptomycin-dependent *Shigella* vaccine, Mel et al.[11] prepared a similar vaccine candidate as a one-step mutant from the pathogenic strain *S. typhi* Ty2. This strain was found to be safe in children and adults at doses of 6.0×10^{10} to 1.8×10^{11} live organisms, but was not evaluated for protective efficacy.

B. ATTENUATED TYPHOID VACCINE BY INTERGENERIC MATING

Dima applied the approach of developing an attenuated live candidate typhoid vaccine through the intergeneric mating of a pathogenic *S. typhi* strain and the nonpathogenic *E. coli* K-12 organism.[12] The resulting undefined hybrid mutant strain was attenuated in animal studies as well as proving to be attenuated in human subjects when evaluated up to doses of 6.6×10^{10} viable organisms. Once again poor serum antibody responses were detected, but on this occasion, coproantibody measurements were made in an effort to determine the presence of local specific antibody. Good antityphoid coproantibody responses were evident in most subjects. In this study, 7 out of the 17 vaccinated subjects were challenged with 1.7×10^5 virulent *S. typhi* Ty1554 (Walter strain). None of the challenged subjects developed clinical or bacteriological evidence of typhoid fever. Unfortunately, this study was uncontrolled, so there is no way of accurately determining the protective efficacy of this particular vaccine strain. In addition, the lack of a defined attenuating marker most likely precluded this organism or any others developed using this approach from being a seriously considered candidate vaccine, there being no guarantees concerning its unlikelihood of reversion to a virulent strain.

C. *SALMONELLA TYPHI* TY21A
1. Development and Protective Efficacy

In 1975, the development of *S. typhi* Ty21a, a potential new candidate live oral typhoid vaccine organism, was described.[13] This candidate vaccine strain was developed through chemical and physical mutagenesis of *S. typhi* Ty2 while grown in the presence of galactose. It was described as differing from pathogenic *S. typhi* Ty2 by being defective in the enzyme uridine diphospho-(UDP)-galactose-4-epimerase (hence described as being a *galE* mutant), as well as having sharply reduced galactokinase and galactose-1-phosphate uridyltransferase activity (only 20% of that of the parent *S. typhi* Ty2 strain). Originally the attenuation of *S. typhi* Ty21a was attributed to the *galE* deletion through the induction of bacteriolysis by the cytoplasmic accumulation of galactose.

2. Clinical Evaluation of *S. typhi* Ty21a

Preliminary human studies performed on a total of 173 human volunteers in Baltimore, who received orally administered doses up to 5×10^{10} live organisms, demonstrated the strain's safety, stability, and relative absence of adverse reactions.[14-16] The protective efficacy of *S. typhi* Ty21a as a live oral vaccine against typhoid in human volunteers was reported by Gilman et al.[15] in 1977. Subjects vaccinated with five to eight doses of 3 to 10×10^{10} live *S. typhi* Ty21a which had been grown in the presence of exogenous galactose (producing a smooth-type LPS) and subsequently challenged with a dose of 10^5 live pathogenic *S. typhi* Quailes strain that caused clinical typhoid fever in 53% of unimmunized controls, were observed to have conferred upon them 87% protection. There was a clinical attack rate of 50% in challenged volunteers who received live *S. typhi* Ty21a grown in the absence of exogenous galactose (producing rough-type LPS), demonstrating the failure of the rough LPS-producing strain to provide significant protection against disease (Table 1).[15,16] The anti-O antigen antibody response was deemed to be low, with very few subjects achieving a four-fold or greater rise in antibody titer; however this response was greater in those subjects receiving "smooth" vaccine organisms than in those receiving "rough" vaccine organisms. This study suggested that the serum anti-H antibody response was not a useful predictor of protection, since there was no difference in the postvaccination anti-H antibody responses, being present in 31% and 33% of subjects ingesting smooth and rough vaccine organisms, respectively, in spite of the significant differences in protection afforded by the two different vaccine preparations.

3. Field Evaluation of *S. typhi* Ty21a

There are several factors that precluded the widespread use of the effective freshly harvested preparation of *S. typhi* Ty21a as used by Gilman et al.[15] These factors include the fact that freshly harvested doses are totally impractical for use in the field, maintenance of the quality control in minimizing batch variation as well as maintaining an effective cold chain being major cost factors, together with the necessity for multiple doses to confer maximal protection. In addition, the cost of commercially producing the

Table 1 **Protective efficacy of "smooth" and "rough"**
***Salmonella typhi* Ty21a in American volunteer subjects**

Group	Number of subjects	Typhoid fever rate (%)
"Smooth"		
Vaccinated	28	7*
Controls	43	53*
"Rough"		
Vaccinated	27	19+
Controls	21	38+

Note: * — Protective efficacy 87%, $p = 0.0002$; + — Protective efficacy 50%, not significant.
Adapted from Gilman, R. H., Hornick, R. B., Woodward, W. E., DuPont, H. L., Levine, M. M., and Libonati, J. P., *J. Infect. Dis.*, 136, 716, 1977.

very large doses of approximately 10^{11} live *S. typhi* Ty21a organisms used is also prohibitive. This is especially so for fresh doses grown in brain-heart infusion broth, since the medium is expensive and the yield poor.[17] The use of lyophilization to reduce dose variation provides the most effective means of preparing, storing, and delivering the vaccine. However, with the streptomycin-dependent strain 27D this was reportedly associated with an adverse effect on the immunogenicity of the live typhoid vaccine.[10]

4. Initial Field Evaluation: Alexandria, Egypt 1978

In 1978 a controlled field trial of *S. typhi* Ty21a was commenced in Alexandria, Egypt.[18] A total of 32,388 school children aged 6 to 7 years was enrolled in the study: 16,486 receiving the oral vaccine; 15,902 receiving an oral placebo using the same schedule as for the vaccinees; and 25,628 remaining as unvaccinated controls. Lyophilized vaccine doses were used comprising 2.7×10^9 live *S. typhi* Ty21a per dose after reconstitution in 20 to 30 ml of diluent. A total of three alternate-day doses was given. Each dose was administered only after the child had chewed a sodium hydrogen carbonate tablet to neutralize gastric acidity. In the ensuing year, not one confirmed or probable case of typhoid fever was identified in the vaccinated group, while 7 confirmed cases and 13 probable cases were identified in the placebo group (incidence 125.7/100,000). This difference was statistically significant. In the unvaccinated group the incidence of confirmed or probable cases was 132.7/100,000. This demonstrated that *S. typhi* Ty21a was a safe and effective vaccine against typhoid fever, providing protection for at least 1 year in the field.

In 1982, Wahdan et al.[19] reported the results of a further 3 years of observation. The attack rate of typhoid fever in the 16,486 vaccinated children was 2 cases per 100,000 children per year, compared to 50 cases per 100,000 children per year in the placebo control group of 15,902 and in the unimmunized group of 25,628. This represented an impressive vaccine protection rate of 96% over a 3-year period following vaccination.

5. Commercial Preparation: "Vivotif", Switzerland 1981

While a lyophilized form of the vaccine given as a reconstituted liquid had been demonstrated to provide substantial protection against typhoid fever in recipients, such a formulation was considered as neither convenient nor practical for commercial manufacture for mass immunization programs. A lyophilized gelatin capsule form of *S. typhi* Ty21a became available in Switzerland in 1981, manufactured by the Swiss Serum Institute, Berne, and marketed under the trade name "Vivotif". Hirschel et al.[20] noted that in their study of Swiss travelers who had taken either the three alternate-day doses of the *S. typhi* Ty21a preparation or the three doses of the oral killed *S. typhi* Ty2 vaccine "Taboral", a typhoid incidence of 11/100,000 doses of *S. typhi* Ty21a sold was observed, which was not significantly different from the incidence of 9/100,000 doses sold of the proven ineffective orally administered killed *S. typhi* Ty2 vaccine. On examination of *S. typhi* Ty21a capsules bought off the shelf in 1983, it was observed that they contained only 6 to 10×10^8 viable bacteria, which declined a further ten-fold following 1 week of storage at room temperature. It appeared that these travelers were receiving substantially less viable *S. typhi* Ty21a organisms than had been used to demonstrate protection in the previous studies. This particular preparation was withdrawn from sale in 1984 and replaced with an enteric-coated lyophilized formulation.

6. Field Evaluation of Enteric-Coated Formulation: Santiago, Chile 1982

In 1982 a comprehensive field study was commenced in Santiago, Chile, to evaluate the protective efficacy of one or two doses of 10^9 viable *S. typhi* Ty21a contained within enteric-coated capsules.[21] In a randomized double-blind study, 91,954 schoolchildren were orally vaccinated on two occasions, 1 week apart with: two vaccine doses; one vaccine dose and one placebo; or two placebos. An additional 45,743 children did not participate in the study. Intensive postvaccination surveillance identified 260 cases of bacteriologically confirmed typhoid fever; the annual incidence rate in the placebo and unvaccinated groups was determined to be in excess of 200/100,000. Over the first 9 months following vaccination, the vaccine efficacy for the two-dose schedule was 67% and for the single dose was 41%. No protective efficacy was found after 9 months in either group. A subsequent study, using two doses of the enteric-coated preparation, given 1 week apart, showed a protective efficacy of 59% over a 2-year period, whereas a single dose only provided 29% protection over the same period. These studies demonstrated the practicality of using an enteric-coated formulation in the field, despite the dose schedule being inadequate.

The likely usefulness of *S. typhi* Ty21a as a public health tool was evaluated further in Santiago, Chile between 1984 and 1987. This large study was conducted over different administrative regions of the city, was larger and more complete than that performed in 1982 and 1983, and utilized both the gelatin capsule form and the enteric-coated gelatin capsule form where the capsules were coated with hydroxyprophymethylcellulose-phthalate.[22] In this study, 109,594 school children 6 to 21 years of age received all three alternate-day doses of the vaccine or the placebo and were placed under surveillance for 3 years. A vaccine efficacy of 67% was observed in the group receiving three alternate-day doses of the enteric-coated vaccine capsules, in contrast to an efficacy of 19% using the gelatin capsules with the same schedule, or 49% with enteric-coated capsules administered 21 days apart. Of the two dosage schedules used, either three alternate-day doses or three doses with 21 days between doses, only the former provided significantly better protection against typhoid regardless of the formulation. The gelatin capsules failed to provide any better protection than placebo, whereas the enteric-coated preparation using either schedule provided significant protection against typhoid.

Therefore the enteric-coated formulation was able to provide at best 67% protection against typhoid fever over a 3-year period. This was markedly better than the two-dose schedule, but was obviously not as good as the 96% protection observed in the Alexandria field study of 1978. This was comparable to that provided by the parenterally administered heat-inactivated typhoid vaccine, although the enteric-coated capsule formulation proved to be a substantially more practical form of vaccine delivery.

The selection of the three-alternate-day-dose regimen as the vaccination schedule had been initially made as a direct result of the success of that schedule in Alexandria, Egypt, and so permitted the comparison of the protective efficacies of the two studies. In two different regions of Santiago from those detailed above, a concurrent study was performed to evaluate the relative effectiveness of differing dose regimens on the protective efficacy of *S. typhi* Ty21a against typhoid fever.[23] This investigation was uncontrolled, there being no placebo group involved apparently as a result of a direct request by the WHO Ethical Review Committee. School children were selected as described previously and received the enteric-coated capsule formulation as above, either as two, three, or four alternate-day doses. Ferreccio et al.[23] observed that as the number of vaccine doses increased, so did the degree of protection afforded by the vaccine.

These extensive field investigations convincingly demonstrated that if long-term protection is necessary in an endemic area of high prevalence, then a four- or possibly more dose vaccination regimen should be employed. However, if short-term incomplete protection would suffice, for example to assist in bringing under control an epidemic situation, then it was be possible to use only the two-dose regimen.[23] In the Santiago study, *S. typhi* Ty21a proved itself to be a highly effective, flexible public health tool in the prevention of typhoid fever, although it did have the inconvenience of requiring multiple doses to achieve a degree of protection.

7. Indonesian Field Evaluation: Plaju, Indonesia 1987

In Plaju, Indonesia, 22,000 persons aged 3 to 44 years received either the vaccine or a placebo administered weekly for 3 weeks.[24,25] The vaccine was prepared as either enteric-coated capsules as used in the Chilean field studies, or as a liquid preparation consisting of lyophilized organisms and buffer salts which was reconstituted in water immediately before use, with each vaccine dose comprising 1 to 4×10^9 viable vaccine organisms. The vaccine was administered orally using a schedule of three weekly doses, a marked departure from the previously utilized schedule. The incidence of blood culture proven typhoid fever in this region was particularly high in children, being between 1,300 to 1,600/100,000 children. The overall rate for the 3- to 44-year age span was 900/100,000; substantially higher than that encountered in Santiago, Chile. During the subsequent 24 months of postvaccination surveillance, the overall efficacy against blood culture proven typhoid fever was 55% for the liquid preparation and 41% for the capsule formulation; with both, vaccine preparation appeared to be more efficacious in adults than in children. The results are detailed in Table 2.

This result was considered disappointing since in a preliminary study in school children in Santiago, Chile, the liquid preparation had a protective efficacy of 80% compared with that of only 45% for the enteric-coated capsules ($p < 0.001$). No satisfactory reason was identifiable for the greater vaccine efficacy of the liquid preparation observed in Chile as compared with Indonesia, although the possibility that vaccine efficacy may be greater where the incidence of typhoid fever is lower was considered as being one possible explanation, and that the dose schedule selected for the Indonesian study was inappropriate was another.

III. CLINICAL INVESTIGATIONS OF THE HUMORAL IMMUNE RESPONSE TO *S. TYPHI* TY21A

Local humoral immunity is considered to be important in contributing to protection against typhoid fever. The live oral typhoid vaccine organism, *S. typhi* Ty21a, has demonstrated an ability to stimulate a degree of protective immunity, albeit of variable consistency and longevity following oral administration. Many clinical studies have been performed in healthy, often previously unexposed, adult volunteer subjects residing in developed countries in an attempt to ascertain the mechanisms involved in the protective immunity observed in the field evaluations and to define conditions which would result in a more consistent and prolonged duration of protection.

Table 2   **Efficacy of *Salmonella typhi* Ty21a in Plaju, Indonesia**

Age of vaccinees	Incidence of typhoid fever[a]	Vaccine formulation	Vaccine efficacy (%)[b]
3–14 years	1,403	Liquid	53
		Capsule	36
15–44 years	382	Liquid	63
		Capsule	60
All ages	896	Liquid	55
		Capsule	41

[a] Cases of typhoid fever per 10^5 persons per years in placebo recipients.

[b] 24 months of observation, all significances $p > 0.05$.

Adapted from World Health Organization Diarrhoeal Diseases Control Programme, Interim Programme Rep. 1988, Report No. WHO/CDD/89.31, 1989, 36.

66

A. DOSE RESPONSE AND KINETICS OF IMMUNE RESPONSE

Investigations into the kinetics and dose response pattern of the local intestinal and serum immune responses in adult volunteer subjects have been conducted in an effort to more accurately define the kinetics of the response and the dose response pattern in order to optimize the delivery and schedule of the vaccine (Figure 1). The short vaccination schedule of three alternate-day doses of $\approx 10^{11}$ live organisms induced significantly greater intestinal IgA antityphoid antibody responses in these volunteers than two comparable doses 21 days apart. The pattern of the serum and intestinal responses differed

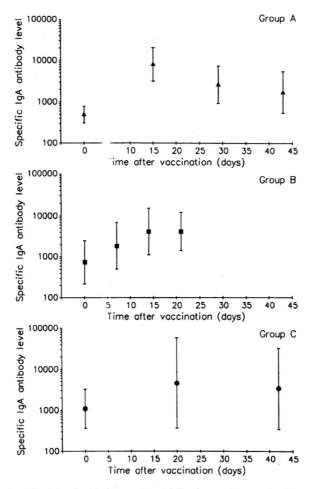

Figure 1 Specific intestinal IgA responses following oral immunization with *Salmonella typhi* Ty21a. Specific intestinal antibody level is the reciprocal of the dilution giving OD = 0.15 units adjusted for total IgA. Responses are geometric mean-adjusted specific antibody level ± 95% confidence interval. Group A, vaccine given on days 0, 2, and 5; group B, days 0, 2, and 4; group C, days 0 and 21. (From Forrest, B. D., LaBrooy, J. T., Beyer, L., Dearlove, C. E., and Shearman, D. J. C., *J. Infect. Dis.,* 163, 336, 1991. With permission.)

only slightly, irrespective of dose schedule. However, the absolute numbers of responders were lower after the first of the two single doses administered 3 weeks apart. Apart from a brief peak in the serum IgG, the second vaccine dose, administered 3 weeks after a primary vaccine dose, did not significantly alter the pattern of the response from that of the three-dose schedule at a similar time point. It appeared that the primary effect of the three-alternate-day-dose schedule was simply to provide additional opportunities for subjects who did not respond to the first or subsequent dose to produce a primary response, a progressive recruitment of responders. This appeared to increase the vaccine "take rate", without having a significant impact on the overall magnitude of the resulting response in that group. This observation was supported by the findings of Black et al.[21], and Ferreccio et al.,[23] both of whom observed that the number of vaccine recipients in the field who were protected against typhoid fever increased with the number of doses administered.

Bartholomeusz et al.[26] observed evidence of long-lasting local immunity in several volunteers who received three doses of the gelatin capsule formulation (containing a minimum of $\approx 10^9$ viable organisms per dose). A striking immune response was evident at 3 weeks, which was still present, though slightly reduced, 1 year after vaccination.[26] In addition, this group observed with fresh vaccine doses that as the vaccine dose was increased ten-fold, both the number of subjects responding, and the magnitude of the intestinal immune responses increased. This study, though dealing with small numbers of subjects, also examined the immunizing potential of an inoculum of $\approx 10^8$ organisms directly placed into the jejunum on two occasions, 14 days apart. It was observed that there was no detectable antityphoid intestinal antibody response evident. Despite this possibly not being the optimal dose schedule, it was suggestive that the minimum dose of *S. typhi* Ty21a required to induce an intestinal immune response in previously unexposed subjects was of the order of 10^8 to 10^9 viable organisms. This would be consistent with the observation made by Hirschel et al.[20] that gelatin capsules containing $\approx 10^8$ viable organisms failed to confer protection in travelers, and is supported by the findings of Forrest et al.[17] However, one report has claimed to be able to identify quite a strong fecal antityphoid LPS antibody response following oral vaccination with either the "Vivotif" gelatin capsules or with the enteric-coated preparation which were both purported to contain $\approx 10^9$ viable organisms.[27]

B. EFFECT OF LYOPHILIZATION ON IMMUNOGENICITY

The effective delivery of a live oral vaccine in the field requires that it be available for distribution in a convenient and stable form. The first step in achieving this is to lyophilize the vaccine doses. The possibility that the process of lyophilization may adversely affect the immunogenicity and protective efficacy of a live bacterial vaccine has been raised earlier following the significant reduction in the ability of an attenuated streptomycin-dependent *S. typhi* typhoid vaccine to stimulate a significant local immune response, or to subsequently confer protection on subjects orally vaccinated with it, when compared to equivalent freshly harvested doses.[10] From the field studies it was impossible to ascertain whether lyophilization adversely affected the immunogenicity of *S. typhi* Ty21a, since at no time did a direct comparison of the two formulations occur, even in small groups. In healthy adult volunteer subjects, using very high doses of $\approx 10^{11}$ viable *S. typhi* Ty21a, it was observed that following lyophilization, *S. typhi* Ty21a retained approximately 50% viability and demonstrated no impairment in its immunogenicity compared to that of an equivalent dose regimen of freshly harvested organisms (Figure 2). The presence of killed organisms was discounted and not regarded as being likely to have contributed significantly to the immune responses observed following vaccination with the lyophilized doses, since the immune responses following the administration of approximately $\approx 10^{11}$ formalin-killed organisms were not significant.[17]

C. IS 10^9 LIVE *S. TYPHI* TY21A AN EFFECTIVE IMMUNIZING DOSE?

Another concern has been with the dose selected for field evaluation. Studies in previously unexposed healthy adult volunteers have failed to demonstrate a measurable intestinal immune response in previously unexposed subjects receiving the three alternate-day doses of $\approx 10^9$ live *S. typhi* Ty21a (Figure 2).[17] The investigators considered it unlikely that this failure to detect a response using this dose regimen reflected any limitations of the assay for intestinal specific antibody, as specific antibody responses were also not identifiable at this dose using a highly sensitive, correlative assay of *in vitro* specific immunoglobulin production using the vaccinated subjects' peripheral blood lymphocytes. It was suggested that the meager response which was observed with the enteric-coated formulation was most likely attributable to the 5×10^{10} killed organisms present, rather than to the 1.1×10^9 viable ones. *S. typhi* Ty21a demonstrated a clearly defined dose-dependent humoral immune response with $\approx 10^{10}$ and $\approx 10^{11}$ live organisms stimulating greater intestinal immune responses than $\approx 10^{11}$ killed organisms, while no responses were evident with either $\approx 10^9$ viable organisms or with the enteric-coated preparation.

The question must then be asked as to why this vaccine preparation, using a three-alternate-day-dose regimen of $\approx 10^9$ viable vaccine organisms, was able to induce any level of protection in the field evaluations? The explanation lies in the basic fact that populations in endemic areas possess a degree of naturally acquired immunity, which has been acquired over many years through repeated subclinical or clinical exposure to the infectious agent in their environment. This is reflected in the observation that attack rates for typhoid fever are much greater in children in these areas than in adults.[28] Therefore, when a new vaccine against typhoid fever is evaluated in adults or older children, the immune responses and protection rates observed are more likely indicative of boosting a lifetime's acquisition of natural immunity rather than a true indicator of vaccine potential. Apart from infants and very young children, these populations cannot in any way be considered comparable to vaccine target groups in countries where the disease is not endemic. This makes equating protection rates in endemic populations with likely protection in the immunologically naive previously unexposed population an extremely difficult exercise.

The protective efficacies demonstrated in the field trials have varied considerably, ranging from 43% to 96%.[19, 22, 25] This variation has been attributed to differences in formulations, vaccination schedules, and infection incidence rates. In fact, there are few consistencies between the studies that would permit any clear conclusion to be drawn, except that *S. typhi* Ty21a is capable of inducing an uncertain degree of immunity in individuals residing in endemic areas. The Indonesian study increased the variables through the utilization of two different preparations and a dose schedule of three alternate weekly doses, such that at least the third dose would have been administered at the time of peak intestinal antibody.[25] This possibly resulted in the exclusion of the third dose through blocking intestinal antibodies.[29, 30] The absence of any knowledge on the prior immune status or the degree of immunological priming of vaccine recipients involved in the many and extensive field trials of *S. typhi* Ty21a conducted in endemic areas would appear to make any sensible extrapolation of the protection data quite difficult.

In the only study which evaluated the protective efficacy of *S. typhi* Ty21a in persons not from or residing in areas endemic for typhoid fever, Gilman et al.[15] demonstrated a protective efficacy of 87% against clinical disease. Not only have vaccine doses of only $\approx 10^9$ viable *S. typhi* Ty21a organisms been demonstrated to be unable to induce immune responses in subjects with no history of prior disease or vaccination as detailed above,[17] but they have also proven to be nonimmunogenic in children <2 years residing in an endemic region, Santiago, Chile.[31] A report from Nepal also suggests that $\approx 10^9$ *S. typhi* Ty21a may not have protected travelers against typhoid while visiting an endemic area.[32]

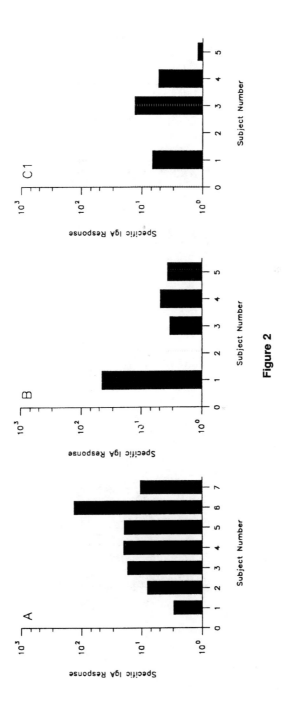

Figure 2

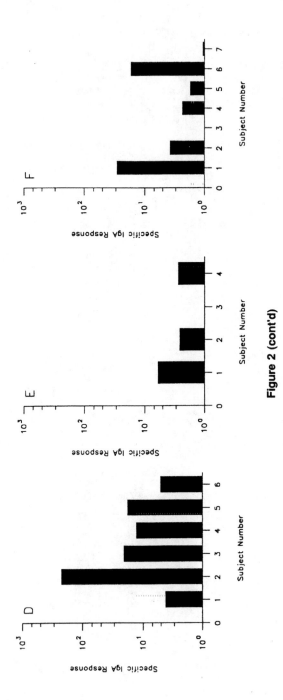

Figure 2 (cont'd)

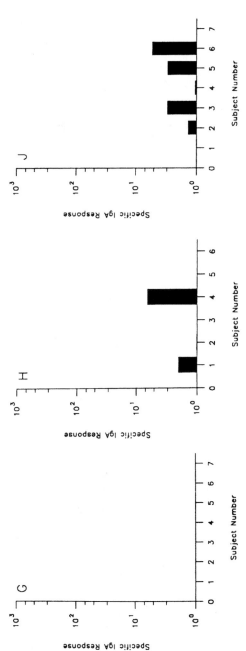

Figure 2 Individual specific intestinal IgA antityphoid lipopolysaccharide antibody responses by typhoid vaccination group. Columns represent the fold rise increase in day 14 (or day 21 for group B, and day 42 for group C1) postvaccination intestinal antityphoid IgA antibody response with respect to day 0 (prevaccination) for an individual subject. Subject groups, vaccines and regimens are as follows: Group A: 1.7×10^{11} live *Salmonella typhi* Ty21a (33% viability), lyophilized and reconstituted organisms, administered on days 0, 2, and 5; group B: 1.7×10^{11} live *Salmonella typhi* Ty21a (33% viability), lyophilized and reconstituted organisms, administered on days 0 only; group C1: 1.7×10^{11} live *Salmonella typhi* Ty21a (33% viability), lyophilized and reconstituted organisms, administered on days 0 and 21; group D: 1.4×10^{11} live *Salmonella typhi* Ty21a (78% viability), freshly harvested organisms, administered on days 0, 2, and 5; group E: 1.3×10^{11} formalin-inactivated *Salmonella typhi* Ty2 (0% viability) organisms, administered on days 0, 2, and 4; group F: 1.7×10^{10} live *Salmonella typhi* Ty21a (33% viability), lyophilized and reconstituted organisms, administered on days 0, 2, and 5; group G: 1.7×10^9 live *Salmonella typhi* Ty21a (33% viability), lyophilized and reconstituted organisms, administered in days 0, 2, and 5; group H: 1.1×10^9 live *Salmonella typhi* Ty21a (2.2% viability), lyophilized organisms in an enteric-coated capsule, administered on days 0, 2, and 4; group J: 5.0×10^8 heat-inactivated phenol-preserved *Salmonella typhi* Ty2 (0% viability) organisms, administered on days 0 and 14.

D. EFFECTS OF PREVIOUS EXPOSURE ON THE IMMUNE RESPONSE TO *S. TYPHI* TY21A

A recent reevaluation of data obtained from clinical studies evaluating *S. typhi* Ty21a in previously unexposed healthy adult volunteers noted that the level of prevaccination cross-reacting background antibodies in the intestine directly reduced the immunogenicity of the live vaccine (Table 3). This occurred irrespective of the magnitude of the dose administered, with the maximal intestinal immune responses only being observed in those subjects with little or no preexisting intestinal antibody, while higher levels of cross-reacting intestinal antibody significantly reduced the immunogenicity of *S. typhi* Ty21a.[29] This was attributed to the blocking effect of these antibodies, consistent with a previous observation that antityphoid LPS IgA antibody prevented boosting of a primary intestinal immune response to *S. typhi* Ty21a with a further oral dose of $\approx 10^{11}$ viable *S. typhi* Ty21a.[30] However, the prevaccination blocking antibodies observed in these studies were considerably lower than those observed following vaccination with $\geq 10^{11}$ viable *S. typhi* Ty21a, with their effect only being evident at the lower vaccine doses of $\approx 10^9$ and $\approx 10^{10}$ viable *S. typhi* Ty21a. The use of the considerably higher doses of $\approx 10^{11}$ were able to overcome the inhibitory effect. It had been anticipated from the limited evidence of Ferguson et al.[33] and from the field observations that the ability of lower doses of *S. typhi* Ty21a should have induced a significant response in those individuals considered partially primed by having moderate levels of background intestinal antibody. However no evidence supporting this was identified. Therefore, it was concluded that in subjects not from typhoid endemic areas, the magnitude of the immune response to a defined dose of orally administered *S. typhi* Ty21a was inversely dependent on the level of preexisting specific intestinal antibody present (Figure 3).

These do not necessarily conflict with the field trial results, with some supporting evidence being available. The Alexandria field trial was conducted in an area with a relatively low incidence of typhoid fever, 44 cases per 100,000, and reported a protective efficacy of 96%,[19] while in the Santiago field trials where the incidence of typhoid fever was >200 cases per 100,000, the protection observed was a considerably lower 67%.[22] It is possible that the increased level of *S. typhi* in the Santiago community resulted in the induction of higher levels of prevaccination intestinal blocking antibodies contributing to the lower efficacy. However, results from other field investigations provide supporting evidence for the augmenting role of previous exposure to *S. typhi* in the resulting induction of a specific immune response to *S. typhi* Ty21a.[31] Therefore it would appear

Table 3 Relationship between jejunal prevaccination *Salmonella typhi* Ty21a-specific IgA antibody and postvaccination mean fold rise

Prevaccination specific antibody level, mean units/mg of total IgA	Viable organisms/vaccine dose		
	10^9 (n = 10)	10^{10} (n = 26)	10^{11} (n = 52)
<500	3.81[a] (5)	14.3 (11)	32.7[b] (22)
95% CI	1.58–6.04	1.30–27.3	19.5–45.9
$\geq$500 to <1000	1.35[a] (5)	4.51 (9)	22.8 (15)
95% CI	0.84–1.86	0.65–8.37	11.7–33.9
$\geq$1000	NS	3.58 (6)	8.30[b] (15)
95% CI		0.36–6.80	2.35–14.3

Note: Data in parentheses are number of subjects included. CI, confidence interval; NS, no subjects.

[a] $p=0.017$; [b] $p=0.0045$.

From Forrest, B. D., *J. Infect. Dis.*, 166, 210, 1992. With permission.

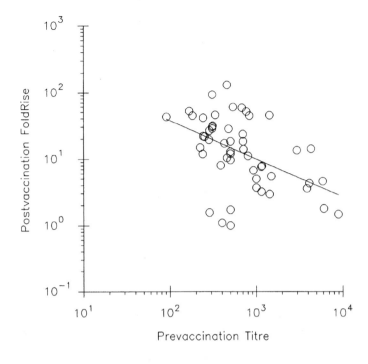

Figure 3 The effect of preexisting intestinal antityphoid lipopolysaccharide IgA antibody on the postvaccination immune response following oral vaccination with 10^{11} live *Salmonella typhi* Ty21a. All prevaccination titers are expressed as specific IgA adjusted for total IgA and are expressed as units of specific activity per mg total IgA. Postvaccination responses are the fold rise in day 14 postvaccination intestinal antityphoid IgA antibody response with respect to day 0 (prevaccination) for an individual subject.

that the induction of an intestinal antibody response to *S. typhi* Ty21a in previously unexposed subjects is inversely proportional to the presence of cross-reacting intestinal secretory immunoglobulin A (sIgA), and that it is likely that the mucosal immune response to *S. typhi* Ty21a in typhoid endemic areas is finely balanced between immunological priming and antigenic exclusion through blocking antibodies, or else involves other mechanisms or antigens not yet investigated.

E. TIMING OF BOOSTER DOSES FOR MAXIMAL EFFECTIVENESS

An outstanding issue concerning the use of *S. typhi* Ty21a concerns the necessity and timing of booster doses. In the adult population of an endemic region, it would appear that the three-alternate-day-dose course is able to provide a satisfactory level of protection for up to 3 years.[19,22] However, as has been discussed, children of these regions and previously unexposed adults in nonendemic regions represent a quite different exposure group. The need for secondary vaccine courses in these populations would appear to be dependent on the duration of the intestinal immune response following the primary vaccination course. Only one study has accurately defined the kinetics of the intestinal immune response following oral vaccination with *S. typhi* Ty21a. Following vaccination with the three-vaccine-dose schedule, a significant increase in jejunal specific antityphoid antibody level was evident as early as day 7 and peaked at 2 weeks, then declining significantly from day 15 to day 43, although the level at 6 weeks still remained elevated above the prevaccination baseline.[17] Allowing for any individual variation as identified by Bartholomeusz et al.,[30] the pattern of response indicated that at 3 months the level of specific IgA antibody would have been expected to be not different from the prevaccination baseline. An attempt to revaccinate during the initial 6 weeks using orally administered doses of ≈10^{11} viable vaccine organisms, failed to significantly alter the decline in specific intestinal IgA antibody noted. However, Dearlove et al.[34] were able to induce specific intestinal IgA immune responses in subjects who had been vaccinated previously with *S. typhi* Ty21a, provided that the initial vaccination course occurred at least 3 months prior to the secondary vaccination course. This finding supports the assertion that specific immunity in the naive subject following oral vaccination with *S. typhi* Ty21a is of short duration, certainly much less than 3 months. However, upon revaccination after that time, an identical intestinal immune response to that seen following primary vaccination is observed.

IV. CLINICAL INVESTIGATIONS OF THE CELLULAR IMMUNE RESPONSE TO S. TYPHI TY21A

S. typhi Ty21a has also been observed to stimulate a significant cell-mediated immune (CMI) response in volunteers ingesting ≈10^9 freshly prepared vaccine organisms, as determined by the lymphocyte migration inhibition assay.[35] However, in common with other investigators using this dose, this group was also unable to detect an antityphoid LPS antibody response in serum or feces following vaccination. In a study comparing CMI responses as determined by a highly sensitive lymphocyte replication assay using whole killed *S. typhi* Ty2 as the antigen, it was shown that 100% of North American volunteer subjects who received the enteric-coated preparation of *S. typhi* Ty21a using the three-dose schedule had a detectable CMI response following vaccination, compared to 92% of typhoid fever patients from Santiago, Chile.[36] The specificity of the assay was shown to be good, with 0% of North American subjects with no known previous exposure to *S. typhi* through disease or previous vaccination having a detectable response. Furthermore, there was no cross-reaction detected against killed *S. enteritidis* or *S. thompson,* when used as antigens.

One study, which evaluated CMI using an assay of antibody-dependent cell cytotoxicity, was able to clearly distinguish differing cellular responses in subjects, depending upon whether they were orally vaccinated with the enteric-coated capsules or received a traditional TAB parenterally administered vaccine (mixed *S. typhi, S. paratyphi* A, and *S. paratyphi* B heat-phenol-inactivated organisms).[37] The subjects receiving the oral typhoid vaccine had distinct cellular responses directed against *S. typhi, S. paratyphi* A, and *S. paratyphi* B, but not against the antigenically unrelated *S. paratyphi* C. None of the subjects parenterally vaccinated with the TAB vaccine had CMI levels as determined using this assay above the natural background against any of the three organisms used above for the vaccination. Since CMI has been suggested to be as important in providing protection against typhoid fever as humoral immunity, the ability of *S. typhi* Ty21a to stimulate a strong CMI response might provide a further contribution of its efficacy as an antityphoid vaccine.

V. *SALMONELLA TYPHI* EX462

Although *S. typhi* Ty21a has been shown to be a useful public health tool in the control of typhoid fever in an endemic region, there are several aspects of it that does not make it the ideal oral typhoid vaccine. The demonstration that the *galE* enzyme deletion was not an attenuating marker of some *Salmonella* strains, including those of *S. cholerasuis* in mice,[38] raised concerns about the actual mechanism of attenuation of *S. typhi* Ty21a. *S. typhi* Ty21a also afforded very little protection when administered as only a single dose;[22] and the method of development of *S. typhi* Ty21a by treating virulent *S. typhi* Ty2 with *N*-methyl-*N'*-nitro-*N*-nitrosoguanidine resulted in a vaccine strain with multiple undefined genetic lesions in addition to the *galE* enzyme defect.[13,39]

Hone et al.[40] described the construction of a *galE* derivative of *S. typhi* Ty2 which had a 0.4 kilobase deletion of the *galE* gene and was sensitive to galactose-induced lysis when cultured with ≥0.06 mmol galactose. Unlike *S. typhi* Ty21a, this strain, designated EX462, contained only an additional deletion in the *via* gene rendering the strain Vi antigen negative. In mouse studies, EX462 demonstrated its high degree of attenuation in the hog gastric mucin-mouse model; however, when orally administered to four healthy adult volunteers using a dose of 7×10^{8} viable organisms following the ingestion of a sodium hydrogen carbonate solution, two developed clinical typhoid fever with the vaccine strain being readily isolated from feces and blood cultures during the illness, which required antimicrobial therapy for resolution.[41] This experiment clearly demonstrated that the *galE* mutation was not an attenuating marker for *S. typhi* Ty2 in humans.

VI. AUXOTROPHIC ATTENUATED TYPHOID VACCINES

In view of the above problems, investigators set about attempting the development of attenuated *S. typhi* strains carrying defined gene deletions in other biochemical pathways[42] as putative candidate vaccine strains. In the early 1950s, it was observed by some investigators that certain strains of *S. typhi* which had sustained one of three biochemical mutations were highly attenuated in the highly artificial mouse typhoid model:[43] the requirement for a purine, such as adenine or adenosine; the requirement for *p*-amino-benzoic acid (PAB); or the requirement for aspartic acid. The aromatic-dependent *S. typhimurium* strains have been demonstrated to be attenuated in mice and calves,[44,45] as have the purine-dependent strains alone.[46] An additional benefit of these aromatic-mutant strains of *Salmonella* may also be as potential carriers of defined protective antigens from foreign organisms, possibly providing a single multivalent attenuated live orally administered vaccine.[47]

A. *AROA PURA S. TYPHI*

A double mutant *S. typhimurium* strain, containing nonreverting *pur*A and *aro*A gene deletions (requiring the exogenous addition of a purine derivative and PAB, respectively, to enable growth) was orally administered to mice and shown to be safe, immunogenic, and protective against virulent challenge.[48] The attenuation of this organism was a result of the absence of appreciable quantities of the required compounds in mammalian tissue.[39]

In a human volunteer study performed in the U.S.,[39] 33 subjects ingested *pur*A *aro*A mutants of either a Vi-negative or Vi-positive *S. typhi* strain in single doses of either 10^{8}, 10^{9}, or 10^{10} viable organisms. Four other subjects ingested two doses of 2×10^{9} viable vaccine organisms 4 days apart. No adverse reactions were observed as a result of orally ingesting the vaccine organism. The humoral immune response to *S. typhi* O, H, Vi, and lysate antigens in both serum and intestinal fluid was poor. However, in most vaccinated subjects CMI responses were demonstrable. In 69% of subjects overall, or 89% of recipients of doses exceeding 10^{9} viable organisms, CMI responses were detectable to *S. typhi* particulate or purified O polysaccharide antigens in lymphocyte replication assays, but not to antigens of other *Salmonella* or *E. coli*.

It was concluded from this study that, despite there being a measure of immunity conferred upon the subjects who were vaccinated, the likelihood of this being protective was considered to be low in view of the absence of humoral immune responses. This is possibly due to the over-attenuation of the vaccine strain by the double mutation. Subsequent studies in mice, using *S. typhimurium* with *purA* alone or *purA aroA* double deletions, demonstrated their ineffectiveness in protection against virulent challenge, and thus their ineffectiveness as orally administrable vaccines.[48]

B. AROC AROD S. TYPHI

As a result of the above findings, investigators have concentrated on developing potential candidate live oral typhoid vaccines by the construction of *S. typhi* strains harboring gene deletions involving two separate genes in the aromatic pathway only.[49] Equivalent *S. typhimurium* strains carrying these gene deletions have been shown to be attenuated and protective against challenge with virulent *S. typhimurium* organisms in mice. Therefore, *aroC aroD* mutants of *S. typhi* Ty2 have been constructed and evaluated in volunteer human subjects.

Two *aroC aroD S. typhi* vaccine strains were developed: CVD906, which was derived from a new Chilean clinical isolate; and CVD908, which was derived from the established *S. typhi* Ty2 strain. The safety and immunogenicity of these two isolates were assessed in two groups of twelve North American volunteer subjects each, who received either a single dose of 5×10^4 or 5×10^5 viable vaccine organisms following ingestion of a sodium hydrogen carbonate solution.[50]

Of the twelve volunteers who received CVD906, fever was observed in one subject at each dose level, and one additional subject had positive blood cultures on two occasions for CVD906 at the lower dose level. Neither fever nor bacteremia was evident in any subject receiving either dose level of CVD908. The local and systemic specific antibody responses are detailed in Table 5.

C. ΔCYA ΔCRP S. TYPHI

Another approach to developing an attenuated *S. typhi* vaccine strain was through the creation of deletions in the genes encoding for adenylate cyclase *(cya)* and cyclic 3′,5′-AMP (cAMP) receptor protein genes *(crp)*. cAMP and its receptor protein are the transcription regulators of many genes concerned with the transport and degradation of catabolites.[51] cAMP is present in mammalian tissue, but at levels believed to be below that required to permit *cya* mutants to exhibit virulence. One Δ*cya* Δ*crp S. typhi* Ty2 strain, designated χ3927, was evaluated for safety and immunogenicity in healthy human subjects in the same study described above, evaluating the auxotrophic strains CVD906 and CVD908.[50] Twelve volunteers received 5×10^5 or 5×10^4 viable χ3927 orally, following the ingestion of a sodium hydrogen carbonate solution. Of the twelve volunteers who received χ3927, two were observed to have fever following vaccination, and χ3927 was isolated from the blood on day 15 and days 8 and 12, respectively, from a further two asymptomatic volunteers. Strain χ3927 was only slightly less immunogenic than either CVD906 or CVD908, with specific anti-LPS serum antibody responses being identifiable in 6/12, compared to 7/12 and 6/12, respectively, for sIgA, and 1/12, compared to 3/12 and 2/12, respectively, for serum IgG. Similarly, there was no difference between the specific anti-LPS jejunal IgA antibody responses between χ3927, CVD906, and CVD908, with responses being identifiable in only 1/12, 1/12, and 2/12 subjects, respectively. Some minor differences were observable using an ELISA for specific antibody-secreting cells secreting with only 5/12 subjects receiving χ3927 achieving an IgA response, while 6/12 and 7/11 subjects who received CVD906 and CVD908, respectively, did so. However, this particular assay as described by these investigators has not been correlated with local or serum immune responses, and so the significance of this result is difficult to interpret.

VII. CLINICAL EVALUATION OF *S. TYPHI* TY21A AS A VECTOR FOR HETEROLOGOUS PROTECTIVE ANTIGENS

Attenuated bacterial vaccine organisms have the additional advantage that they can act as carriers of defined protective antigens of other organisms. Therefore, a bacterial strain developed as an attenuated vaccine against a particular disease can be used as a delivery system for a range of protective antigens relevant to an unrelated disease. The use of attenuated bacteria to carry and express the genes of heterologous organisms is gradually increasing in importance.[52] Essentially, this development has focused on the use of the oral route to vaccinate against the specifically targeted organisms. As a result, it is mainly attenuated enteric bacterial pathogens that have been used as vectors to deliver the foreign antigen(s) to the immune system. Recently attention has been drawn to the use of attenuated *S. typhi* strains as vectors,[53-56] due to the strong intestinal and systemic immune responses that are frequently initiated following infection with the pathogenic parent strain. This includes marked CMI responses, orally administered *Salmonella* strains carrying defined antigens having also been used to protect animals against diseases where the CMI response is considered to be more important, such as malaria.[57,58] Since the oral route of vaccination offers considerable advantages over other delivery routes, such as ease of administration and reduction in side effects, this approach will continue to be further developed.

B. *SALMONELLA TYPHI-SHIGELLA* HYBRID VACCINES

The mobilization of the 120-MDa plasmid of *Shigella sonnei*, which carries the genes for the O-specific side chain, into *S. typhi* Ty21a resulted in an hybrid expressing the *Shigella* group D somatic antigen.[59] This strain, labeled 5076-1C, was demonstrated to be both safe and immunogenic in healthy North American volunteer subjects, and a three-alternate-day-dose schedule of 10^9 viable organisms was demonstrated to confer 40% protection against *Shigella sonnei* challenge in such volunteers.[60] However, this vaccine strain failed to demonstrate a consistent level of efficacy, with considerable interbatch variation being evident,[61,62] which was attributed to the unstable association of the group D antigen with the bacterial surface.[62]

C. *SALMONELLA TYPHI* TY21A-*VIBRIO CHOLERAE* HYBRID VACCINES

Since cholera stimulates poor systemic immunity but excellent protective local intestinal immunity,[63] research has focused upon development of improved vaccines suitable for oral administration. One approach to the development of an oral cholera vaccine involved the cloning of protective antigens from *V. cholerae* into *S. typhi* Ty21a. The rationale for this approach was that:

1. Studies demonstrated the feasibility of bivalent oral vaccines; for example, immunization of mice with a *S. typhimurium/E. coli* hybrid resulted in protection against *S. typhimurium* challenge as well as stimulating a good anti-*E. coli* O8 lipopolysaccharide IgA antibody response.[64] This indicated that the hybrid strain not only retained its status as a vaccine against *S. typhimurium* but also stimulated a specific antibody response against expressed foreign antigens. This was supported by studies in other laboratories which confirmed that attenuated *S. typhimurium* strains could present cloned determinants to the humoral and cellular immune systems.[65]

2. *S. typhi* Ty21a is a safe, effective, live orally administrable vaccine which has shown itself able to act successfully as a vector for foreign putative protective antigens;

3. The correlation of anticholera LPS antibodies in the field with protection against disease,[66] and the finding that anti-LPS antiserum is protective in the infant mouse model[67] and in rabbits,[68, 69] together support a major role for anti-LPS antibodies in providing protection against cholera. In support, it has been demonstrated that anti-LPS

antibody contributes significantly to the serum vibriocidal antibody response (in fact, the entire vibriocidal antibody response can be removed by absorption of the serum with purified LPS)[70,71] which has been shown to correlate with protection; and

4. As discussed previously, locally produced specific antibody is the most effective mechanism of providing protection against enteric pathogens.[72-74]

For these reasons, the localization and subsequent transfer of the genes encoding the O antigen polysaccharide of the cholera LPS into potential carrier organisms was initiated. The genes required for the biosynthesis of the O antigens of the Inaba and Ogawa serotypes of *V. cholerae* were initially transferred into *E. coli* K-12. The anti-Inaba O antigen antiserum raised in rabbits using this *E. coli*/Inaba hybrid was demonstrated to provide the same degree of protection against classical *V. cholerae* Inaba 569B challenge in the baby mouse protection test as the antiserum raised using the parent cholera strain.[75]

Subsequently a series of hybrid *S. typhi* Ty21a-*Vibrio cholerae* hybrid vaccines have been produced and evaluated for safety and immunogenicity in immunologically naive adult volunteer subjects. These vaccine strains were all based on a rifampicin-resistant *S. typhi* Ty21a into which a plasmid was conjugated carrying genes encoding for the *V. cholerae* Inaba O antigen. The resulting strains were all shown *in vitro* to produce *V. cholerae* O antigen, when grown in the absence of exogenous galactose, and both *V. cholerae* and *S. typhi* O antigens, when grown in the presence of exogenous galactose.[76-79] The immunogenicity of one of these hybrid vaccines, EX645, is presented in Tables 4 and 5.

Of these many candidate vaccines, only two were evaluated for their ability to confer a degree of protection on volunteer subjects against challenge with virulent *V. cholerae*. The study evaluating the protective efficacy of EX880 was inconclusive, due to the failure of the control subjects to develop disease following the administration of the challenge inoculum.[80] EX645 was demonstrated to be both safe and immunogenic when administered to subjects in doses up to 6×10^{10} viable organisms,[81] despite the viability of the vaccine strain and its plasmid retention being considerably adversely affected by the process of lyophilization.

However, EX645 was unable to confer a significant degree of protection upon recipients of three alternate-day oral doses of 6×10^{10} viable organisms, when challenged with 1.1×10^9 viable pathogenic *V. cholerae* Inaba strain N16961. The protective

Table 4 Summary of EX645 serum antilipopolysaccharide immune responses

Serum	Typhoid	Cholera
IgA		
Pre (day 0)[a]	44.4	17.9
(95% CI)	(17.7–111)	(9.30–34.6)
Post (day 14)[a]	338	27.1
(95% CI)	(96.1–1,190)	(10.5–69.4)
Fold rise	7.61	1.51
Significance	0.00029	0.16
IgG		
Pre (day 0)[a]	39.7	15.7
(95% CI)	(34.5–45.7)	(9.05–27.1)
Post (day 14)[a]	660	19.3
(95% CI)	(283–1,540)	(8.46–44.0)
Fold rise	16.6	1.23
Significance	0.00022	0.31
IgM		
Pre (day 0)[a]	117	162
(95% CI)	(56.4–244)	(76.3–344)
Post (day 14)[a]	306	234
(95% CI)	(145–644)	(121–452)
Fold rise	2.62	1.44
Significance	0.029	0.18

Note: Fold rises expressed as geometric mean fold rises. Significance values expressed as *p* value only following ln(x) transformation of data and analysis by Student's paired *t*-test for sera.

[a] Reciprocal of geometric mean titers.

From Forrest, B. D., The Effective Delivery of a Bivalent Vaccine against Diarrhoeal Disease, M.D. thesis, University of Adelaide, Adelaide, South Australia, 1990.

efficacy was determined to be 25%, which was not found to be statistically significant ($p = 0.13$, Fisher's exact test, 2-tailed), although the vaccine did significantly reduce the mean stool volume of the vaccinated subjects with respect to the control subjects ($p = 0.0013$) (Table 6), with maximal protection being afforded against moderate (>2.0 l) to moderately-severe (>3.0 l) diarrhea. There was no statistical difference in the incubation periods between the control or vaccinated subjects, nor was there a statistically significant reduction in the peak number of challenge organisms fecally excreted ($p = 0.053$) (Table 6).[82] The failure of the vaccine to protect against clinical cholera most likely reflected the low

Table 5 Summary of EX645 jejunal IgA antilipopolysaccharide immune responses

Jejunal	Typhoid	Cholera
Pre (day 0)[a]	224	142
(95% CI)	(337–2,200)	(68.1–297)
Post (day 14)[a]	5,781	383
(95% CI)	(1,406–23,760)	(69.8–2,096)
Fold rise	25.8	2.70
Significance	0.00047	0.23

Note: Fold rises expressed as geometric mean fold rises. Significance values expressed as p value only following $\ln(x)$ transformation of data and analysis by Student's paired t-test for jejunal fluid.
[a] Reciprocal of geometric mean titers following correction for total class-specific immunoglobulin.
From Forrest, B. D., The Effective Delivery of a Bivalent Vaccine against Diarrhoeal Disease, M.D. thesis. University of Adelaide, Adelaide, South Australia, 1990.

cholera O antigen load presented to the small intestine as supported by the very low levels of cholera O antigen-specific antibody detected, with the number of viable vaccine organisms upon reconstitution found to be only 11%, in comparison to the 63% viability found in a freshly harvested vaccine preparation. Plasmid retention was also quite low, with only 50% of the viable reconstituted organisms retaining the plasmid, where in the fresh doses 92% retention was obtained. As a result, the number of viable vaccine organisms in the reconstituted lyophilized vaccine doses that were capable of producing cholera O antigen was less than 10% of that found in the freshly harvested doses (lyophilized 5.5%, fresh 58%).[83]

Therefore, although the use of *S. typhi* Ty21a as a vector for the carriage of heterologous protective antigens has provided a degree of promise, to date these attempts have resulted in equivocal outcomes.

VIII. CONCLUSION

Considerable advances have been made in the technology that allows the development of potentially new vaccines based on live attenuated orally administrable *S. typhi* strains. The past 20 years have, more than anything else, demonstrated the difficulty of using the outcomes of laboratory experiments as predictors of clinical outcome. The clinical evaluation of *S. typhi* vaccines has complimented the molecular biology. With the mouse model being rendered meaningless as a predictor of likely safety in human subjects of attenuated *S. typhi* strains, the need to evaluate laboratory developments in volunteer subjects has made this almost a mandatory exercise. However, it is apparent that there is still considerable work necessary for the development of an attenuated *S. typhi* strain that is sufficiently attenuated to pose little or no health risk to the recipient, while retaining sufficient ability to colonize and replicate and so induce an effective immune response. The issue which needs to be addressed through the clinical evaluations of candidate live *S. typhi* vaccines, is what degree of concern should be placed on the brief fevers and occasional bacteremia seen in subjects who are unlikely ever to come into risk of naturally acquired infection, compared to these same minor adverse effects in populations with a substantial risk of naturally acquired infection.

Table 6. **Clinical and bacteriological responses of vaccinated and control subjects following challenge with *V. cholerae* El Tor Inaba N16961**

Subjects	Diarrheal stool volume (ml)	Number of diarrheal stools	Incubation period (h)	Peak *V. cholerae* excretion ($\times 10^7$)
Vaccinees				
11001-4	956	7	17.0	10
11001-5	497	2	25.5	1.5
11001-9	2,053	9	20.0	7.5
11001-10	784	7	53.0	0.065
11001-12	0	0	—	0.002
11001-13	0	0	—	0.00027
11001-14	312	5	16.0	11
11001-17	602	6	22.0	5
Mean	867[a]	6	25.6	3.5[b]
Controls				
11002-1	2,054	10	31.5	12
11002-2	1,168	8	22.0	10
11002-3	889	8	22.0	7.5
11002-6	4,399	17	16.5	15
11002-9	1,819	13	13.5	30
11002-12	1,597	6	16.0	0.5
11002-15	4,619	12	17.5	0.8
11002-17	3,405	11	21.0	10
11002-19	906	8	32.0	10
11002-20	622	3	27.5	1
11002-21	3,294	20	22.0	10
11002-22	2,634	13	5.5	10
11002-23	6,434	22	20.0	13
Mean	2,603[a]	11.6	20.5	6.2[b]

Note: [a] $p = 0.0013$, Wilcoxon rank sum test; [b] $p = 0.053$, Wilcoxon rank sum test.
From Forrest, B. D., The Effective Delivery of a Bivalent Vaccine against Diarrhoeal Disease, M.D. thesis, University of Adelaide, Adelaide, South Australia, 1990.

It is clear from the experience with *S. typhi* Ty21a that overattenuation results in a strain of erratic and controversial efficacy, whereas underattenuation as seen with EX462 results in a strain that retains full virulence. It is likely that any of the vaccine strains that have intermediate immunogenicity and retain a very slight virulence are likely to be satisfactory choices as vaccines. However, if attenuated *S. typhi* strains are to be considered as vectors for the carriage of heterologous antigens, especially for diseases where typhoid is not endemic, then the retention of any degree of virulence probably becomes unacceptable.

Wherever the development of attenuated typhoid vaccines leads us, the need for continued development and expansion of the experimental human model has a critical role to play, providing the only true indicator of the likely safety, immunogenicity, and efficacy of a possible vaccine candidate.

REFERENCES

1. Edelman, R. and Levine, M. M., Summary of an international workshop on typhoid fever, *Rev. Infect. Dis.*, 8, 329, 1986.

2. Levine, M. M., Kaper, J. B., Herrington, D., Ketley, J., Losonsky, G., Tacket, C. O., Tall, B., and Cryz, S., Safety, immunogenicity, and efficacy of recombinant live oral cholera vaccines, CVD103 and CVD103-HgR, *Lancet,* 2, 467, 1988.
3. World Health Organization, Intestinal immunity and vaccine development: a WHO memorandum, *Bull. WHO,* 57, 719, 1988.
4. Iverson, W. P. and Waksman, S. A., Use of streptomycin-dependent strains of bacteria for demonstrating ability of microorganisms to produce streptomycin, *Science,* 108, 382, 1948.
5. Reitman, M., Infectivity and antigenicity of streptomycin-dependent *Salmonella typhosa, J. Infect. Dis.,* 117, 101, 1967.
6. Cvjetanovic, B., Mel, D. M., and Felsenfeld, O., Study of live typhoid vaccine in chimpanzees, *Bull. WHO,* 42, 499, 1970.
7. DuPont, H. L., Hornick, R. B., Snyder, M. J., Libonati, J. P., and Woodward, T. E., Immunity in typhoid fever: evaluation of live streptomycin-dependent vaccine, *Antimicrob. Agents Chemother. — 1970,* p. 236, 1971.
8. DuPont, H. L., Hornick, R. B., Snyder, M. J., Libonati, J. P., Formal, S. B., and Gangarosa, E. J., Immunity in shigellosis. I. Response of man to attenuated strains of shigella, *J. Infect. Dis.,* 125, 5, 1972.
9. DuPont, H. L., Hornick, R. B., Snyder, M. J., Dawkins, A. T., Heiner, G. G., and Woodward, T. E., Studies of immunity in typhoid fever. Protection induced by killed antigens or by primary infection, *Bull. WHO,* 44, 667, 1971.
10. Levine, M. M., DuPont, H. L., Hornick, R. B., Snyder, M. J., Woodward, W., Gilman, R. H., and Libonati, J. P., Attenuated, streptomycin-dependent *Salmonella typhi* oral vaccine: potential deleterious effects of lyophilization, *J. Infect. Dis.,* 133, 424, 1976.
11. Mel, D. M., Arsic, B. L., Radovanovic, M. L., Kaljalovic, R., and Litvinjenko, S., Safety tests in adults and children with live oral typhoid vaccine, *Acta Microbiol. Acad. Sci. Hung.,* 21, 161, 1974.
12. Dima, V. F., Volunteer studies in the development of a live oral typhoid vaccine, *Arch. Roum. Path. Exp. Microbiol.,* 42, 191, 1983.
13. Germanier, R. and Furer, E., Isolation and characterization of galE mutant Ty21a of *Salmonella typhi:* a candidate strain for a live, oral typhoid vaccine, *J. Infect. Dis.,* 131, 553, 1975.
14. Germanier, R., Vaccination against typhoid fever with a live oral vaccine, *Dev. Biol. Stand.,* 33, 85, 1976.
15. Gilman, R. H., Hornick, R. B., Woodward, W. E., DuPont, H. L., Levine, M. M., and Libonati, J. P., Evaluation of a UDP-glucose-4-epimeraseless mutant of *Salmonella typhi* as a live oral typhoid vaccine, *J. Infect. Dis.,* 136, 716, 1977.
16. Hornick, R. B., DuPont, H. L., Levine, M. M., Gilman, R. H., Woodward, W. E., Snyder, M. J., and Woodward, T. E., Efficacy of a live oral typhoid vaccine in humans, *Dev. Biol. Stand.,* 33, 89, 1976.
17. Forrest, B. D., LaBrooy, J. T., Beyer, L., Dearlove, C. E., and Shearman, D. J. C., The human humoral immune response to *Salmonella typhi* Ty21a, *J. Infect. Dis.,* 163, 336, 1991.
18. Wahdan, M. H., Serie, C., Germanier, R., Lackany, A., Cerisier, Y., Guerin, N., Sallam, S., Geoffroy, P., Sadel el Tantawi, A., and Guesry, P., A controlled field trial of live oral typhoid vaccine Ty21a, *Bull. WHO,* 58, 469, 1980.
19. Wahdan, M. H., Serie, C., Cerisier, Y., Sallam, S., and Germanier, R., A controlled field trial of live *Salmonella typhi* strain Ty21a oral vaccine against typhoid: three-year results, *J. Infect. Dis.,* 145, 292, 1982.
20. Hirschel, B., Wuthrich, R., Somaini, B., and Steffen, R., Inefficacy of the commercial live oral Ty21a vaccine in the prevention of typhoid fever, *Eur. J. Clin. Microbiol.,* 4, 295, 1985.

21. Black, R. E., Levine, M. M., Ferreccio, C., Clements, M. L., Germanier, R., and the Chilean Typhoid Committee, Field trials of the efficacy of Ty21a attenuated *Salmonella typhi* oral vaccine in Santiago, Chile, 11th Int. Congr. Tropical Medicine and Malaria, September 16 to 22, 1984, Calgary, Canada, 15.

22. Levine, M. M., Ferreccio, C., Black, R. E., Germanier, R., and the Chilean Typhoid Committee, Large-scale field trial of Ty21a live oral typhoid vaccine in enteric-coated capsule formulation, *Lancet*, 1, 1049, 1987.

23. Ferreccio, C., Levine, M. M., Rodriguez, H., Contreras, R., and the Chilean Typhoid Committee, Comparative efficacy of two, three, or four doses of TY21a live oral typhoid vaccine in enteric-coated capsules: a field trial in an endemic area, *J. Infect. Dis.*, 159, 766, 1989.

24. World Health Organization Diarrhoeal Diseases Control Programme, Programme for control of diarrhoeal diseases, Interim Programme Rep. 1988, Rep. No. WHO/CDD/89.31, 1989, 36.

25. Simanjuntak, C. H., Paleologo, F. P., Punjabi, N. H., Darmowigoto, R., Totosudirjo, S. H., Haryanto, P., Suprijanto, E., Witham, N. D., and Hoffman, S. L., Oral immunisation against typhoid fever in Indonesia with Ty21a vaccine, *Lancet*, 338, 1055, 1991.

26. Bartholomeusz, R. C. A., LaBrooy, J. T., Johnson, M., Shearman, D. J. C., and Rowley, D., Gut immunity to typhoid: the immune response to a live oral typhoid vaccine Ty21a, *J. Gastroenterol. Hepatol.*, 1, 61, 1986.

27. Cancellieri, V. and Fara, G. M., Demonstration of specific IgA in feces after immunization with live Ty21a *Salmonella typhi* vaccine, *J. Infect. Dis.*, 151, 482, 1985.

28. Yugoslav Typhoid Commission, A controlled field trial of the effectiveness of acetone-dried and inactivated and heat-phenol-inactivated typhoid vaccines in Yugoslavia. Report, *Bull. WHO*, 30, 623, 1964.

29. Forrest, B. D., LaBrooy, J. T., Dearlove, C. E., and Shearman, D. J. C., Effect of parenteral immunization on the intestinal immune response to *Salmonella typhi* Ty21a in humans, *Infect. Immun.*, 60, 465, 1992.

30. Forrest, B. D., Impairment of immunogenicity of *Salmonella typhi* Ty21a due to pre-existing cross-reacting intestinal antibodies, *J. Infect. Dis.*, 166, 210, 1992.

31. Murphy, J. R., Grez, L., Schlesinger, L., Ferreccio, C., Baqar, S., Munoz, C., Wasserman, S. S., Losonsky, G., Olson, J. G., and Levine, M. M., Immunogenicity of *Salmonella typhi* Ty21a for young children, *Infect. Immun.*, 59, 4291, 1991.

32. Schwartz, E., Shlim, D. R., Eaton, M., Jenks, N., and Houston, R., The effect of oral and parenteral typhoid vaccination on the rate of infection with *Salmonella typhi* and *Salmonella paratyphi A* among foreigners in Nepal, *Arch. Intern. Med.*, 150, 349, 1990.

33. Ferguson, A. and Sallam, J., Mucosal immunity to oral vaccines, *Lancet*, 339, 179, 1992.

34. Dearlove, C. E., Forrest, B. D., van den Bosch, L., and LaBrooy, J. T., The antibody response to an oral Ty21a-based typhoid-cholera hybrid is unaffected by prior vaccination with Ty21a, *J. Infect. Dis.*, 165, 182, 1992.

35. Sirianni, M. C., Turbessi, G., Scarpati, B., Russo, G., Mascellino, M. T., and Aiuti, F., A preliminary report on the immunological responses after oral vaccine (Ty21a), *Boll. Ist. Sieroter Milan*, 63, 352, 1984.

36. Murphy, J. R., Baqar, S., Munoz, C., Schlesinger, L., Ferreccio, C., Lindberg, A. A., Svenson, S., Losonsky, G., Koster, F., and Levine, M. M., Characteristics of humoral and cellular immunity to *Salmonella typhi* in residents of typhoid-endemic and typhoid-free regions, *J. Infect. Dis.*, 156, 1005, 1987.

37. D'Amelio, R., Tagliabue, A., Nencioni, L., Di Addario, A., Villa, L., Manganaro, M., Boraschi, D., Le Moli, S., Nisini, R., and Matricardi, P. M., Comparative analysis of

immunological responses to oral (Ty21a) and parenteral (TAB) typhoid vaccines, *Infect. Immun.,* 56, 2731, 1988.

38. Nnalue, N. A. and Stocker, B. A. D., Some *galE* mutants of *Salmonella choleraesuis* retain virulence, *Infect. Immun.,* 54, 635, 1986.

39. Levine, M. M., Herrington, D., Murphy, J. R., Morris, J. G., Losonsky, G., Tall, B., Lindberg, A. A., Svenson, S., Baqar, S., Edwards, M. F., and Stocker, B., Safety, infectivity, immunogenicity, and in vivo stability of two attenuated auxotrophic mutant strains of *Salmonella typhi,* 541Ty, and 543Ty, as live oral vaccines in humans, *J. Clin. Invest.,* 79, 888, 1987.

40. Hone, D., Morona, S., Attridge, S., and Hackett, J., Construction of defined galE mutants of Salmonella for use as vaccines, *Infect. Immun.,* 156, 167, 1987.

41. Hone, D., Attridge, S. R., Forrest, B. D., Morona, R., Daniels, D., LaBrooy, J.T., Bartholomeusz, R. C. A., Shearman, D. J. C., and Hackett, J., A *galE, via* (Vi-antigen negative) mutant of *Salmonella typhi* Ty2 retains virulence in humans, *Infect. Immun.,* 56, 1326, 1988.

42. Stocker, B. A. D., Auxotrophic *Salmonella typhi* as live vaccine, *Vaccine,* 6, 141, 1988.

43. Bacon, G. A., Burrows, T. W., and Yates, M., The effect of biochemical mutation on the virulence of *Bacterium typhosum*: the loss of virulence of certain mutants, *Br. J. Exp. Pathol.,* 32, 85, 1951.

44. Hoiseth, S. K. and Stocker, B. A. D., Aromatic-dependent *Salmonella typhimurium* are nonvirulent and effective as live vaccines, *Nature,* 291, 238, 1981.

45. Stocker, B. A. D., Hoiseth, S. K., and Smith, B. P., Aromatic-dependent *Salmonella* sp. as live vaccine in mice and calves, *Dev. Biol. Stand.,* 53, 47, 1983.

46. McFarland, W. C. and Stocker, B. A. D., Effect of different purine auxotrophic mutations on mouse virulence of a Vi-positive strain of *Salmonella dublin* and of two strains of *Salmonella typhimurium, Microb. Pathogen.,* 3, 129, 1987.

47. Maskell, D. J., Sweeney, K. J., O'Callaghan, D., Hormaeche, C. E., Liew, F. Y., and Dougan, G., *Salmonella typhimurium aroA* mutants as carriers of the *Escherichia coli* heat-labile enterotoxin B subunit to the murine secretory and systemic immune systems, *Microb. Pathogen.,* 2, 211, 1987.

48. O'Callaghan, D., Maskell, D., Liew, F. Y., Easmon, C. S. F., and Dougan, G., Characterization of aromatic- and purine-dependent *Salmonella typhimurium*: attenuation, persistence, and ability to induce protective immunity in BALB/c mice, *Infect. Immun.,* 56, 419, 1988.

49. Dougan, G., Chatfield, S., Pickard, D., Bester, J., O'Callaghan, D., and Maskell, D., Construction and characterization of vaccine strains of *Salmonella* harboring mutations in two different *aro* genes, *J. Infect. Dis.,* 158, 1329, 1988.

50. Tacket, C. O., Hone, D. M., Curtiss, R., Kelly, S. M., Losonsky, G., Guers, L., Harris, A. M., Edelman, R., and Levine, M. M., Comparison of the safety and immunogenicity of ΔaroC ΔaroD and Δcya Δcrp *Salmonella typhi* strains in adult volunteers, *Infect. Immun.,* 60, 536, 1992.

51. Curtiss, R., III and Kelly, S. M., *Salmonella typhimurium* deletion mutants lacking adenylate cyclase and cyclic AMP receptor protein are avirulent and immunogenic, *Infect. Immun.,* 55, 3035, 1987.

52. Levine, M. M., Woodward, W. E., Formal, S. B., Gemski, P., DuPont, H. L., Hornick, R. B., and Snyder, M. J., Studies with a new generation of oral attenuated shigella vaccines: *Escherichia coli* bearing surface antigens of *Shigella flexneri, J. Infect. Dis.,* 136, 577, 1977.

53. Stocker, B. A. D., Auxotrophic *Salmonella typhi* as live vaccine, *Vaccine,* 6, 141, 1988.

84

54. Clements, J. D., Use of attenuated mutants of *Salmonella* as carriers for delivery of heterologous antigens to the secretory immune system, *Pathol. Immunopathol. Res.,* 6, 137, 1987.
55. Yamamoto, T., Tamura, Y., and Yokota, T., Enteroadhesion fimbriae and enterotoxin of *Escherichia coli:* genetic transfer to a streptomycin-resistant mutant of the galE oral-route live-vaccine *Salmonella typhi* Ty21a, *Infect. Immun.,* 50, 925, 1985.
56. Clements, J. D. and El-Morshidy, S., Construction of a potential live oral bivalent vaccine for typhoid fever and cholera-*Escherichia coli*-related diarrheas, *Infect. Immun.,* 46, 564, 1984.
57. Sadoff, J. C., Ballou, W. R., Baron, L. S., Marajian, W. R., Brey, R. N., Hockmeyer, W. T., Young, J. F., Cryz, S. J., Ou, J., Lowell, G. H., and Chulay, J. D., Oral *Salmonella typhimurium* vaccine expressing circumsporozoite protein protects against malaria, *Science,* 240, 336, 1988.
58. Aggarwal, A., Kumar, S., Jaffe, R., Hone, D., Gross, M., and Sadoff, J., Oral *Salmonella:* malaria circumsporozoite recombinants induce specific cytotoxic T cells, *J. Exp. Med.,* 172, 1083, 1990.
59. Formal, S. B., Baron, L. S., Kopecko, D. J., Washington, O., Powell, C., and Life, C. A., Construction of a potential bivalent vaccine strain: introduction of *Shigella sonnei* Form I antigen genes into the *galE Salmonella typhi* Ty21a typhoid vaccine strain, *Infect. Immun.,* 34, 746, 1981.
60. Black, R. E., Levine, M. M., Clements, M. L., Losonsky, G., Herrington, D., Berman, S., and Formal, S. B., Prevention of shigellosis by a *Salmonella typhi-Shigella sonnei* bivalent vaccine, *J. Infect. Dis.,* 155, 1260, 1987.
61. Herrington, D., van der Verg, L., Formal, S. B., Hale, T. L., Tall, B. D., Cryz, S. J., Tramont, E. C., and Levine, M. M., Studies in volunteers to evaluate candidate *Shigella* vaccines: further experience with a bivalent *Salmonella typhi-Shigella sonnei* vaccine and protection conferred by previous *Shigella sonnei* disease, *Vaccine,* 8, 353, 1990.
62. Hale, T. L. and Formal, S. B., Oral shigella vaccines, *Curr. Top. Microbiol. Immunol.,* 146, 205, 1989.
63. Levine, M. M., Immunity to cholera as evaluated in volunteers, in *Cholera and Related Diarrheas,* 43rd Nobel Symp. 1978, Ouchterlony, O. and Holmgren, J., Eds., Karger, Basel, 1980, 195.
64. Hohman, A. W., Schmidt, G., and Rowley, D., Intestinal colonization and virulence of *Salmonella* in mice, *Infect. Immun.,* 22, 763, 1978.
65. Dougan, G., Hormaeche, C. E., and Maskell, D. J., Live oral *Salmonella* vaccines: potential use of attenuated strains as carriers of heterologous antigens to the immune system, *Parasite Immunol.,* 9, 151, 1987.
66. Mosley, W. H., Woodward, W. E., Aziz, K. M. A., Rahman, A. S. M. M., Chowdhury, A. K. M. A., Ahmed, A., and Feeley, J. C., The 1968–1969 cholera field trial in rural East Pakistan. Effectiveness of monovalent Ogawa and Inaba vaccines and purified Inaba antigen, with comparative results of serological and animal protective tests, *J. Infect. Dis.,* 121 (Suppl.), S1, 1970.
67. Watanabe, Y., Verwey, W. F., and MacDonald, E. M., Protective antigen from El Tor vibrios. II. Responses in animals and man to partially purified Ogawa lipopolysaccharide antigen, *Bull. WHO,* 32, 823, 1965.
68. Svennerholm, A.-M., Experimental studies on cholera immunization. IV. The antibody response to formalinized *Vibrio cholerae* and the purified endotoxin with special reference to protective capacity, *Int. Arch. Allergy Appl. Immunol.,* 49, 434, 1975.
69. Watanabe, Y., Verwey, W. F., Guckian, J. C., Williams, H. R., Phillips, P. E., and Rocha, S. S., Some of the properties of mouse protective antigens derived from *Vibrio cholerae, Texas Rep. Biol. Med.,* 27 (Suppl. 1), 275, 1969.

70. Jertborn, M., Svennerholm, A.-M., and Holmgren, J., Gut mucosal, salivary and serum antitoxic and antibacterial antibody responses in Swedes after oral immunization with B subunit-whole cell cholera vaccine, *Int. Arch. Allergy Appl. Immunol.*, 75, 38, 1984.

71. Neoh, S. H. and Rowley, D., Protection of infant mice against cholera by antibodies to three antigens of *Vibrio cholerae*, *J. Infect. Dis.*, 126, 41, 1972.

72. Rowley, D., Immune responses to enterobacteria presented by various routes, *Prog. Allergy*, 33, 159, 1983.

73. Welliver, R. C. and Ogra, P. L., Importance of local immunity in enteric infection, *J. Am. Vet. Med. Assoc.*, 173, 560, 1978.

74. Targan, S. R., Immunologic mechanisms in intestinal diseases, *Ann. Intern. Med.*, 106, 853, 1987.

75. Manning, P. A., Heuzenroeder, M. W., Yeadon, J., Leavesley, D. I., Reeves, P. R., and Rowley, D., Molecular cloning and expression in *Escherichia coli* K-12 of the O antigens of the Inaba and Ogawa serotypes of the *Vibrio cholerae* O1 lipopolysaccharides and their potential for vaccine development, *Infect. Immun.*, 53, 272, 1986.

76. Forrest, B. D., The development of a bivalent vaccine against diarrhoeal disease, *Southeast Asian J. Trop. Med. Public Health*, 19, 449, 1988.

77. Forrest, B. D. and LaBrooy, J. T., *In vivo* evidence of immunological masking of the *Vibrio cholerae* O antigen of a hybrid *Salmonella typhi* Ty21a-*Vibrio cholerae* oral vaccine in humans, *Vaccine*, 9, 515, 1991.

78. Attridge, S. R., Daniels, D., Morona, J. K., and Morona, R., Surface co-expression of *Vibrio cholerae* and *Salmonella typhi* O-antigens on Ty21a clone EX210, *Microb. Pathogen.*, 8, 177, 1990.

79. LaBrooy, J. T., Forrest, B. D., and Bartholomeusz, R. C. A., Immunization against cholera with a Ty21a-cholera hybrid, *Ann. Sclavo Collagano Monogr.*, 1–2, 143, 1987.

80. Attridge, S. R., Dearlove, C., Beyer, L., van den Bosch, L., Howles, A., Hackett, J., Morona, R., LaBrooy, J., and Rowley, D., Characterization and immunogenicity of EX880, a *Salmonella typhi* Ty21a-based clone which produces *Vibrio cholerae* O antigen, *Infect. Immun.*, 59, 2279, 1991.

81. Forrest, B. D., LaBrooy, J. T., Attridge, S. R., Boehm, G., Beyer, L., Morona, R., Shearman, D. J. C., and Rowley, D., Immunogenicity of a candidate live oral typhoid/cholera hybrid vaccine in humans, *J. Infect. Dis.*, 159, 145, 1989.

82. Tacket, C. O., Forrest, B., Morona, R., Attridge, S. R., LaBrooy, J. T., Tall, B. D., Reymann, M., Rowley, D., and Levine, M. M., Safety, immunogenicity, and efficacy against cholera challenge in humans of a typhoid-cholera hybrid vaccine derived from *Salmonella typhi* Ty21a, *Infect. Immun.*, 58, 1620, 1990.

83. Forrest, B. D., The Effective Delivery of a Bivalent Vaccine against Diarrhoeal Disease, M.D. thesis, University of Adelaide, Adelaide, South Australia, 1990.

Chapter 3

Multivalent BCG Vaccines

**Jeremy W. Dale, Odir A. Dellagostin, Elizabeth Norman,
Alan D. T. Barrett, and Johnjoe McFadden**

TABLE OF CONTENTS

I. MYCOBACTERIAL DISEASES AND VACCINES

Mycobacteria are responsible for two of the most important diseases to afflict mankind: tuberculosis (TB) and leprosy. Described by John Bunyan as "captain of all those men of death", tuberculosis was responsible for 20% of all deaths in 19th century England. Although TB declined in the west, it has remained one of the world's most serious health problems affecting an estimated 20 millions worldwide and responsible for three million deaths annually. It has recently been estimated that tuberculosis accounts for 26% of avoidable adult deaths in the developing world — the largest cause of death in the world from a single infectious agent.

Mycobacteria belong in the actinomycete branch of Gram-positive bacteria, a group that includes *Nocardia, Corynebacterium,* and *Streptomyces* species. These bacteria share a number of common properties, including a tendency for mycelial growth, aerobic metabolism, and DNA with a high (55 to 70%) G + C content. The tubercle bacillus was isolated by Robert Koch in 1882 and shown to be the causative agent of both human and bovine tuberculosis. The generic name *Mycobacterium* was introduced in 1896 on account of the tendency for the tubercle bacillus to grow as a fungal-like pellicle in liquid

0-8493-4866-8/94/$0.00+$.50
© 1994 by CRC Press Inc.

media. At first only human and bovine forms of the bacillus were recognized, but by the middle of the 20th century it was clear that the genus contained many saprophytic species and many species, such as *Mycobacterium avium*, that are specific animal pathogens. The mycobacteria may be divided into two groups, fast and slow growers, on the basis of their growth rate in culture. Most of the pathogens, including *Mycobacterium tuberculosis*, are slow growing with a doubling time of 10 to 24 hours.

Many of the properties of mycobacteria such as their antigenicity, adjuvanticity, virulence, and antitumor activity, are thought to involve components of the mycobacterial cell wall. The structure of the cell wall consists of a peptidoglycan backbone covalently linked to branched chains of arabinogalactan esterified at their termini by mycolic acids (α-branched β-hydroxy fatty acids with long alkyl chains). Several unusual lipids and glycolipids may also be associated with the cell wall, including trehalose-containing lipooligosaccharide, mannophosphoinositides, glycopeptidolipids, phenolic glycolipids, and cord factor (α-α-D-trehalose 6,6,'-dimycolate). The high lipid content of the cell wall also accounts for the hydrophobic properties of mycobacteria. Proteins are also present in the cell wall, but as yet they have not been characterized.

The term "tubercle bacillus" was used for human and bovine variants of the species that caused tuberculosis, but in 1970 the latter variant was given separate species status as *Mycobacterium bovis*. However, *M. bovis* is very closely related to *M. tuberculosis* and its separate species status remains controversial. Both *M. tuberculosis* and *M. bovis* cause pulmonary tuberculosis in humans. In order to understand the mechanisms of protection afforded by BCG vaccination it is useful to examine the pathogenesis of tuberculosis.[1]

A. TUBERCULOSIS

Infection with *M. tuberculosis* most commonly occurs by inhalation of small droplets containing only a few live tubercle bacilli. The primary focus of infection is usually therefore the middle or lower zones of the lung. Abdominal tuberculosis may be associated with ingestion of tubercle bacilli, indicating that the pathogen is also infectious via the oral route. In the lung, the bacilli are readily phagocytosed by alveolar macrophages, but pathogenic mycobacteria are able to resist killing by macrophages and replicate efficiently within the cytoplasm of macrophages at this site to form the primary focus of infection. Extracellular and intracellular bacilli may then enter the local lymphatics and, thereafter, the lymphatic and blood circulation to disseminate widely through the body. This stage of disease is usually clinically silent, and in most cases immunity develops within a few weeks. However about 5% of those initially infected will develop primary tuberculosis soon after infection. In the remainder who develop immunity at this stage, replication of the pathogen is curtailed, and the primary lesion heals to form a granuloma that walls off the mycobacteria from the surrounding tissue. The majority of these individuals will remain free of tuberculosis throughout their lives, indicating that the normal immune response is capable of containing the infection. Indeed, there is evidence that these individuals are immune to superinfection. However, a minority (about 5%) will at some stage in their lives, usually many years later, develop postprimary tuberculosis due to loss of host immunity associated with, e.g., illness or malnutrition (HIV infection is now the most important factor leading to progression to this stage of disease). Clearly the tubercle bacillus is capable of remaining dormant but viable in the host for many years.

Mycobacteria such as *M. tuberculosis* are intracellular pathogens and in the host are usually found in phagocytic cells such as macrophages. The finding of high levels of antibody but cellular anergy associated with the uncontrolled replication of *Mycobacterium leprae* in lepromatous leprosy patients suggests that as with other intracellular pathogens, protection against mycobacterial disease is principally cell mediated rather than humoral.[2] Reactivation of tuberculosis associated with HIV infection also indicates the importance of T cells in controlling the infection. Immunity is thought to involve the action of antigen-specific T lymphocytes that activate the nonspecific microbiocidal functions of infected macrophages. Antigen must be presented to T lymphocytes by antigen-presenting cells in association with MHC class I or class II proteins. It is not known which mycobacterial antigens are responsible for inducing a protective T cell response, but much work in mycobacterial immunology and genetics is directed towards this question. Macrophage killing of pathogenic bacteria, even when activated, is however relatively inefficient and a role for cytotoxic T lymphocytes in protection is presently envisaged. In any case, to survive, mycobacteria must resist intracellular killing. The mechanism by which *M. tuberculosis* survives within phagocytic cells is unclear, but may involve interference with activation, resistance to oxidative killing systems, and inhibition of phagosome-lysosome fusion. Additionally, mycobacteria and mycobacterial components have been shown to induce or interfere with cytokine release by mechanisms that may be important in both survival of the pathogen in the host and also the immunopathology and immunostimulation that accompany mycobacterial infection.[2]

B. HISTORY OF BCG

The BCG vaccine (bacille Calmette-Guérin) was developed at the Institut Pasteur in Lille from a strain originally isolated from a cow with tuberculous mastitis; although BCG is usually referred to as an attenuated strain of *M. bovis,* it is bacteriologically distinct from *M. bovis.* Unfortunately, the original strain was lost during the 1914–1918 war, and its identity cannot be confirmed (see Grange et al.[3]).

Attenuation was achieved by 230 subcultures of this strain on glycerol-bile-potato medium, during the years from 1908 to 1921. Many daughter strains have subsequently been derived from this original isolate; these are commonly identified by the country of manufacture or the production laboratory. Neither designation is completely reliable because some countries or laboratories have changed vaccine strains while still retaining the same designation. Many research reports, and even vaccine trials, do not specify adequately the source of the BCG strain used, as there has been an implicit assumption that all BCG strains are identical (despite much anecdotal evidence of different immunological responses). It is now clear that BCG strains can be divided into two major groups on the basis of three characteristics: secretion of a specific protein antigen (MPB70), cell wall lipid composition, and DNA fingerprinting.[4] One group, which includes BCG Japan (BCG Tokyo), secretes MPB70 in large amounts, possesses methoxymycolates in the cell wall, and carries two copies of the insertion sequence IS986/IS6110. The original seed cultures for these strains were all derived from the Institut Pasteur between 1925 and 1928.

The second group of strains, which includes the Glaxo and Pasteur strains, does not secrete MPB70, does not possess methoxymycolates, and has only a single copy of IS986/IS6110; these strains are all derived from seed lots obtained after 1932. Initially, there were three different lines of BCG maintained at the Institut Pasteur on different media, but two of these lines were discarded in 1932. It is possible that BCG Japan, and the other members of the former group, were derived from one of the two discontinued lines. (See Fomukong et al.[4] for original references.) The characteristics used for distinguishing the two groups of BCG strains are not thought to be directly related, but are separate genetic markers reflecting the different history of these strains. It is likely, therefore, that there will be many other differences between these strains, and these differences may be expected to affect the efficacy and safety of the vaccine. Furthermore, repeated subculture of each strain over a number of years means that the strains within each of the two main groups cannot be expected to be completely homogeneous, and a preliminary study with additional gene probes has disclosed restriction fragment length polymorphisms between strains of the second group (N. G. Fomukong and J. W. Dale, unpublished).

C. USE OF BCG

Since *M. bovis* commonly infects via the ingestion of contaminated milk, setting up an initial focus of infection in the gut, it is to be expected that the attenuated strain BCG could also be used as a vaccine via the same route — and indeed the earliest uses of BCG were as an oral vaccine, with it being first administered orally to human infants in 1921. The use of BCG as a vaccine received a severe setback when 73 children at Lübeck (Germany) died in 1930 following vaccination. This incident was not due to reversion of BCG to virulence, but was a consequence of accidental administration of virulent tubercle bacilli instead of the attenuated strain. Nevertheless, it was not until the 1950s that BCG again became widely acceptable as a vaccine.

However, although originally administered orally, the more familiar use now is as an intradermal vaccine given to persons who are skin test negative by the tuberculin test. In this form, live BCG is the most widely used human vaccine in the world and is the only vaccine recommended to be given at birth. In addition to tuberculosis prophylaxis, BCG also appears in some studies to confer a degree of protection against leprosy. The immunostimulatory properties of BCG are also exploited in the treatment of bladder cancer.

However, the protection against tuberculosis engendered by BCG appears to vary greatly in different areas of the world from 70 to 80% in trials conducted among North American Indians and in Great Britain to 0 to 30% in trials conducted in South India, Uganda, and in Georgia, U.S.[5,6] The reasons for the varying efficacy are unknown but may include genetic differences in the host population, natural infection with environmental mycobacteria interfering with the protection afforded by BCG, and differences between the vaccines used and vaccination schedule.

A critical question is the duration of protection afforded by BCG vaccination. Cell-mediated immunity (CMI) to tuberculoproteins can be demonstrated for 5 to 50 years following vaccination suggesting that immunity may be similarly long-lived. It is thought that, as with virulent *M. tuberculosis*, BCG persists in a dormant state within the vaccinated host, maintaining immunity by continually presenting the immune system with small amounts of antigen. However, repeated BCG vaccination to boost immunity is standard policy in many countries although its efficacy has never been assessed.

Killed BCG does not induce substantial levels of CMI unless incorporated in a water-in-oil type of emulsion (complete Freund's adjuvant, CFA) — preparations too toxic for use in humans. Replication of BCG is therefore essential for development of effective immunity and can be demonstrated in vaccinated experimental animals. From studies in animals, it has been proposed that the protection induced by BCG vaccination stems from its interference with the hematogenous spread of tubercle bacilli. The corollary of this hypothesis is that vaccination would not prevent either the establishment of natural primary infection with *M. tuberculosis* or interfere with repeated vaccination. The molecular basis of attenuation in BCG is completely unknown. Fortunately, there is no evidence of it ever having reverted to virulence in any host. The safety of BCG vaccination in HIV-infected individuals is more uncertain. Anecdotal reports describe lymphadenitis and disseminated BCG disease in HIV-seropositive individuals following BCG vaccination; however, a study in Kinshasa found no difference in complications following BCG vaccination in HIV-seropositive children compared to HIV-seronegative children. WHO presently recommends that BCG should not be given to symptomatic HIV-infected children or adults, or asymptomatic children or adults in areas where the risk of TB is low. However, in areas where the risk of TB is high, BCG can be given to asymptomatic HIV-infected children, since the risk of TB is greater than the risk of complications.

The potential value of BCG as a recombinant multivaccine is due to the well-known immunostimulatory and adjuvant properties of mycobacteria.[7] CFA, a killed and dried suspension of *M. tuberculosis* cells in a water-in-oil emulsion, exerts a profound effect on the immunological response of the host against unrelated antigens included in the oil phase. High levels of both cellular immunity and serum antibody directed against the foreign antigen are obtained and maintained for extended periods. CFA may also break tolerance in experimental animals — thyroiditis, allergic encephalomyelitis, and adrenalitis can be induced in experimental animals by injection of CFA with homologous antigen. CFA alone, without antigen, may also have powerful nonspecific immunostimulatory effects and can in some experimental systems induce various immune disorders such as adjuvant arthritis, generalized granulomatous lesions, and amyloidosis. Heat-killed BCG in mineral oil has similar adjuvant and immunostimulatory properties. However, it should be emphasized that none of these disorders are associated with BCG vaccination in man.

The potent immunostimulatory activities of mycobacteria have suggested their use as immunotherapeutic agents. Injection of a mixture of live BCG plus killed *M. leprae* has been shown to convert a proportion of skin test-negative lepromatous leprosy patients (with cellular anergy to *M. leprae*) to lepromin skin test positive.[8] Similar immunotherapeutic intervention has shown to be successful in the treatment of cutaneous leishmaniasis using BCG plus killed *Leishmania mexicana*.[9] Injection with both CFA and vaccination with live BCG enhances the resistance of experimental animals to a variety of unrelated pathogens including *Brucella, Bacillus anthracis,* staphylococci, salmonellae, *Toxoplasma,* and other pathogens.[7,10] Both live and killed BCG have been shown to exert potent antitumor activities in man and animals.[10] Growth of tumor cells in mice is strongly inhibited if the mice are pretreated with either live or killed BCG. Both live and killed BCG have been used as therapeutic agents for cancer therapy in man.[10]

II. GENE CLONING SYSTEMS FOR MYCOBACTERIA

A. SHUTTLE PLASMIDS

The development of an effective gene cloning system for a specific bacterial host requires (1) the ability to introduce DNA into the host, (2) replication and inheritance of the inserted DNA, often by the use of plasmid or bacteriophage vectors, and (3) the availability of selectable markers for identification or selection of transformed cells. The ability to express the inserted genes and to control that expression is a further consideration that will be dealt with subsequently.

The difficulty with these parameters is that all three have to be available simultaneously; the absence of known plasmid-mediated antibiotic resistance in mycobacteria or of established transformation systems proved a considerable obstacle. Although there were reports of transformation and transfection of mycobacteria, and also of conjugal transfer (reviewed by Grange[11]), these proved difficult to reproduce. One strategy that has proved useful on many occasions when working with mycobacterial systems is to draw on experience gained with *Streptomyces* — and this was one of those occasions. Jacobs et al.[12] adapted *Streptomyces* techniques for preparation of spheroplasts and the use of PEG-mediated spheroplast transformation to introduce DNA into *M. smegmatis.*

In the absence of mycobacterial plasmids carrying resistance markers, these initial experiments were performed with bacteriophage DNA, including shuttle phasmids that replicated as ColE1-based plasmids in *E. coli* and as phages in *M. smegmatis* (or subsequently in BCG). Later, Snapper et al.[13] used shuttle plasmids based on a temperate mycobacteriophage L1 and carrying a kanamycin resistance gene to establish stable lysogens of *M. smegmatis.*

At the same time, the development of the first mycobacterial shuttle plasmids represented an important advance. Tobias Kieser from the John Innes Institute in Norwich took the naturally occurring plasmid pAL5000 from a strain of *M. fortuitum*[14-16] randomly linearized it by partial digestion with *Mbo*I and ligated it with an *E. coli* vector, pIJ666, carrying chloramphenicol acetyltransferase (from pACYC184) and the Tn5 phosphotransferase gene[13] (Figure 1). A plasmid mixture was isolated from pooled *E. coli* transformants and used to transform *M. smegmatis* with selection for kanamycin resistance. Several different constructs were isolated, of which one (pYUB12) has been widely used subsequently (Figure 2). pAL5000 still provides the basis for most of the shuttle plasmids used in mycobacteria, which are derived either from pYUB12 or directly from pAL5000 — such as pAL8 and pRR3 (Figure 2).[17]

Based on the original sequence data for pAL5000,[16] attempts were made to identify the origin of replication and hence the minimum region necessary for construction of a functional replicon; Ranes et al.[17] identified a 2.5-kb fragment and Stover et al.[18] used a smaller (1.8 kb) fragment. The sequence of pAL5000 has recently been redetermined,[14] and it is to be expected that this will lead to a reevaluation of the functional analysis of pAL5000.

Other shuttle plasmids have been constructed, based on the *Corynebacterium* plasmid pNG2,[19] or using the replication origin from the mycobacteriophage D29.[20,21] In addition, the broad host-range plasmid RSF1010 can be transferred by conjugation from *E. coli* to *M. smegmatis,* if mobilized by the conjugative plasmid RP4.[22]

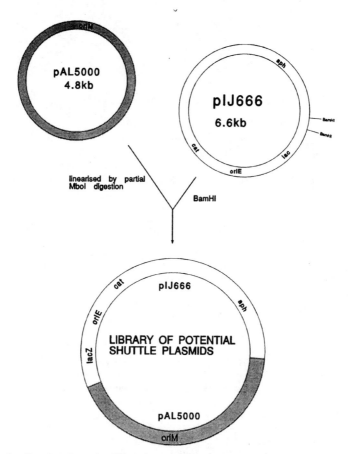

Figure 1 Construction of a library of potential mycobacterial shuttle plasmids, by fusion of a mycobacterial plasmid pAL5000 with an *E. coli* plasmid vector.

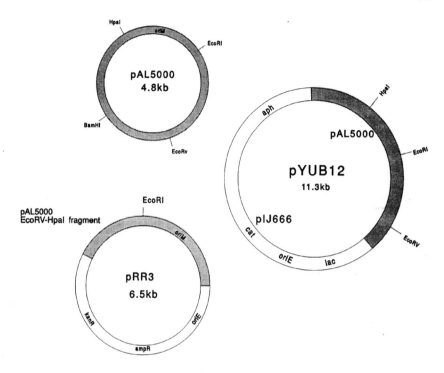

Figure 2 Structure of two mycobacterial shuttle vectors. pYUB12 was formed by complete fusion of the naturally occurring mycobacterial plasmid pAL5000 with an *E. coli* plasmid (see Figure 1), while pRR3 contains part of pAL5000.

The use of shuttle plasmids has also been facilitated by the development of electroporation as a more efficient alternative to spheroplast transformation and by the use of mutant strains of *M. smegmatis* such as mc²155 that are more efficiently transformed[23] — although it should be noted that the increased transformation refers to electroporation with pYUB12 and does not affect, for example, transfection with bacteriophage DNA or transformation with a vector (pY6002) that integrates by homologous recombination[24] (see below).

Although shuttle plasmids are convenient for laboratory-scale work, several workers have encountered problems of stability with pYUB12 and related plasmids, and have therefore searched for ways of integrating the foreign DNA into the mycobacterial chromosome. This strategy also has the potential advantage of dispensing with the need for antibiotic selection, since the presence of resistance genes is likely to cause regulatory problems for the use of a live vaccine. These integrative vectors fall into three classes: (1) integration by homologous recombination, (2) integration by transposition (or transpositional cointegrate formation), and (3) site-specific integration, using integrative phage or plasmid.

B. INTEGRATION BY HOMOLOGOUS RECOMBINATION

Husson et al.[24] constructed a genomic library of *M. smegmatis* using pUC19 as the vector; from a pool of *E. coli* transformants, plasmid DNA was extracted and used for transformation of uracil auxotrophic *(pyrF)* strains of *E. coli* in order to identify recombinant

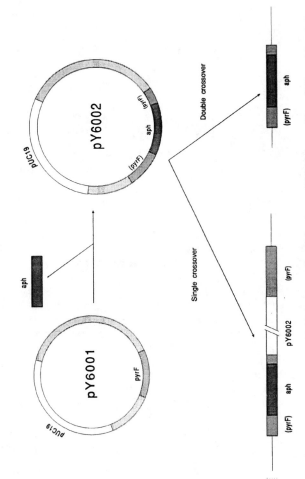

Figure 3 Integration by homologous recombination. pY6002 is an *E. coli* plasmid carrying mycobacterial DNA including the *pyrF* gene; in pY6002 this gene is disrupted by insertion of an *aph* (kanamycin resistance) gene. Kanamycin-resistant mycobacterial transformants arise either by a single recombinational event, leading to insertion of the complete plasmid and retention of one functional copy of *pyrF*, or by a double crossover, which replaces the functional *pyrF* gene with the disrupted one.

plasmids carrying the *M. smegmatis pyrF* gene by complementation. The plasmid pY6001 (Figure 3) was shown to possess an insert containing the *M. smegmatis pyrF* gene which enables positive selection (by complementation of uracil auxotrophy) and negative selection (since a functional *pyrF* gene confers sensitivity to 5-fluoroorotic acid, 5-FOA). The *aph* gene from Tn903 was inserted into the *Bam*H1 site of pY6001, disrupting the *pyrF* gene, and creating plasmid pY6002 (Figure 3). It should be noted that these plasmids do not have a functional mycobacterial replicon and are therefore not expected to replicate independently in *M. smegmatis*.

When wild-type, prototrophic *M. smegmatis* was electroporated with pY6002, with selection for kanamycin resistance, two classes of transformants were obtained. The first type were uracil prototrophs and sensitive to 5-FOA, and Southern blots revealed the integration of the entire plasmid via a single homologous recombination event. The second class of transformants were uracil auxotrophs and resistant to 5-FOA, with Southern blots showing that the intact parental *pyrF* gene had been replaced by the disrupted gene from the pY6002 plasmid, presumably by a double cross-over event (Figure 3).

By inserting additional genes into pY6002, it is possible to use this approach to insert these genes into the *M. smegmatis* chromosome. Husson et al.[24] demonstrated the feasibility of this using the gene for the 65-kDa antigen of *M. leprae*, which was successfully expressed in *M. smegmatis*.

This procedure can be useful for obtaining mutants of *M. smegmatis*, by subjecting the plasmid library to transposon mutagenesis in *E. coli*.[25] However, a major limitation of this approach for vaccine construction is that it appears to be unsuccessful in BCG. For unknown reasons, the recombinants obtained in BCG do not have the predicted structure but appear to arise from less specific recombination events, referred to as "illegitimate recombination" by Kalpana et al.[25]

C. TRANSPOSITIONAL INTEGRATION

Several insertion sequences have been characterized from various mycobacterial species, although until recently there has been little direct evidence of their mobility. One of these elements, IS900 (see Reference 26), is found in *M. paratuberculosis* and is an unusual element in that it lacks terminal inverted repeats, does not appear to generate target-site duplications, and shows a degree of target-site specificity and orientation. It seems to have some relationship with elements from other bacterial species (and *Streptomyces* in particular), including IS110, IS116, and the minicircle IS117.

England et al.[27] created an artificial composite transposon by placing two copies of IS900 flanking a kanamycin resistance gene (*aph* from Tn903) in pUC18. Since this plasmid, pUS701 (Figure 4) is not expected to replicate in a mycobacterial host, electroporation followed by selection for kanamycin resistance should yield cells in which the *aph* gene has become integrated into the chromosome. Kanamycin-resistant colonies were obtained at a frequency about 10^{-3} of that shown with the autonomously replicating shuttle plasmid pYUB12, giving an estimate of the efficiency of transposition. Southern blots showed that most of the products were cointegrates with an extra copy of IS900, implying a replicative transposition. These transformants were considerably more stable than those obtained with the shuttle plasmid pYUB12. We have successfully used this system for expression of foreign antigens in *M. smegmatis* and in BCG (see below and Reference 53).

M. tuberculosis and related organisms, including BCG, contain a more typical insertion sequence known as IS986[28-31] or IS6110.[32] This element is a member of the IS3 family and has 38-bp inverted repeat ends, and (usually) generates a target site duplication,

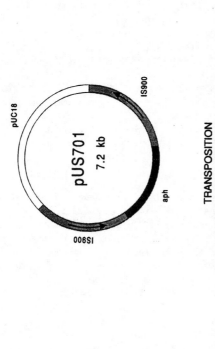
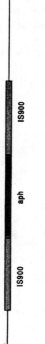

Figure 4 Integration by transposition. pUS701 is an *E. coli* plasmid carrying an artificial composite transposon formed by two copies of IS900 flanking an *aph* (kanamycin resistance) gene. Kanamycin-resistant mycobacterial transformants arise either by transposition of the composite transposon, or by cointegrate formation in which the entire plasmid is integrated, accompanied by replication of one copy of IS900.

although with very little specificity. It is in widespread use for molecular epidemiology of *M. tuberculosis*, due to the extensive polymorphism generated.[28,30]

We have recently demonstrated transposition and cointegrate formation with IS986, using the same approach as England et al.[27] used with IS900.[54] Although this system is attractive for transposon mutagenesis, due to the near-random insertions, it is at present less useful for inserting foreign antigens since the efficiency is somewhat lower than that seen with IS900. The availability of more effective delivery systems for insertion sequences and transposons, such as the temperature-sensitive derivatives of pAL5000 recently described,[33] will greatly enhance the usefulness of both IS900 and IS986/IS6110.

D. SITE-SPECIFIC INTEGRATION

Lysogenic bacteriophages commonly integrate into the chromosome of the infected bacterium by site-specific recombination between specific attachment sites on the phage DNA *(attP)* and bacterial chromosome *(attB)*. Integration is mediated by the product of a phage gene *(int)*. Since *attP* and *attB* are similar but not identical, the resulting sequences at either end of the integrated phage DNA *(attL* and *attR)* are not substrates for the action of the Int protein by itself. Excision requires an additional phage product, Xis. A vector carrying *attP* and *int*, but not *xis*, should therefore result in stable integration of the required genes into the bacterial chromosome.

Mycobacteriophage L5 is a temperate phage that infects *M. smegmatis* and some strains of BCG and forms stable lysogens by site-specific integration. The complete DNA sequence of L5 has been determined in Graham Hatfull's laboratory at the University of Pittsburgh, and an analysis of the sequence data showed that it contains a region identified as a putative integrase gene on the basis of the similarity of its predicted amino acid sequence with those of known integrases from other bacteriophages.[34] Cloning and sequencing of the attachment junctions *(attL* and *attR)* from an L5 lysogen, and of the *M. smegmatis* attachment site *(attB)* revealed that integration occurs within a 43-bp core region that is identical in *attP* and *attB*. A virtually identical sequence (with a single base change) occurs in the genome of BCG Pasteur.[34]

Cloning of a 2-kb *Sal*I fragment carrying *attP* and *int* into a pUC vector carrying the kanamycin resistance gene from Tn903 resulted in an integration proficient plasmid, pMH94[34] (Figure 5). This plasmid was able to transform the high efficiency transformation strain of *M. smegmatis*, mc²155, at a similar frequency to pYUB12. The parent strain of *M. smegmatis*, mc²6, was also transformed efficiently by pMH94, although this strain yields few transformants with the autonomously replicating plasmid pYUB12. BCG Pasteur and *M. tuberculosis* H37Ra were also transformed to kanamycin resistance by pMH94, although somewhat less efficiently than was *M. smegmatis*, and at a lower frequency than seen with pYUB12. Hybridization analysis confirmed that the plasmid was integrated site specifically in all isolates tested. The integrated plasmid was stably maintained in *M. smegmatis* through 30 generations of nonselective growth, while 35% loss of the extrachromosomal plasmid pYUB12 was observed under the same conditions. Interestingly, another construct with a larger fragment of L5 (pMH5) was less stable than pMH94, suggesting that pMH5 may contain the *xis* gene necessary for excision of the integrated fragment.

An alternative approach using the site-specific integrative ability of bacteriophages is to construct transducing phages. Anes et al.[35] cloned a fragment of the temperate mycobacteriophage Ms6 in a derivative of pUC19 containing the *aph* gene from Tn5 and transformed a lysogen of *M. smegmatis* with selection for kanamycin resistance; presumed homologous recombination between the phage sequences generated a transducing

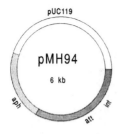

Figure 5 An integrative vector using the mycobacterio-phage L5 attachment system. pMH94 is an *E. coli* vector carrying the L5 attachment site and integrase gene, enabling the plasmid to integrate into a specific site on the mycobacterial chromosome.

phage capable of transferring kanamycin resistance. The kanamycin-resistant transductants were stable for 150 generations, despite evidence of structural instability in the transducing phage. This approach is likely to be useful for genetic analysis and manipulation of mycobacteria for research purposes, but seems to offer little advantage in potential vaccine construction when compared to the integrative L5 vectors described above.

The integrative behavior of temperate bacteriophages is mimicked by some plasmids from *Streptomyces* species, such as pSAM2, originally isolated from *Streptomyces ambofaciens*. This plasmid can replicate autonomously in several *Streptomyces* species, or can undergo integration into the chromosome by site-specific recombination between *att* sequences on the plasmid and chromosome. The plasmid contains sequences coding for potential products with homology to the Int and Xis proteins of lambda and related phages. Mazodier et al.[36] showed that several mycobacterial species contained sequences related to the pSAM2 *attB* site in *Streptomyces*, which indicated that vectors based on pSAM2 could be used as integrative vectors in mycobacteria. This was confirmed by Martin et al.[37] who constructed a vector (pTSN39) containing an *E. coli* origin of replication (pBR322) and the *aph* gene from Tn903. This vector generated kanamycin-resistant transformants of *M. smegmatis* mc²155 at a frequency of 5 to 100 per μg of DNA, compared to 10^5/μg for the shuttle plasmid pRR3. Southern blotting indicated that all the transformants contained the plasmid integrated at a unique site, suggesting that integration was dependent on site-specific recombination between the *attP* and *attB* sites. Kanamycin resistance was stably maintained for about 50 generations, and no extrachromosomal plasmid forms were detected, despite the presence of the pSAM2 *xis* gene.

III. EXPRESSION OF FOREIGN GENES IN MYCOBACTERIA

Exploitation of BCG for recombinant vaccine production demands not only stable inheritance of the cloned gene, but also formation of a product in a suitable form and at an appropriate level for generation of the required immune response. This will require both transcriptional and translational signals, as well as, in some cases, appropriate posttranslational modification.

A. MYCOBACTERIAL GENE EXPRESSION
1. Transcriptional Control

Some information on the nature of mycobacterial promoters can be gleaned by inference from known DNA sequences in comparison with other bacteria and *E. coli* in particular;[38] this analysis identifies the presence in many cases of promoter-like sequences related to the consensus prokaryotic promoter or to *E. coli* heat-shock promoters. However, very few of these promoters have been confirmed by direct evidence. Some mycobacterial genes are able to function in *E. coli*, apparently from their own promoters, but the prevailing view is that most mycobacterial promoters are not efficiently recognized in

E. coli. The reverse situation, the recognition of foreign promoters by mycobacteria, is even less clear, although some foreign genes (notably the kanamycin resistance genes of Tn5 and Tn903) are expressed from their own promoters in mycobacteria. The development of expression systems in mycobacteria has therefore largely been empirical, using sequences derived from the region upstream from characterized mycobacterial genes to provide the required signals.

2. Translational Control

Sequence analysis of mycobacterial genes has identified in most cases a likely ribosome binding site (Shine-Dalgarno sequence) close to the putative start codon; in this respect, translational control in mycobacteria appears to be similar to other bacteria, although the start codon is commonly GUG rather than AUG.[38] Most expression systems used in mycobacteria supply translation initiation signals derived from the original mycobacterial gene as well as a promoter, so that an in-frame insertion of the required gene will be translated. However, codon usage has also to be taken into account. Mycobacterial genes commonly show a high degree of codon bias, most obviously in the preference for G or C at the third position (as expected from the high G+C content of mycobacterial DNA). Some codons are particularly uncommon, such as the AGA and AGG codons for arginine, which are very rarely used in *M. tuberculosis.*[38] This may reflect a scarcity of the appropriate tRNA, which would pose a limitation if high levels of expression of a heterologous gene are required.

B. EXPRESSION SYSTEMS

Among the first mycobacterial genes to be cloned and sequenced were those coding for the 65-kDa and 72-kDa antigens of *M. tuberculosis,* which are two of the dominant antigens in mycobacterial infections. The sequence of these genes revealed that they are members of the highly conserved *hsp*60 and *hsp*70 families of stress proteins, and both genes have been used to provide signals for expression of cloned genes in BCG. Other expression systems have been based on the *M. leprae* gene coding for an 18-kDa protein antigen (a member of the alpha-crystallin family of stress proteins[39]), the secreted α-antigen from *M. kansasii,* and a promoter region from *M. paratuberculosis.*[40]

1. Expression Systems Based on *hsp*60

The most extensive results have come from a collaboration between Stover, de la Cruz, Fuerst, and co-workers of Medimmune Inc, Hatfull and others from the University of Pittsburgh, and Jacobs and Bloom and co-workers from the Albert Einstein School of Medicine.[18,41-44]

Stover et al.[18] described the construction of an expression cassette containing 404 bp of the 5′ regulatory region of the BCG *hsp*60 gene (including the first six codons of the translated region) together with a multiple cloning site and transcriptional terminator, in both an extrachromosomal vector (pMV261) based on the mycobacterial origin of replication from pAL5000 and an integrative vector (pMV361) based on the L5 integration system (Figure 6). This system was evaluated using the *E. coli lacZ* gene, which was expressed constitutively at a high level in BCG containing the extrachromosomal pMV261 construct, with β-galactosidase constituting up to 15% of total cell protein. However, in the integrative single copy vector, pMV361, expression was 5- to 10-fold lower.[41,42] Interestingly, under stress induction, β-galactosidase synthesis was unchanged using pMV261, while synthesis increased from the integrative vector.[18]

A number of HIV-1 and SIV antigens have been successfully expressed in these two systems. However, no viable constructs of HIV-1 gp160 could be obtained, and expression of HIV-1 gp120 or SIV gag in the extrachromosomal vector was lethal and the gene could only be cloned successfully using the single copy integrative vector.[43] Even then

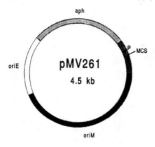

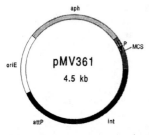

Figure 6 Structure of two mycobacterial expression vectors. pMV261 is an extrachromosomal shuttle plasmid containing *oriM* derived from pAL5000, while pMV361 is an integrative vector incorporating the attachment and integrase regions from the mycobacteriophage L5. Both plasmids carry the heat shock promoter from the mycobacterial *hsp*60 gene, allowing expression of foreign DNA inserted at the multiple cloning site (MCS).

expression was low, representing only 0.5% of the β-galactosidase product for gp120. Interestingly, HIV-1 gag was expressed to similar levels by both the extrachromosomal and integrative vectors.[18] The authors have speculated that the HIV-1 env gene product is cytotoxic and can only be successfully expressed at low concentrations. Both the hsp60 and hsp70 promoters have been used to express HIV and SIV antigens, but none of these antigens have been produced in quantities as great as that seen for β-galactosidase.[41] However, HIV-1 pol (minus the protease activity) was expressed at sufficiently high levels to be detected by coomassie blue-stained SDS-PAGE.[43] SIV gag, gp120 and gp40 (envelope glycoproteins), and HIV-1 gag, RT (reverse transcriptase), pol (minus the protease activity), gp120 and gp41 (an envelope glycoprotein), and fragment C of the *Clostridium tetani* toxin have all been successfully expressed by these workers.

In an analogous study, Winter et al.[45,46] used an expression cassette carrying the heat shock promoter of the *groES/groEL1* operon of *Streptomyces albus*, together with a synthetic ribosome binding site, to express the HIV-1 *nef* gene (a 27-kDa regulatory protein) in BCG, using the shuttle plasmid vector pRR3. Western blotting demonstrated a high level of nef product, constituting approximately 1% of total BCG protein.

2. Expression Systems Based on *hsp70*

Aldovini and Young[47] used a 155-bp upstream sequence from the *M. tuberculosis hsp*70 gene (including the start codon) in the high copy number shuttle plasmid pYUB12, to express the HIV-1 proteins gag, pol (polymerase), and gp120 in BCG, and showed that expression was constitutive — although quoting unpresented data indicating that a lower level of expression from an integrative vector was inducible by heat shock. They estimated that gag constituted approximately 0.1% of total BCG protein.

Stover et al.[18] have also referred to the successful use of the hsp70 promoter, in addition to the fuller account of the hsp60 system as described above.

3. Secretion Systems

Other workers have argued that secretion of the foreign antigen will be advantageous for development of an effective immune response. Matsuo et al.[48] therefore cloned a gene from *M. kansasii* that codes for the secreted α-antigen, using a shuttle plasmid (pIS18) derived independently from the same pIJ666-pAL5000 library as pYUB12.

When this plasmid was introduced into BCG Tokyo, the transformants were shown to secrete the α-antigen. Introduction of a synthetic oligonucleotide coding for a B cell epitope (amino acids 12 to 19) of HIV-1 gag p17 (a 17,000-mol wt internal protein of the virus) into a site close to the 3′-end of the α-antigen gene (Figure 7) resulted in a fusion protein that was also secreted from BCG transformants. The fusion protein was recognized by rabbit anti-alpha-K polyclonal antisera and an anti-gag monoclonal antibody in western blotting of culture media, showing that the fusion protein had been synthesized and secreted from the recombinant BCG. However, the concept that secretion is necessary for this purpose must be debatable, as many nonsecreted mycobacterial antigens are known to produce a strong immune response in infected individuals.

4. Systems Based on the *M. leprae* 18-kDa Gene

At the University of Surrey, we have designed a series of integrative expression vectors (based on the IS900 integration system) that facilitate the cloning and expression of synthetic epitopes, as well as complete genes, as fusion proteins. We have used the *M. leprae* 18-kDa antigen as the basis of the expression system, rather than the *hsp*60 or *hsp*70 genes, for several reasons. The antigen is well characterized[49,50] and known to contain T-helper cell determinants that stimulate human *M. leprae*-specific T cell clones;[51] immunological responses are detected in patients with leprosy, indicating that it is effectively presented to the immune system by the infected cells. At the same time, it can be readily distinguished from the equivalent *M. tuberculosis*/BCG antigen, using a specific monoclonal antibody. It is also advantageous to use a heterologous gene for this purpose, since this reduces the risk of complications arising from homologous recombination (as well as facilitating characterization of transformants). Finally, the small size of the gene facilitates the construction of vectors of a manageable size and with useful unique restriction sites.

We have therefore constructed vectors that include the 18-kDa gene, with its upstream regulatory sequence, and the Tn903 *aph* gene between two copies of IS900, an insertion

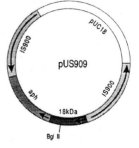

Figure 7 Structure of a mycobacterial shuttle plasmid allowing secretion of a fusion protein carrying a synthetic gag epitope. The shuttle plasmid is formed from fusion of pAL5000 and pIJ666 (Figure 1); the synthetic oligonucleotide coding for the gag epitope is inserted at the 3′ end of the gene coding for the secreted alpha antigen from *M. kansasii* (alpha-K).

Figure 8 Structure of an insertional expression vector. pUS909 is an *E. coli* plasmid carrying a composite transposon formed by two copies of IS900, flanking an *aph* gene and the *M. leprae* gene coding for an 18-kDa protein antigen. Expression of foreign genes, as fusion proteins, is achieved by insertion at the *Bgl*II site within the 18-kDa gene.

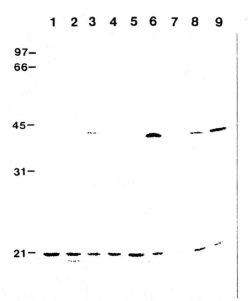

Figure 9 Expression of foreign genes in mycobacteria using a transpositional insertion vector. Extracts of mycobacterial clones were run on SDS-PAGE and Western blotted; production of the *M. leprae* 18-kDa antigen, or 18-kDa-SIV gag P27 fusion proteins, was detected using an 18-kDa-specific monoclonal antibody. Lanes: 1: *M. smegmatis* host; 2: *M. smegmatis* transformed with the transpositional insertion vector pUS909 (see Figure 8); 3 through 9: *M. smegmatis* clones transformed with pUS909 containing the gag P27 gene inserted into the *Bgl*I site (within the 18-kDa gene). The *M. leprae* 18-kDa antigen itself is detected in lane 2, while lanes 3 through 9 show varying levels of expression of a fusion protein of the expected size. The band at 21 kDa in all lanes is an *M. smegmatis* protein detected with this antibody.

sequence originating from *M. paratuberculosis,*[26] using a pUC-based vector that is not expected to replicate in a mycobacterial host (Figure 8). Transformation of *M. smegmatis* or BCG with selection for kanamycin resistance results in integration of the entire plasmid or the composite transposon into the mycobacterial chromosome. Using these constructs, we have shown expression of the *M. leprae* 18-kDa antigen, from its own promoter, in *E. coli, M. smegmatis,* and BCG Pasteur.

These vectors have a unique *Bgl*II restriction site towards the 3′ end of the 18-kDa gene, into which heterologous genes can be inserted (Figure 8). The complete SIV gene coding for the gag p27 protein has been inserted at this position and expressed in *E. coli, M. smegmatis,* and BCG Pasteur. Southern blotting has shown that the vector is stably integrated into the chromosome in a mycobacterial host, and Western blotting (Figure 9) has demonstrated the presence of a fusion protein that is recognized by an anti-18-kDa antigen monoclonal antibody[52] and sheep anti-gag polyclonal antisera. In common with Fuerst et al.[42] we were unable to get viable constructs of vector containing the entire HIV-1 gp120 gene.

Further work has involved constructing vectors which express fusion proteins of the 18-kDa antigen with virus B cell epitopes. These studies have included inserting the major neutralizing antigenic site from foot-and-mouth-disease virus (FMDV) (amino acids 140 to 160 from virus protein 1 [VP1]) which has been expressed as a fusion protein with the 18-kDa antigen. This fusion protein is recognized in Western blots by anti-18-kDa monoclonal antibody L5 and rabbit polyclonal anti-FMDV VP1 antisera.

5. Use of the P_{AN} Promoter from *M. paratuberculosis*

Murray et al.[40] identified a putative promoter region, P_{AN}, adjacent to the 3' end of one copy of the insertion sequence IS900 in *M. paratuberculosis*.[26] Fusion of this sequence to a promoterless β-galactosidase gene, using the mycobacterial shuttle plasmid pRR3, resulted in the expression of β-galactosidase in both *M. smegmatis* and BCG. High resolution S1 nuclease mapping confirmed that transcription in *M. smegmatis* was initiated from the expected site adjacent to the promoter.

IV. IMMUNITY INDUCED BY RECOMBINANT BCG

Despite evidence that shuttle plasmids are unstable in mycobacteria, Ranes et al.[17] showed that an *E. coli*-mycobacterial shuttle vector was stable for 3 months in mice, in the absence of antibiotic selection. Thus, the potential existed for administering live recombinant BCG to animals that would be stable and express foreign antigens *in vivo*.

Some studies have used BCG expressing β-galactosidase (rBCG/β-gal) as a model system. de la Cruz et al.[44] inoculated 6-week-old Balb/c mice with rBCG/β-gal by the intradermal (ID), intravenous (IV) and intraperitoneal (IP) routes of inoculation. All three routes resulted in the induction of anti-β-galactosidase antibodies that were retained for at least 8 weeks. The best results were obtained with the IV route where only 200 CFU were required to induce high levels of antibody (anti-β-galactosidase ELISA titers of 1 in 30,000 were observed after only one inoculation of recombinant), whereas 10^4 CFU were required to give an antibody response following inoculation by the ID route.[18] Not surprisingly, antibody levels increased slowly in comparison to administration of rBCG/β-gal and incomplete Freund's adjuvant by any of the three routes.

Cellular immune responses have been analyzed in the C57BL/6 (H-2^b) and Balb/c (H-2^d) inbred strains of mice. Splenocytes from C57BL/6 mice given rBCG/β-gal by the ID route produced gamma interferon in response to stimulation with β-galactosidase, while control mice did not. Similarly, interleukin 2 (IL-2), but not IL-5, was also induced on stimulation with antigen. Taken together, the above data would suggest that the Th1 subset of T-helper cells was being stimulated specifically. The rBCG/β-gal has also been shown to induce a cytotoxic T lymphocyte response. Balb/c mice inoculated with either 200 or 2×10^6 CFU by the IV route gave high levels of cytotoxic T lymphocyte activity. In contrast, following IP inoculation, cytotoxic T lymphocyte activity was greater following inoculation of 2×10^6 CFU than with 200 CFU, which was consistent with the difference in antibody levels following these inocula and this route of inoculation. No cytotoxic T lymphocyte activity was detected following ID inoculation of rBCG/β-gal. Recombinant BCG, expressing β-galactosidase and kanamycin resistance, could be found in the spleen at 2 to 4 weeks postinoculation.

Murray et al.[40] used rBCG expressing a β-galactosidase fusion protein, driven by the P_{AN} promoter on a shuttle plasmid, to immunize BALB/c mice (10^7 CFU, subcutaneously), and demonstrated a proliferative response of lymph node cells to β-galactosidase. A significant production of gamma interferon was detected after stimulation with β-galactosidase. An antibody response was also observed, following IV administration of 10^7 CFU, but only after several booster doses (10^6 CFU, IV).

The stability of their construct *in vivo* was examined by recovering BCG bacilli from spleen homogenates 2 months after IV inoculation with 10^7 CFU. Of the organisms recovered, 46% retained the kanamycin resistance marker, but only 26% also expressed β-galactosidase. The partial instability of the shuttle plasmid used underlines the potential advantage of using integrative vectors, although it appears that in this case enough cells retained the plasmid for a sufficient length of time to stimulate an immunological response.

Several studies have investigated immune responses to BCG recombinants expressing HIV or SIV antigens. Stover et al.[18] and Fuerst et al.[42] described the ID inoculation of

Balb/c mice with 10^6 CFU of recombinant BCG expressing gp41, which induced a slowly developing antibody response that was none the less significant by 16 weeks postinoculation. In comparison, a BCG recombinant expressing gp120 (rBCG/gp120) induced no significant antibody titers after one inoculation, although there was a cytotoxic T-lymphocyte response following IP inoculation of 10^6 CFU. However, there was no gamma interferon induced by stimulation of splenocytes with gp120 peptide following IP inoculation of rBCG/gp120.[18,42]

Studies by Aldovini and Young[47] were less impressive. They inoculated Balb/c with one dose of 5×10^6 CFU of rBCG/gag or rBCG/gp120 by either the subcutaneous or IV routes. ELISA analysis of sera at 5 weeks postinoculation showed that three out of five rBCG/gag and only one out of five rBCG/gp120 mice had antiviral antibodies, at low levels (<1:50); control BCG gave no detectable antiviral antibody. Cellular immune responses were examined in rBCG/gag-immunized mice after two boosts of 5×10^6 CFU by the IV route at weeks 4 and 8 postinoculation. Splenocytes from immunized mice produced gamma interferon in response to stimulation with HIV-1 gag or gag peptides. Also, IL-2 was synthesized as measured in a proliferation assay. Chromium release assays indicated that most of the antigen-specific cytotoxic cells from the spleen of immunized mice express CD8. Taken together, the studies of Aldovini and Young[47] would suggest that mice immunized with recombinant BCG induce a poor antibody response but a significant CMI response in terms of cytotoxic T cells and Th1 lymphocytes. Stimulation by the gag peptides suggests that the immune response is recognizing different portions of the gag protein.

Winter et al.[45,46] inoculated female Balb/c mice subcutaneously with 10^7 CFU of BCG expressing nef at the base of the tail; at 14 days postinoculation, lymph nodes were found to contain viable rBCG/nef. Unfortunately the authors coinoculated mice with incomplete Freund's adjuvant which will potentiate the immune response. Thus, it is difficult to assess how good an immunogen the recombinant BCG was. Nonetheless, lymph node cells taken from the immunized mice proliferated in response to stimulation with nef protein, showing that there was a strong T cell response.

Stover et al.[18] and Fuerst et al.[42] compared immunity induced by live or dead recombinant BCG expressing a fragment of tetanus toxin (ToxC, fragment C of the tetanus toxin of molecular weight 50-kDa and lacking toxic activity). Outbred swiss NIH mice were inoculated either IP or ID with 10^6 CFU of live or dead rBCG/ToxC in pMV261. Those mice given live rBCG/ToxC by the IP or ID routes were protected against challenge by 100 LD of toxin. In comparison, heat-killed rBCG/ToxC did not induce any detectable antitoxin antibody, and the mice were not protected against challenge.

Overall, these studies in mice show that live recombinant BCG is required to stimulate the immune response and that immunity is not short-lived. One immunization by different routes with live recombinant BCG is sufficient to enable continued expression of a foreign antigen and stimulation of an antibody response. Immunity appears to be due to the continued growth of recombinant BCG in the mice. Unfortunately, some antigens are not good inducers of antibody, but all the foreign antigens stimulate a cellular immune response. These results are consistent with the known biology of BCG where BCG induces a strong cellular immune response and increases in titer *in vivo* for the first 4 weeks postimmunization and then gradually declines thereafter. Much remains to be investigated *in vivo*. To date, only the mouse model system has been studied and in only a few genetic backgrounds. This is important in view of the good cellular immune response mounted by BCG. Clearly, other animal systems need to be analyzed. Although the induction of immunity against foreign antigens has been demonstrated, little is known about the important issue of protective immunity. Even though protection against challenge by a toxin has been shown, this is not the same as challenge by a multiplying infectious agent.

V. FUTURE DIRECTIONS

One of the problems in the exploitation of recombinant BCG is the difficulty of working with mycobacteria. Many mycobacteria, including BCG, grow slowly and may take several weeks to form a colony. Accordingly, good bacteriological techniques are required and work proceeds slowly in comparison to other bacterial systems. Nevertheless, knowledge of the molecular biology of mycobacteria is expanding exponentially, although we still need a better understanding of the control of gene expression, especially in mycobacteria that are growing in an intracellular environment.

However, the biggest problems will be in devising the best method of presenting the recombinant BCG to the host immune system. The pilot studies in mice to date have concentrated on administration by routes such as intravenous, intraperitoneal, or intradermal. However, for many vaccines, oral administration would be preferable, not only on grounds of cost and ease of use, but also because of the possibility of stimulating protective mucosal immunity. Since it is known that BCG can be successfully administered orally, the possibility exists for the development of multivalent vaccines that can be produced cheaply for use in developing countries. However, much remains to be learned about the mechanisms of immunity induced by intracellular BCG as viable organisms can be recovered from phagocytes *in vivo*. Therefore, processing and presentation of antigens to the immune system in the correct conformation will be critical to the success of potential recombinant BCG vaccines. In this context, it would be extremely helpful to understand the nature of the attenuation of BCG, as well as the significance of the variation between BCG strains.

Secretion of antigen by the recombinant BCG may be advantageous in such a situation, but is probably not necessary, since in natural mycobacterial infections an immune response is developed to a wider range of nonsecreted antigens. This may reflect leakage from damaged cells. In such a situation, the factor of prime importance in the stimulation of a cellular immune response is the presentation to the immune system in BCG-infected phagocytes. However, for certain antigens that are toxic for BCG, the use of signals for the secretion of expressed foreign antigens may prevent them from being toxic to host cells.

Further information is also required on the likely duration of a response to recombinant BCG vaccines and the effect of prior BCG immunization. Although there is some controversy over the effectiveness of BCG vaccination against tuberculosis, in situations where a protective effect has been demonstrated it appears to be long lasting. However, revaccination is used routinely in some countries and results in stimulation of the host immune response. Thus, even those people already vaccinated with BCG should be suitable for immunization using a recombinant BCG vaccine. At the same time, it should be noted that the use of BCG as a recombinant vaccine has to be considered separately from the controversy over the effectiveness of BCG as a vaccine against tuberculosis; it is conceptually possible for a recombinant BCG vaccine to protect against another disease without offering protection against tuberculosis.

Overall, due to the excellent ability of BCG to stimulate the immune system, recombinant BCG has great potential for the development of multivalent vaccines. Whether or not this promise is achieved remains to be seen.

ACKNOWLEDGMENTS

The work at the University of Surrey is funded by the Science and Engineering Research Council, the Medical Research Council AIDS Directed Programme, the Wellcome Trust, the Commission of the European Communities, and studentships from the Brazilian and Cameroon governments.

The HIV and SIV reagents used were generously provided by the MRC AIDS reagent project and the SIV p27 gene in pKA27 by Dr. Peter Kitchin.

REFERENCES

1. Patel, A. M. and Abrahams, E. W., Pulmonary tuberculosis, in *The Biology of the Mycobacteria, Vol. 3*, Ratledge, C., Stanford, J., and Grange, J. M., Eds., Academic Press, London, 1989, 179.
2. Dannenberg, A. M., Immune mechanisms in the pathogenesis of pulmonary tuberculosis, *Rev. Infect. Dis.*, 2 (Suppl. 2), S369, 1989.
3. Grange, J. M., Gibson, J., Osborn, T. W., Collins, C. H., and Yates, M. D., What is BCG?, *Tubercle*, 64, 129, 1983.
4. Fomukong, N. G., Dale, J. W., Osborn, T. W., and Grange, J. M., Use of gene probes based on the insertion sequence IS986 to differentiate between BCG vaccine strains, *J. Appl. Bacteriol.*, 72, 126, 1992.
5. Smith, D. W., BCG, in *The Mycobacteria: a Sourcebook*, Kubica, G. P. and Wayne, L. G., Eds., Marcel Dekker, New York, 1984, 1057.
6. Fine, P. E. M., The BCG story: lessons from the past and implications for the future, *Rev. Infect. Dis.*, 2 Suppl. 2, S353, 1989.
7. Bekierkunst, A., Adjuvanticity of mycobacteria and their glycolipid components, wax D and cord factor, in *The Mycobacteria: a Sourcebook*, Kubica, G. P. and Wayne, L. G., Eds., Marcel Dekker, New York, 1984, 761.
8. Convit, J., Aranzazu, N., Ulrich, M., Pinardi, M. E., Reyes, O., and Alvarado, J., *Int. J. Leprosy*, 50, 415, 1982.
9. Convit, J., Castellanos, P. L., Rondon, A., Pinardi, M. E., Ulrich, M., Castes, M., Bloom, B. R., and Garcia, L., *Lancet*, i, 401, 1993.
10. Weiss, D. W., Nonspecific immunity and cancer, in *The Mycobacteria: a Sourcebook*, Kubica, G. P. and Wayne, L.G., Eds., Marcel Dekker, New York, 1984, 863.
11. Grange, J. M., The genetics of mycobacteria and mycobacteriophages, in *The Biology of the Mycobacteria*, Ratledge, C. and Stanford, J., Eds., Academic Press, London, 1982, 309.
12. Jacobs, W. R., Tuckman, M., and Bloom, B. R., Introduction of foreign DNA into mycobacteria using a shuttle phasmid, *Nature*, 327, 532, 1987.
13. Snapper, S. B., Lugosi, L., Jekkel, A., Melton, R. E., Kieser, T., Bloom, B. R., and Jacobs, W. R., Lysogeny and transformation in mycobacteria: stable expression of foreign genes, *Proc. Natl. Acad. Sci. U.S.A.*, 85, 6987, 1988.
14. Labidi, A., Mardis, E., Roe, B. A., and Wallace, R. J., Jr., Cloning and DNA sequence of the *Mycobacterium fortuitum* var. *fortuitum* plasmid pAL5000, *Plasmid*, 27, 130, 1992.
15. Labidi, A., David, H. L., and Roulland-Dussoix, D., Cloning and expression of mycobacterial plasmid DNA in *Escherichia coli*, *FEMS Microbiol. Lett.*, 30, 221, 1985.
16. Rauzier, J., Moniz-Pereira, J., and Gicquel-Sanzey, B., Complete nucleotide sequence of pAL5000, a plasmid from *Mycobacterium fortuitum*, *Gene*, 71, 315, 1988.
17. Ranes, M. G., Rauzier, J., Lagranderie, M., Gheorghiu, M., and Gicquel, B., Functional analysis of pAL5000, a plasmid from *Mycobacterium fortuitum:* Construction of a "mini" mycobacterium-*Escherichia coli* shuttle vector, *J. Bacteriol.*, 172, 2793, 1990.
18. Stover, C. K., de la Cruz, V. F., Fuerst, T. R., Burlein, J. E., Benson, L. A., Bennett, L. T., Bansal, G. P., Young, J. F., Lee, M. H., Hatfull, G. F., Snapper, S. B., Barletta, R. G., Jacobs, W. R., Jr., and Bloom, B. R., New use of BCG for recombinant vaccines, *Nature*, 351, 456, 1991.

19. Radford, A. J. and Hodgson, A. L. M., Construction and characterization of a *Mycobacterium-Escherichia coli* shuttle vector, *Plasmid,* 25, 149, 1991.
20. Lazraq, R., Houssaini-Iraqui, M., Clavel-Sérès, S., and David, H. L., Cloning and expression of the origin of replication of mycobacteriophage D29 in *Mycobacterium smegmatis, FEMS Microbiol. Lett.,* 80, 117, 1991.
21. David, M., Lubinsky-Mink, S., Ben-Zvi, A., Ulitzur, S., Kuhn, J., and Suissa, M., A stable *Escherichia coli-Mycobacterium smegmatis* plasmid shuttle vector containing the mycobacteriophage D29 origin, *Plasmid,* 28, 267, 1992.
22. Gormley, E. P. and Davies, J., Transfer of plasmid RSF1010 by conjugation from *Escherichia coli* to *Streptomyces lividans* and *Mycobacterium smegmatis, J. Bacteriol.,* 173, 6705, 1991.
23. Snapper, S. B., Melton, R. E., Kieser, T., Mustafa, S., and Jacobs, W. R., Isolation and characterization of efficient plasmid transformation mutants of *Mycobacterium smegmatis, Mol. Microbiol.,* 4, 1911, 1990.
24. Husson, R. N., James, B. E., and Young, R. A., Gene replacement and expression of foreign DNA in mycobacteria, *J. Bacteriol.,* 172, 519, 1990.
25. Kalpana, G. V., Bloom, B. R., and Jacobs, W. R., Jr., Insertional mutagenesis and illegitimate recombination in mycobacteria, *Proc. Natl. Acad. Sci. U.S.A.,* 88, 5433, 1991.
26. Green, E. P., Tizard, M. L. V., Moss, M. T., Thompson, J., Winterbourne, D. J., McFadden, J. J., and Hermon-Taylor, J., Sequence and characteristics of IS900, an insertion element identified in a human Crohn's disease isolate of *Mycobacterium paratuberculosis, Nucleic Acids Res.,* 17, 9063, 1989.
27. England, P. M., Wall, S., and McFadden, J., IS900-promoted stable integration of a foreign gene into mycobacteria, *Mol. Microbiol.,* 5, 2047, 1991.
28. Zainuddin, Z. F., Mycobacterial Plasmids and Related DNA Sequences, Ph.D. thesis, University of Surrey, Guildford, U.K., 1988.
29. Zainuddin, Z. F. and Dale, J. W., Polymorphic repetitive DNA sequences in *Mycobacterium tuberculosis* detected with a gene probe from a *Mycobacterium fortuitum* plasmid, *J. Gen. Microbiol.,* 135, 2347, 1989.
30. Hermans, P. W. M., Van Soolingen, D., Dale, J. W., Schuitema, A. R. J., McAdam, R. A., Catty, D., and van Embden, J. D. A., Insertion element IS986 from *Mycobacterium tuberculosis:* a useful tool for diagnosis and epidemiology of tuberculosis, *J. Clin. Microbiol.,* 28, 2051, 1990.
31. McAdam, R. A., Hermans, P. W. M., Van Soolingen, D., Zainuddin, Z. F., Catty, D., van Embden, J. D. A., and Dale, J. W., Characterization of a *Mycobacterium tuberculosis* insertion sequence belonging to the IS3 family, *Mol. Microbiol.,* 4, 1607, 1990.
32. Thierry, D., Brisson-Noël, A., Vincent-Lévy-Frébault, V., Nguyen, S., Guesdon, J.-L., and Gicquel, B., Characterization of a *Mycobacterium tuberculosis* insertion sequence, IS6110, and its application in diagnosis, *J. Clin. Microbiol.,* 28, 2668, 1990.
33. Guilhot, C., Gicquel, B., and Martín, C., Temperature-sensitive mutants of the *Mycobacterium* plasmid pAL5000, *FEMS Microbiol. Lett.,* 98, 181, 1992.
34. Lee, M. H., Pascopella, L., Jacobs, W. R., Jr., and Hatfull, G. F., Site-specific integration of mycobacteriophage L5: integration-proficient vectors for *Mycobacterium smegmatis, Mycobacterium tuberculosis,* and bacille Calmette-Guérin, *Proc. Natl. Acad. Sci. U.S.A.,* 88, 3111, 1991.
35. Anes, E., Portugal, I., and Moniz-Pereira, J., Insertion into the *Mycobacterium smegmatis* genome of the *aph* gene through lysogenization with the temperate mycobacteriophage Ms6, *FEMS Microbiol. Lett.,* 95, 21, 1992.
36. Mazodier, P., Thompson, C., and Boccard, F., The chromosomal integration site of the *Streptomyces* element pSAM2 overlaps a putative tRNA gene conserved among actinomycetes, *Mol. Gen. Genet.,* 222, 431, 1990.

37. Martin, C., Mazodier, P., Mediola, M. V., Gicquel, B., Smokvina, T., Thompson, C. J., and Davies, J., Site-specific integration of the *Streptomyces* plasmid pSAM2 in *Mycobacterium smegmatis, Mol. Microbiol.,* 5, 2499, 1991.
38. Dale, J. W. and Patki, A., Mycobacterial gene expression and regulation, in *Molecular Biology of the Mycobacteria,* McFadden, J., Ed., Surrey University Press/Academic Press, London, 1990, 173.
39. Verbon, A., Hartskeerl, R. A., Schuitema, A., Kolk, A. H. J., Young, D. B., and Lathigra, R., The 14,000-molecular-weight antigen of *Mycobacterium tuberculosis* is related to the alpha-crystallin family of low-molecular-weight heat shock proteins, *J. Bacteriol.,* 174, 1352, 1992.
40. Murray, A., Winter, N., Lagranderie, M., Hill, D. F., Rauzier, J., Timm, J., Leclerc, C., Moriarty, K. M., Gheorghiu, M., and Gicquel, B., Expression of *Escherichia coli* β-galactosidase in *Mycobacterium bovis* BCG using an expression system isolated from *Mycobacterium paratuberculosis* which induced humoral and cellular immune responses, *Mol. Microbiol.,* 6, 3331, 1992.
41. Stover, C. K., Burlein, J. E., Bennett, L. T., de la Cruz, V. F., Young, J. F., Fuerst, T. R., Hatfull, G. F., Lee, M. H., Jacobs, W. R., and Bloom, B. R., Development of BCG as a live recombinant vaccine vehicle, in *Vaccines 91,* Cold Spring Harbor Laboratory Press, Cold Spring Harbor, NY, 1991, 393.
42. Fuerst, T. R., de la Cruz, V. F., Bansal, G. P., and Stover, C. K., Development and analysis of recombinant BCG vector systems, *AIDS Res. Hum. Retroviruses,* 8, 1451, 1992.
43. Fuerst, T. R., Stover, C. K., and de la Cruz, V. F., Development of BCG as a live recombinant vector system: potential use as an HIV vaccine, *Biotechnol. Ther.,* 2, 159, 1991.
44. de la Cruz, V. F., Stover, C. K., Benson, L. A., Palasynski, S. R., Fuerst, T. R., Young, J. F., Pearce, E., Jacobs, W. R., Jr., and Bloom, B. R., Humoral and cellular immune response to recombinant Mycobacteria (BCG), in *Vaccines 91,* Cold Spring Harbor Laboratory Press, Cold Spring Harbor, NY, 1991, 399.
45. Winter, N., Lagranderie, M., Rauzier, J., Timm, J., Leclerc, C., Guy, B., Kieny, M. P., Gheorghiu, M., and Gicquel, B., Expression of heterologous genes in *Mycobacterium bovis* BCG: induction of a cellular response against HIV-1 Nef protein, *Gene,* 109, 47, 1991.
46. Winter, N., Lagranderie, M., Rauzier, J., Timm, J., Leclerc, C., Gheorghiu, M., Gicquel, B., Guy, B., and Kieny, M. P., Expression of the HIV-1 *nef* gene in *Mycobacterium bovis* BCG and induction of a T-cell response against the Nef antigen, in *Vaccines 92,* Cold Spring Harbor Laboratory, Cold Spring Harbor, NY, 1992, 373.
47. Aldovini, A. and Young, R. A., Humoral and cell-mediated immune responses to live recombinant BCG-HIV vaccines, *Nature,* 351, 479, 1991.
48. Matsuo, K., Yamaguchi, R., Yamazaki, A., Tasaka, H., Terasaka, K., Totsuka, M., Kobayashi, K., Yukitake, H., and Yamada, T., Establishment of a foreign antigen secretion system in mycobacteria, *Infect. Immun.,* 58, 4049, 1990.
49. Harris, D. P., Bäckström, B. T., Booth, R. J., Love, S. G., Harding, D. R., and Watson, J. D., The mapping of epitopes of the 18-kDa protein of *Mycobacterium leprae* recognized by murine T cells in a proliferation assay, *J. Immunol.,* 143, 2006, 1989.
50. Booth, R. J., Harris, D. P., Love, J. M., and Watson, J. D., Antigenic proteins of *Mycobacterium leprae.* Complete sequence of the gene for the 18-kDa protein, *J. Immunol.,* 140, 597, 1988.
51. Mustafa, A. S., Gill, H. K., Nerland, A., Britton, W. J., Mehra, V., Bloom, B. R., Young, R. A., and Godal, T., Human T-cell clones recognize a major *M. leprae* protein antigen expressed in *E. coli, Nature,* 319, 63, 1986.

52. Doherty, T. M., Bäckström, B. T., Prestidge, R. L., Love, S. G., Harding, D. R. K., and Watson, J. D., Immune responses to the 18-kDa protein of *Mycobacterium leprae*: Similar B cell epitopes but different T cell epitopes seen by inbred strains of mice, *J. Immunol.*, 146, 1934, 1991.

53. Dellagostin, O. A., Wall, S., Norman, E., O'Shaughnessey, T., Dale, J. W., and McFadden, J., Construction and use of integrative vectors to express foreign genes in mycobacteria, *Mol. Microbiol.*, in press.

54. Fomukong, N. G. and Dale, J. W., Transpositional activity of IS986 in *Mycobacterium smegmatis*, *Gene*, 130, 99, 1993.

Chapter 4

Oral Recombinant Adenovirus Vaccines

Michael D. Lubeck, Bheem M. Bhat, Alan R. Davis, and Paul P. Hung

TABLE OF CONTENTS

I. INTRODUCTION

A. ADENOVIRUS STRUCTURE/CLASSIFICATION

Adenoviruses were first isolated in 1953 from human tissue explants (tonsil and adenoid) and shown 1 year later to be associated in military recruits with an epidemic form of acute respiratory disease (ARD). Soon thereafter, adenovirus isolates were obtained from individuals with a variety of other clinical syndromes. At present more than 40 different human adenovirus serotypes have been described.[1] Over 55 nonhuman adenovirus serotypes are also known. Adenoviruses (for review, see Reference 2) are nonenveloped DNA-containing viruses that possess an icosahedral capsid. Fibers extend from the 12 vertices of the icosahedral capsid and serve as attachment proteins. Although the capsid structures of adenoviruses are similar morphologically, differences between some strains occur due to variation in the length of the fibers. The family Adenoviridae is divided into two genera: Mastadenovirus, which encompasses all mammalian adenoviruses, and Aviadenovirus, which consists of the avian adenoviruses. These two groups are antigenically unrelated, but members within groups share common antigens. Shortly after their isolation and early characterization, certain human adenoviruses were shown to be capable of inducing tumors in newborn rodents[3] and of transforming cells in tissue culture.[4] One of the early classification schemes for adenoviruses was based on their oncogenic and transforming potential, whereby group A adenoviruses exhibit the highest oncogenic potential, group B adenoviruses are moderately oncogenic, and groups C, D, and E adenoviruses exhibit no oncogenic potential and minimal transformation potential (Table 1). Analyses of the G + C content and DNA homologies among viruses have confirmed the genetic relatedness of viruses within groups. The implications of adenovirus oncogenesis and transforming potential as they relate to vaccine safety are addressed later in this review.

B. CLINICAL DISEASE

Adenoviruses most commonly produce diseases of the respiratory tract, the gastrointestinal tract, and the eye (Table 2) (for review, see Reference 3). These diseases are generally mild, although serious complications are occasionally seen. The majority of the infections in humans is caused by a minority of the adenovirus serotypes, of which Ad3 and Ad7 are most frequently implicated. Infants, children, and immunocompromised individuals, in addition to military recruits, are all extremely susceptible to adenovirus infections.

Respiratory diseases are the most common clinical manifestation associated with adenoviruses. The symptoms produced include malaise, headache, chills, fever, and myalgia. Adenoviruses frequently cause milder symptoms, (nasal congestion, coryza, and cough), similar to those associated with the common cold. Among the most severe respiratory manifestations are pharyngitis and tonsillitis. An epidemic form of ARD has been found in the military and is usually caused by adenovirus types 4 and 7, although outbreaks caused by types 3, 14, and 21 have also been reported. A fairly high proportion of military recruits (up to 80%) contract ARD caused by adenovirus, and of these about 20% require hospitalization. This high incidence of serious incapacitating illness stimulated interest in the development of vaccines to control disease caused by Ad4 and Ad7 (see below).

Adenovirus respiratory infections are occasionally associated with inflammation of the conjunctiva, including a severe form involving both the cornea and the conjunctiva. These infections, which may also occur in an epidemic form, are caused mainly by Ad8

Table 1 **Classification of adenovirus based on oncogenicity**

Group	Serotypes	Oncogenicity (rodents)	G+C (%)
A	12, 18, 31	High	48–49
B	3, 7, 11, 14, 21	Weak	49–52
C	1, 2, 5, 6	None	57–59
D	8–10, 13, 15, 33, 37	None	58–59
E	4	None	High

Table 2 **Major diseases induced by adenovirus**

Illness	Serotype
Acute respiratory disease	3, 4, 7, 21
Acute pharyngitis	1, 2, 3, 5, 6, 7
Pneumonia	1, 2, 3, 4, 7
Epidemic keratoconjunctivitis	8, 11, 19, 37
Gastroenteritis	40, 41

and Ad19. In addition, adenovirus types 40 and 41 are often found in association with infantile gastroenteritis.

II. HISTORY OF ADENOVIRUS VACCINES

A. VACCINE EFFICACY

Shortly after the etiologic association of adenovirus with epidemic ARD was established, efforts were initiated to develop an effective vaccine (for review, see Reference 6). An initial focus on killed and subunit adenovirus vaccine development eventually shifted to live adenovirus, based in part on the observation that adenoviruses can replicate in the intestines without causing clinical disease. Subsequent studies demonstrated that Ad4 and Ad7 adapted to growth in WI-38 human diploid lung fibroblasts were effective at inducing protective immune responses in military recruits when administered orally in enteric-coated capsules or tablets.[7,8] During the past 13 years of use since their licensure (1980), these Ad4 and Ad7 vaccines have been shown in extensive clinical testing to be clearly attenuated, although it has been unclear whether the attenuation phenotype resulted solely from administration by the oral route or whether the vaccine strains became genetically attenuated during the extensive process of adaptation to growth in WI-38 cells.[6] Because no animal model is available to evaluate the level of attenuation of adenovirus vaccines, it has not been possible to distinguish between these two possibilities. However, the complete absence of induction of any ARD by Ad4 and Ad7 vaccine following administration to millions of recruits (including associated horizontal spread to family members without disease induction[9,10]) suggests that attenuation may have occurred during adaptation in tissue culture.[4]

Early studies revealed some variability in efficacy rates which was later shown to be related to the timing of the administration of the vaccines; vaccines administered within 2 hours of arrival at the training base had consistent efficacy rates of 95% at doses of $10^{4.8}$ $TCID_{50}$,[11] whereas later administration was associated with variability. Ad4 and Ad7 vaccines are coadministered without interstrain interference and have now been administered to more than 100 million military recruits, exhibiting high efficacy and safety.

B. INDUCTION OF MUCOSAL IMMUNITY

Early clinical studies indicated that protection against ARD was correlated with induction of serum neutralizing antibodies but not secretory antibody responses. Thus, induction of secretory responses by Ad4 and Ad7 vaccines was not examined in detail in expanded clinical studies. However, it is evident from the available data that adenovirus is capable of inducing immune responses at secretory sites.[12] Oral administration of adenovirus vaccines results in the induction of secretory responses in the gut by 2 to 4 weeks postinoculation.[13] However, secretory responses in the upper respiratory tract develop later and at a lower frequency than responses observed in the gut.[13] Data are not available regarding induction of secretory responses in the male or female genital tracts following oral administration of Ad4 and Ad7 vaccines.

III. USE OF ADENOVIRUS VECTORS FOR RECOMBINANT VACCINES

A. ADVANTAGES

Adenoviruses appear to be attractive recombinant vaccine vectors[14,15] for a number of reasons. Based on the extensive experience obtained with adenovirus vaccines in the military, it seems probable that live oral recombinant adenovirus vaccines can achieve similar records of safety and possibly efficacy. In addition, as observed in other live vector systems, live recombinant adenovirus vaccines would be expected to induce long-lived immune responses to heterologous proteins, including possible induction of cellular immunity. Moreover, since adenoviruses replicate at mucosal surfaces, repeated immunizations with recombinant adenoviruses would be expected to induce significant secretory immunity. For this reason, adenovirus-vectored vaccines may be particularly effective against pathogens that infect or gain entry at mucosal surfaces. Other advantages of adenoviruses as vectors include the well-established molecular biology of adenoviruses.[2] The expression of proteins by adenoviruses is understood in detail, allowing for high level expression of heterologous genes. Construction of recombinants is relatively straightforward and predictable, due in part to the high frequency of recombination in cell culture. In addition, expressed proteins have been shown to undergo normal posttranslational processing.[16,17] The use of adenovirus mutants deleted in the E3 region allows the introduction of up to 7.5 kb of foreign DNA, taking into consideration the capacity of adenovirus virus to package recombinant genomes that exceed the adenovirus genome (36 kb) by 5% (see below). Recombinant adenoviruses have also been shown to be quite stable genetically (unpublished observations). As live oral vaccines, recombinant adenovirus vaccines would be relatively inexpensive to produce and easy to administer and would thus likely be ideal for mass immunization programs. Finally, the highly restricted host range of human adenoviruses precludes spread of recombinant virus to animal reservoirs.

B. POTENTIAL DIFFICULTIES/UNRESOLVED ISSUES
1. Oncogenicity

Concerns over the potential oncogenicity of Ad4 and Ad7 vaccines in humans significantly delayed their acceptance for use in the military. It thus seems of interest to review the possible oncogenicity of adenoviruses being developed as vectors for construction of recombinant vaccines. In this regard, it should be noted that although Ad7 was initially classified as a group B adenovirus on the basis of moderate oncogenicity in rodents, more extensive analysis of several Ad7 strains has demonstrated great differences in oncogenicity among these strains. The Ad7 strain used for vaccine production was selected in part on the basis of a complete lack of oncogenicity in hamsters (no tumors in over 300 hamsters observed for 700 days), as compared with other Ad7 strains which did induce tumors.[6] Ad4 (group E) is nononcogenic in newborn rodents and has low transformational potential. Ad5, which is also being developed as a vaccine vector, has been classified as a group C adenovirus (nononcogenic in rodents).

Extensive analyses of the oncogenic potential of adenoviruses in humans have thus far failed to establish a link between the presence of adenovirus sequences and human cancer.[18] Cell transformation by human adenovirus was originally detected in rodent cells,[4] which are not productively infected. Human cells were later shown to be transformed by human adenovirus DNA.[19] However, transformation of human cells also occurs only under conditions of nonpermissivity, and is achieved only using viral DNA fragments but not infectious virus. This latter observation underscores the improbability of tumor induction by Ad in humans.

2. Role of E3 Region

Due to the limited capacity of Ad to package excess foreign DNA, introduction of deletions into the Ad vector has been used as a strategy to allow accommodation of larger amounts of foreign genetic material. Since the adenovirus E3 region has been shown to be nonessential for virus replication *in vitro*, many early recombinant viruses were constructed using E3-deleted vectors. However, recently emerging evidence indicates that the E3 region may play an important role in the persistence of infection in humans. Insights into these findings are summarized in the following paragraphs of this section.

The adenovirus E3 region is one of four early complex transcription units and is located between map units (m.u.) 75 and 89 in the linear double-stranded adenovirus genome.[20] The E3 promoter, which is active during early stages of viral infection, generates about nine overlapping mRNAs that are self-regulated quantitatively by alternative splicing.[21] The E1A-responsive E3 promoter is unique among adenoviral promoters in that it contains binding sites for the NFkB transcription factor, which allows for E1A-independent transcription of E3 in lymphoid cells.[22] Since certain E3 proteins appear to enable adenovirus-infected cells to evade immune surveillance and also prepare infected cells for efficient virus replication, these features might explain the persistence of Group C adenoviruses in lymphoid tissue.[23]

Among the 47 known adenovirus serotypes, the E3 region seems to be universally conserved.[23] There are nine predicted E3 proteins in group C adenoviruses (Ad2 and Ad5), of which six have been identified in infected cells.[23] These are the 6.7K, 11.6K, 10.4K, 14.5K, 14.7K, and gp19K proteins.[23,24] All of the genes encoding these proteins are also found in group B adenoviruses (Ad3, Ad7, Ad35) which also encode two additional E3 proteins, 20.1K and 20.4K.[25,26]

Interestingly, none of the E3 proteins are required for adenovirus replication in cultured cells or in acute lower respiratory tract infections of hamsters[27] or cotton rats.[28] Even though E3-deleted virus is occasionally isolated from tissue culture passages,[29] no such natural isolates have been reported in humans.[30] This implies that adenovirus E3 proteins provide a critical function during interactions with their natural host.

Functions associated with the E3 proteins gp19K, 10.4K, 14.5K, and 14.7K have been revealed by various *in vitro* experiments.[23] The first indication pointing to the function of gp19K came from the demonstration that it binds to class I antigens of the major histocompatibility complex (MHC) in Ad2-transformed rat cells.[31] Similar interactions were later observed in human and mouse cells.[32] gp19K molecules from various serotypes of groups B, C, D, and E have also been shown to bind to MHC class I antigens. gp19K binds to these antigens in the endoplasmic reticulum, where the complex is retained.[32,33] Cell surface expression of class I antigens complexed with small viral peptide antigens is required for recognition and lysis of virus-infected cells by virus-specific cytotoxic T cells (CTLs).[34] Thus by preventing class I antigen expression at the cellular surface, gp19K alone among E3 proteins prevents lysis of adenovirus-infected cells by adenovirus-specific CTLs.[23] Note that gp19K exhibits different affinities for different class I molecules, raising the possibility that susceptibility to adenovirus infection in humans may be related to the affinity of an individual's class I antigens to the gp19K of the infecting adenovirus.[23] Further, when the generality of gp19K-class I MHC interactions was tested in a variety of human cell lines, various degrees of inhibition of cell surface expression of class I antigens was observed after infection with adenovirus.[35] This suggests that CTL recognition and lysis may not be limited by class I MHC antigen interactions for most human cell types.

The E3 14.7K protein appears to be a general inhibitor of lysis of mouse as well as some human cells by tumor necrosis factor (TNF),[23] a multifunctional cytokine secreted by activated macrophages that regulates a wide variety of immune responses. This inhibition is also exerted by the E3 10.4K/14.5K complex and the E1B-19K protein.[23] Collectively, these proteins counteract the susceptibility to lysis by TNF induced by the adenovirus E1A proteins. Thus, E3 may be a cassette of genes dedicated to helping the virus directly or indirectly evade immune surveillance.[23] The E3 10.4K and 14.5K proteins can also function in concert to down-regulate the EGF receptor (EGF-R) in adenovirus-infected cells, which in turn decreases EGF-R-mediated stimulation of kinase activity and results in the lack of induction of DNA synthesis and mitosis.

3. Preexisting Immunity

The impact of preexisting immunity to adenovirus on the efficacy of orally administered recombinant adenovirus is a critical issue that is poorly understood. It is presently unclear whether preexisting immunity in the general population to an adenovirus serotype precludes its use as a live virus vector. Available clinical data do not permit conclusions on whether preexisting systemic antibody prevents significant enteric replication of adenovirus and thus might block effective primary or booster responses to heterologous proteins. However, a recent Ad-human immunodeficiency virus (HIV) vaccine study in chimpanzees[36] indicates that recombinant adenovirus vaccines can successfully initiate infection of the gut in the presence of moderate levels of serum antibody to adenovirus. In that study, which is discussed in more detail later in this review, primary oral inoculations of chimpanzees with Ad7-HIV gp160 resulted in the induction of serum antibody to Ad7. Approximately 1 year later, an intranasal booster with Ad7-HIV gp160 was administered and resulted in significant enteric virus replication and in the induction of a booster response to gp160. These data are encouraging with regard to the prospects of using commonly circulating adenoviruses as vectors. However, only the examination of recombinant adenovirus vaccines in clinical studies will resolve this question. If such analyses determine that commonly circulating adenoviruses are unsuitable vectors, then the use of less prevalent strains as vectors would be required. Further, in the event common adenoviruses are not suitable for general use, Ad5 may yet be suitable for recombinant vaccine use in infants,[14] since infants do not generally develop antibodies to Ad5 until a few years after birth and because this adenovirus serotype is not associated in infants with serious illness. It is unlikely that humoral immunity to one strain would prevent the use of an alternative strain as a vector because Ad serotyping is based on neutralization criteria. We have successfully immunized primates using a sequential immunization protocol using three serotypically distinct Ad vectors (Ad4, Ad5, Ad7; see below).

C. STRATEGIES FOR RECOMBINANT VECTOR DEVELOPMENT

Recombinant adenovirus types 2, 5, 4, and 7 have been developed as high level expression vectors using several approaches.[14,37,38,39] Broadly, these recombinants are categorized as either replication defective or replication competent, as compared to the wild-type virus in tissue culture.

1. Replication-Defective Recombinants[14,37,40]

In these types of recombinants, a foreign gene is inserted by replacing the essential adenoviral major late promoter (MLP) or E1 regions. In the earliest of such vectors, a portion of the MLP was deleted and the gene for simian virus 40 T antigen was expressed under the control of the MLP.[40] Due to the partial deletion of the essential MLP, such recombinants require wild-type helper virus. However, recombinant adenoviruses with a deletion in the E1 region can be cultivated without helper virus in the 293 cell line, which constitutively expresses E1 proteins.[41] In such recombinants, a foreign gene is inserted as an independent expression cassette containing MLP, tripartite leader (TPL) (including intervening sequences), and polyadenylation sequences. However, despite their production of high levels of a given protein in the 293 cell line, such replication-defective recombinants have limited potential as live oral vaccines because they are unable to replicate productively in primary cells and *in vivo*. Nonetheless, recent animal experiments indicate that recombinant adenovirus containing such a defect produce significant antigen when introduced intranasally into the lungs of cotton rats, as shown for the cystic fibrosis gene,[42] or may induce significant immune responses, as demonstrated for recombinants expressing hepatitis B virus (HBV) surface antigen (HBsAg).[43]

2. Replication-Competent Recombinants[14,37,39]

The adenovirus E3 region has also been utilized for insert sites for foreign gene(s) to facilitate generation of replication-competent adenoviruses. Following the demonstration that E3-deleted viruses were viable in tissue culture,[29] various genes have been expressed downstream of the E3 promoter, either by deleting or by retaining some or all of the E3 open reading frames.[27] A given gene may also be inserted along with late stage-specific regulatory elements, such as synthetic TPL[40] or strong splice acceptor sequences (unpublished observations), to maximize expression at early and late stages. In the adenoviral replication cycle, abundant late stage transcripts arising from the MLP contain multiple spliced TPL sequences that increase translation of late genes.[16,37] Incorporation of such sequences in the E3 region increases the expression of various genes of interest since late stage mRNAs pass through the E3 region, while E3 promoter-derived transcripts are present only during early times. Deletion of a part of the E3 region (80 to 88 m.u. or 3 kb) greatly increases the capacity of the vector to accommodate a larger sized foreign gene. Without deletion of inessential sequences, the recombinant genome may carry only about 5% more than its normal size of 36,000 base pair sequences.[14,37] Therefore most recombinant expression vectors are constructed to contain an E3 deletion that allows them to accommodate more foreign DNA in the form of a single or multiple immunogen gene(s). On the other hand, retention of all or most of the E3 region proteins might be beneficial, since accumulating experimental evidence suggests that these proteins contribute to the persistence of adenoviral infection *in vivo* by masking the infected cell from immune surveillance.

Foreign genes have also been inserted in the E4 region, a strategy that allows normal expression of the entire E3 region. However, the E4 insertion site is situated between the E4 promoter and the right inverted terminal repeat at map unit 100,[44,45] and since this region is transcriptionally inactive, expression of foreign gene products has been achieved by using an independent expression cassette. Typically, a high level of late stage expression is obtained when a gene is inserted within a cassette having an adenoviral MLP, TPL (including intervening sequences), and hexon polyadenylation signal sequences.[45] This type of cassette has also been successfully inserted at deletion sites within the E1 and E3 regions.[16,37] Since these cassettes are independent units, they can be inserted in either orientation to alter gene expression (unpublished observations). In such types of E4 region recombinant viruses, it is important to evaluate viral growth in diploid cell culture (e.g., WI-38), since any interference with the essential E4 transcripts or proteins might decrease virus production.

3. Construction of Recombinant Viruses

Different approaches have been implemented for construction of recombinant viruses depending upon the site of insertion and the type of expression cassette used.[14,16,37,39,40] After selection of an adenovirus vector, a portion of the adenovirus genome is cloned into a plasmid vector based on restriction enzyme patterns. For a previously unstudied serotype, the DNA sequence may be determined and compared with that of a known genome to precisely define an insertion site. Heterologous DNA can be inserted as part of an expression cassette or under the control of an endogenous adenoviral promoter, either alone or with some specific synthetic regulatory sequences for efficient gene expression. Once a recombinant adenovirus genome-containing plasmid has been cloned, it can be used to generate a recombinant adenovirus *in vivo* by transfecting the linearized plasmid into cultured cells together with a purified homologous adenoviral DNA fragment that overlaps the cloned adenoviral sequence so that the transfected fragments together include the entire genome (0 to 100 m.u.).[46]

Homologous recombination *in vivo* at overlapping sequences generates infectious recombinant adenovirus containing the foreign gene.[46] An alternative approach exploits available specific restriction sites, in which two or three fragments are ligated *in vitro* and then transfected into cells, resulting in the generation of recombinant virus and reducing the background wild-type virus.[14,37] Typically, infectious recombinants are obtained as plaques in tissue culture monolayer, after which the plaques are amplified to generate higher viral titers, and the viruses are then analyzed for expression of a given protein by various immunological or labeling techniques. Viral DNA structure must always be analyzed (by Hirt DNA extraction and further restriction enzyme digestion)[37] to confirm the location of the foreign DNA as well as the structural integrity of the recombinant viral genome.

D. PRECLINICAL STUDIES
1. Animal Models
Identification of animal models to evaluate recombinant adenovirus vaccines has been difficult due to the highly restricted host range of human adenoviruses. Among small laboratory animals, only the hamster[27,47] and cotton rat[48] have been shown to sustain permissive lung infections by some human adenoviruses. These models have consequently found use in immunogenicity studies involving Ad5-vectored vaccines. Other small animal models have been identified that are nonpermissive for adenovirus replication but that express heterologous proteins during abortive infections by recombinant Ad5 (e.g., rabbit[17] and mouse[49]). These models have also been used with success in immunogenicity studies. Immunization regimens consisting of sequential administration of Ad4, Ad5, and Ad7 vectors have been evaluated in the dog,[50,51] which sustains abortive infections with these viruses. Monkeys are abortively infected with Ad5 and have been used occasionally to evaluate recombinant adenovirus vaccines.[52] The single permissive model that has been identified to date for Ad4, Ad5, and Ad7 vaccine vectors is the chimpanzee.[53] Oral administration of recombinant vaccines results in the enteric replication of these recombinant viruses and the induction of seroresponses to heterologous proteins.[53] However, the limited availability of these animals and associated costs have greatly restricted studies in this model. Thus initial immunogenicity studies of recombinant adenovirus vaccines are routinely conducted in the less desirable subprimate models before testing in the chimpanzee model.

2. Immunogenicity and Efficacy Studies
Several recombinant adenovirus vaccines have been prepared that express individual or multiple genes from viral pathogens. Examination of some of these recombinants in animal models for immunogenicity has demonstrated protective efficacy in some cases (Table 3). Ad5 recombinant viruses expressing hepatitis B virus (HBV) genes were the first recombinant adenovirus vaccines to be constructed and tested in animals. Early studies in rabbits and hamsters confirmed the immunogenic potential of HBsAg produced *in vivo* by Ad5 vectors.[50] The dog model was later used to evaluate the immunogenicity of sequentially administered heterotypic adenovirus vectors containing the HBV major S gene.[50] To overcome anticipated problems of induced immunity to the Ad vector used for primary immunization, Ad7-HBV was used for primary immunizations and Ad4-HBV for booster vaccinations. In this study, responses generally greater than 1000 milli-international units (mIU) were induced following the booster immunizations (responses greater than 10 mIU are considered protective in humans). In the permissive chimpanzee model, sequential oral administration of Ad7- and Ad4-HBV recombinant viruses expressing the HBV major S antigen induced low anti-HBs responses following the booster immunization (a transient anti-HBs response was detected in one animal following

Table 3 Immunogenicity of recombinant adenovirus vaccines in animals

Inserted gene	Ad vector(s)	Animal model	Dose (pfu)	Route[a]	Immunogenicity[b]	Protection from live virus challenge	Ref.
Hepatitis B virus							
Middle S (S2)	Ad5	Rabbit	10^9	IV	+RIA	NA	17
Middle S (S2)	Ad5 (E1A defective)	Chimpanzee	10^9	IV	+RIA(1/2)	1 partial, 1 no protection	43
Major S	Ad5, Ad5 E3 deletion	Hamster	10^{7-9}	IN	+RIA	NA	27
Major S	Ad7[c]	Dog	10^{7-10}	IT	+RIA	NA	50
	Ad4[c]	Dog	10^9	IT	+RIA	NA	50
HBcAg/major S	Ad5	Dog	10^{8-10}	IT	+/+RIA	NA	54
HBprecAg/major S	Ad5	Dog	10^{8-10}	IT	+/+RIA	NA	54
Major S	Ad7[c]	Chimpanzee	10^7	PO	1°:+RIA(1/2)	1 partial,	53
	Ad4[c]	Chimpanzee	10^{10}	PO	2°:+RIA(2/2)	1 complete	53
	Ad4	Chimpanzee	10^{10}	PO	-RIA(1/1)	No	53
Herpes Simplex Virus Glycoprotein B							
	Ad5	Mice	5×10^7	IP	-	+	49
		Monkeys		PO	+	Variable	55
Human immunodeficiency virus							
gp160	Ad5	Cotton rats	10^8	IN	+ ELISA,WB	NA	56
gag(p24)	Ad5	Mice	$10^{7,8}$	IP	+ WB	NA	52
		Monkeys	10^8	SC	+WB(3/4)	NA	52
gp160	Ad4, Ad5, Ad7	Dogs	10^9	IT	+ WB,ELISA,N	NA	57
gp160, gag(p55)	Ad7, Ad4, Ad5[d]	Chimpanzee	10^{7-10}	PO	+WB(3/3), ELISA(3/3), N(1/3)	NA	36

Table 3 (continued) **Immunogenicity of recombinant adenovirus vaccines in animals**

Inserted gene	Ad vector(s)	Animal model	Dose (pfu)	Route[a]	Immunogenicity[b]	Protection from live virus challenge	Ref.
gp160	Ad7	Chimpanzee	10^8	IN	+WB(3/3), ELISA(3/3), N(1/3)	NA	36
Epstein-Barr virus							
gp340, gp220	Ad5 (E1A defective)	Rabbits	10^{10}	IV, IM	+IFA, N	NA	58
Respiratory syncytial virus							
F glycoprotein	Ad5	Cotton rats	10^8	IN	+ELISA	+	59
			10^8	ID	+ELISA	±	
F,G, and F/G glycoproteins	Ad4, Ad5 Ad7	Dogs	10^{7-9}	IT	–	+	60
F glycoprotein	Ad7, Ad4 Ad5	Chimpanzee	10^9	PO	+ELISA,±N	NA	60
Parainfluenza virus 3							
F and HN	Ad5	Mice	10^7	IP	–	NA	61
Human cyto-megalovirus							

Major envelope glycoprotein (gB) Tick-borne encephalitis virus	Ad5	Hamsters	10^9	IN	–, IFA	NA	62
NS1 protein	Ad5	Mice	10^7	IP	+WB	±	63
Pseudorabies							
Glycoprotein gp50	Ad5 (E1A defective)	Mice	10^7	IP	+ELISA,±N	weak	64
		Rabbits	10^9	IV, IM,	+ELISA,±N	±	64
Rabies virus							
Glycoprotein	Ad5	Mice	10^{4-7}	IP, PO	–	+	65
		Dogs	5×10^5	IN, SC	–	NA	65
Glycoprotein	Ad5	Skunks	10^{7-10}	baits, PO, IM	–	+	66
		Foxes	$10^{8,9}$	PO	–	+	66

[a] ID: intraduodenal; IM: intramuscular; IN: intranasal; IP: intraperitoneal; IT: intratracheal; IV: intravenous; SC: subcutaneous; PO: oral.

[b] N: neutralization, IFA: immunofluorescence, WB: Western blot, (number positive/total number).

[c] Primary immunization: Ad7 recombinant; booster immunization: Ad4 recombinant.

[d] Primary immunizations: Ad7-env and Ad7-gag; first booster: Ad4 env and Ad4 gag; second booster: Ad5 env and Ad5 gag.

primary immunization[53]). Following challenge with infectious HBV, one animal was fully protected from HBV-induced disease and the second animal showed modified hepatic disease. A control chimpanzee and a chimpanzee inoculated sequentially with Ad7 (vaccine strain) and the Ad4-HBV recombinant virus both experienced acute infections upon HBV challenge. This study demonstrated for the first time that enteric replication of recombinant adenovirus elicits immune responses to expressed heterologous viral proteins and that such responses may result in protection upon experimental challenge. In a second chimpanzee study,[43] an Ad5 (E1A-defective) recombinant expressing middle S antigen (S plus preS2) did not elicit detectable anti-HBs seroresponses following intravenous inoculation but did confer partial protection upon HBV challenge in one of two immunized chimpanzees.

Recombinant adenoviruses expressing the human immunodeficiency virus (HIV) gp160 likewise have been evaluated in small animals and in chimpanzees. An initial study of an Ad5-gp160 recombinant demonstrated immunogenicity in cotton rats.[56] A later study conducted in dogs showed that sequential immunizations with heterotypic adenovirus vectors (Ad7 and Ad4) induced high HIV neutralizing antibody titers that were effectively boosted by administration of an HIV envelope subunit vaccine.[57] Sequential oral administration of Ad7, Ad4, and Ad5 recombinant viruses expressing gp160 (lyophilized virus contained in gelatin capsules enteric-coated with cellulose acetate phthalate) to chimpanzees[36] demonstrated the induction of neutralization antibodies in one of three chimpanzees following the second oral booster. However, enteric replication of the Ad-HIV recombinants in this study was generally poor. Subsequent intranasal inoculation of these three chimpanzees with the Ad7-gp160 recombinant used for the primary oral inoculations resulted in better enteric replication of the virus (infection of the intestines probably occurred from ingestion of infected nasal or pharyngeal secretions) and in the induction of neutralizing antibodies in all three chimpanzees.[36] Secretory antibody responses in the upper respiratory tract were also induced following the intranasal inoculations. Strong proliferative responses by chimpanzee peripheral blood leukocytes (PBLs) were induced upon incubation with recombinant HIV antigens following oral administration of the Ad-HIV vaccines. The reason for the poor virus replication following oral administration in this study is not presently understood. However, since Ad7 recombinants administered intranasally showed improved replication in the chimpanzee gut, it may be that oral delivery by enteric-coated gelatin capsules is not optimal for enteric inoculation and that an improved oral delivery system will be required for recombinant adenovirus. In a study of Ad5-HIV gag recombinants, immunization of mice and monkeys induced serum antibody responses to the gag protein.[52]

Significant immune responses and in some instances, significant levels of protection against live viral challenge have been induced in nonprimate species by recombinant adenovirus vaccines containing genes from herpes simplex virus,[49,55] Epstein-Barr virus,[58] respiratory syncytial virus,[59,60] parainfluenza virus 3,[61] human cytomegalovirus,[62] tick-borne encephalitis virus,[63] pseudorabies virus,[64] and rabies virus[65,66] (Table 3). Together these data confirm the potential of recombinant adenovirus to induce appropriate systemic immune responses.

However, the greatest hope for recombinant adenovirus vaccines might reside in their potential to induce secretory and possibly cellular immune responses. In the oral primate Ad-HIV vaccine study[36] described above, secretory responses were induced even though enteric virus replication was relatively poor. A subsequent study conducted in chimpanzees has shown improved enteric replication of recombinant Ad-HIV vaccines and substantially enhanced responses at secretory sites (upper respiratory tract, female genital tract, intestinal tract) to HIV proteins (unpublished observations). Although PBLs showing strong proliferative responses to recombinant HIV antigens have been induced in chimpanzees by Ad-HIV vaccines, there are at present no reports regarding the induction of CTLs. This is due at least in part to the technical difficulties involved in analyzing cellular responses in the animal models used for evaluation of adenovirus vaccines. However, it seems likely that demonstration of CTL induction by recombinant adenoviruses will be forthcoming.

E. CLINICAL STUDIES

Thus far there has been but a single clinical evaluation of an oral recombinant adenovirus vaccine in humans.[67] In that study, the Ad7 vaccine routinely administered to military recruits was constructed to express the hepatitis B surface antigen. This vaccine, termed Ad7HZ6-1, was shown in a preclinical chimpanzee study to be immunogenic and to induce protection when used with an Ad4-HBV heterotypic booster[53] (see above). In this clinical study, three volunteers per group received oral immunization of either Ad7HZ6-1 at a dose of 1.6×10^7 plaque forming units (pfu), Ad7 vaccine at a dose of 1.0×10^6 pfu, or a placebo. Surprisingly, the titer of virus shed in stools of Ad7HZ6-1 recipients was approximately 100-fold less than that of Ad7 vaccine, even though the dose of Ad7HZ6-1 administered was more than ten times higher. Only the adenovirus isolated from stools of Ad7HZ6-1 recipients expressed HBsAg, and the recovered adenovirus had a restriction endonuclease digestion pattern equivalent to that of Ad7HZ6-1, indicating genetic stability of the recombinant adenovirus. Seroconversion to Ad7, as assessed by serum neutralizing antibody titers, ranged from 32 to 64 for those volunteers given Ad7 and from <4 (one volunteer) to 16 (two volunteers) for those given Ad7HZ6-1. An antibody response to HBsAg was not observed, but a booster dose of vaccine was not administered in this study. Both the Ad7 and the Ad7HZ6-1 vaccines were well tolerated, and no adverse reactions were noted. A transient elevation in hepatic transaminase levels was observed among both vaccinees and controls at levels similar to those seen in other phase I vaccine trials. However, these were not considered to be of clinical significance.

Although Ad7HZ6-1 replicated very poorly in volunteers that were seronegative for Ad7 antibodies, the use of higher dosages of vaccine or multiple doses might enhance the viral replication and immune responses. In addition, Ad7HZ6-1 contains a deleted E3 region, and although E3 region gene products are not essential for replication of adenovirus in tissue culture, they are thought to be important in protection of virus-infected cells from immune destruction (see above). Thus, in this study, E3-deleted Ad7HZ6-1 was shown to be attenuated relative to the parent virus in that it was shed at a far lower titer and stimulated less potent anti-adenovirus immune responses. This suggests that future recombinant adenoviruses designed for oral administration may need to contain either all or a portion of the E3 region for optimal replication *in vivo*.

IV. CONCLUSIONS

During the past several years considerable progress has been made in optimizing strategies for construction of recombinant adenoviruses and in evaluating recombinant adenovirus vaccines in newly developed animal models. The capacity of recombinant adenoviruses to induce systemic immune responses that are protective has been demonstrated. In addition, the use of multiple serotypically distinct adenovirus vectors for sequential booster immunizations has been demonstrated in the dog and in the chimpanzee models. The availability of multiple adenovirus strains as potential vectors, many of which have not been associated with serious disease, may also help to address the problem of preexisting immunity to adenovirus. Many adenovirus serotypes are rare and the incidence of antibodies to these strains in the general population is very low. Such strains may represent ideal candidates as vaccine vectors. However, despite significant recent advances, several critical questions persist that must be answered before the true potential of the adenovirus vector system is established. Although the induction by adenovirus of secretory immunity and cell-mediated immunity to heterologous proteins has recently come to light, more extensive data are clearly required in both areas. Especially useful would be CTL and additional secretory immunity data generated in the oral primate model. The poor enteric replication of the Ad-HBV construct Ad7HZ6-1 in humans as well as the poor replication of Ad-HIV vaccines in chimpanzees following oral immunization suggest that some recombinant adenoviruses may have decreased replication competency when administered orally as enteric-coated capsules or tablets. Whether the poor replication of these viruses resulted from the absence of the adenovirus E3 region or to a suboptimal means of vaccine delivery is not understood. However, indications are that improved vaccine delivery to the gut is desirable. Finally, combination vaccination protocols using live recombinant adenovirus for primary immunizations and subunit vaccines for final booster immunizations may be effective at inducing enhanced immune responses. Such regimens may be particularly effective for vaccination against diseases that are transmitted across mucosal barriers.

REFERENCES

1. Hierholzer, J. C., Wigand, R., Anderson, L. J., Adrian, T., and Gold, J. W. M., Adenoviruses from patients with AIDS: a plethora of serotypes and a description of five serotypes of subgenus D (types 43–47), *J. Infect. Dis.,* 158, 804, 1988.
2. Ginsberg, H. S., Ed., *The Adenoviruses,* Plenum Press, New York, 1984.
3. Huebner, R. J., Rowe, W. P., and Lane, W. T., Oncogenic effects in hamsters of human adenovirus type 12 and 18, *Proc. Natl. Acad. Sci. U.S.A.,* 48, 2051, 1962.
4. Trentin, J. J., Yabe, Y., and Taylor, G., The quest for human cancer viruses, *Science,* 137, 835, 1962.
5. Horwitz, M. S., Adenoviruses, *Virology,* 2nd ed., Fields, B. N. and Knipe, D. M., Eds., Raven Press, New York, 1990, 1723.
6. Rubin, B. A. and Rorke, L. B., Adenovirus vaccines, *Vaccines,* Plotkin, S. A. and Mortimer, E. A., Jr., Eds., W. B. Saunders, Philadelphia, 1988, 492.
7. Top, F. H., Jr., Control of adenovirus acute respiratory disease in U.S. Army trainees, *Yale J. Biol. Med.,* 48, 185, 1975.
8. Chaloner-Larsson, G., Contreras, G., Furesz, J., Boucher, D. W., Krepps, D., Humphreys, G. R., and Mohanna, S. M., Immunization of Canadian armed forces personnel with live types 4 and 7 adenovirus vaccines, *Can. J. Public Health,* 77, 367, 1986.
9. Meuller, R. E., Muldoon, R. L., and Jackson, G. E., Spread of enteric live adenovirus type 4 vaccine in married couples, *J. Infect. Dis.,* 119, 51, 1969.
10. Meuller, R. E., Muldoon, R. L., and Jackson, G. E., Communicability of enteric live adenovirus type 4 vaccine in families, *J. Infect. Dis.,* 119, 60, 1969.
11. Dudding, B. A., Top, R. H., and Winter, P., Acute respiratory disease in military trainees. The adenovirus surveillance program 1966–1971, *Am. J. Epidemiol.,* 97, 187, 1973.
12. Natuk, R. N., Lubeck, M. D., Davis, A. R., Chengalvala, M., Chanda, P. K., Mizutani, S., Eichberg, J. W., and Hung, P. P., Adenovirus as a vector system for induction of secretory immunity, *Vaccine Res.,* 1, 275, 1992.
13. Scott, R. M., Dudding, B. A., Romano, S. V., and Russell, P. K., Enteric immunization with live adenovirus type 21 vaccine. II. Systemic and local immune responses following immunization, *Infect. Immun.,* 5, 300, 1972.
14. Graham, F. L. and Prevec, L., Adenovirus-based expression vectors and recombinant vaccines, *Biotechnology,* 20, 363, 1992.
15. Chengalvala, M. V. R., Lubeck, M. D., Selling, B. J., Natuk, R. J., Hsu, K.-H. L., Mason, B. B., Chanda, P. K., Bhat, R. A., Bhat, B. M., Mizutani, S., Davis, A. R., and Hung, P. P., Adenovirus vectors for gene expression, *Curr. Opin. Biotech.,* 2, 178, 1991.

16. Davis, A. R., Kostek, B., Mason, B. B., Hasio, C. L., Morin, J., Dheer, S. K., and Hung, P. P., Expression of hepatitis B surface antigen with a recombinant adenovirus, *Proc. Natl. Acad. Sci. U.S.A.*, 82, 7560, 1985.

17. Ballay, A., Levrero, M., Buendia, M.-A., Tiollais, P., and Perricaudet, M., *In vitro* and *in vivo* synthesis of the hepatitis B virus surface antigen and of the receptor for polymerized human serum album from recombinant adenovirus, *EMBO J.*, 4, 3861, 1985.

18. Green, M., Wold, W. S. M., Mackey, J. K., and Rigden, P., Analysis of human tonsil and cancer DNAs and RNAs for DNA sequences of group C (serotypes 1, 2, 5, and 6) human adenoviruses, *Proc. Natl. Acad. Sci. U.S.A.*, 76, 6606, 1979.

19. Graham, F. L., Smiley, J., Russell, W. C., and Nairn, R., Characteristics of a human cell line transformed by DNA from human adenovirus type 5, *J. Gen. Virol.*, 36, 59, 1977.

20. Chow, L. T., Broker, T. R., and Lewis, J. B., Complex splicing patterns of RNAs from the early regions of adenovirus 2, *J. Mol. Biol.*, 134, 265, 1979.

21. Bhat, B. M., Brady, H. A., Pursley, M. H., and Wold, W. S. M., Deletion mutants that alter the differential RNA processing in E3 complex transcription unit of adenovirus, *J. Mol. Biol.*, 190, 543, 1986.

22. Williams, J. R., Garcia, J., Harrich, D., Pearson, L., Wu, F., and Gynor, R., Lymphoid specific gene expression of the adenovirus early region 3 promoter is mediated by NF-kB binding motifs, *EMBO J.*, 9, 4435, 1990.

23. Wold, W. S. M. and Gooding, L. R., Region E3 of adenovirus: a cassette of genes involved in host immunosurveillance and virus-cell interactions, *Virology*, 184, 1, 1991.

24. Petersson, H., Jornvall, H., and Zabielski, J., Multiple mRNA species for the precursor to an adenovirus-encoded glycoprotein: Identification and structure of the signal sequence, *Proc. Natl. Acad. Sci. U.S.A.*, 77, 6349, 1980.

25. Signäs, C., Akusjärvi, G., and Petersson, V., Region E3 of human adenoviruses: differences between the oncogenic adenovirus-3 and the nononcogenic adenovirus-2, *Gene*, 50, 173, 1986.

26. Flomenberg, P. R., Chen, M., and Horwitz, M. S., Sequence and genetic organization of adenovirus type 35 early region 3, *J. Virol.*, 62, 4431, 1988.

27. Morin, J. E., Lubeck, M. D., Barton, J. E., Conley, A. J., Davis, A. R., and Hung, P. P., Recombinant adenovirus induces antibody response to hepatitis B virus surface antigen in hamsters, *Proc. Natl. Acad. Sci. U.S.A.*, 84, 4626, 1987.

28. Ginsberg, H. S., Lundholm-Beauchamp, U., Horstwood, R. L., Pernis, B., Wold, W. S. M., Chanock, R. M., and Prince, G. A., Role of early region 3 (E3) in pathogenesis of adenovirus disease, *Proc. Natl. Acad. Sci. U.S.A.*, 86, 3823, 1989.

29. Jones, N. and Shenk, T., Isolation of deletion and substitution mutants of adenovirus type 5, *Cell*, 13, 181, 1978.

30. Adrian, T., Becker, M., Hierholzer, J. C., and Wigand, R., Molecular epidemiology and restriction site mapping of adenovirus 7 genome types, *Arch. Virol.*, 106, 73, 1989.

31. Kvist, S., Ostberg, L., Persson, H., Philipson, L., and Peterson, P. A., Molecular association between transplantation antigens and cell surface antigen in adenovirus-transformed cell line, *Proc. Natl. Acad. Sci. U.S.A.*, 75, 5674, 1978.

32. Pääbo, S., Nilsson, T., and Peterson, P. A., Adenoviruses of subgenera B, C, D, and E modulate cell-surface expression of major histocompatibility complex class I antigens, *Proc. Natl. Acad. Sci. U.S.A.*, 83, 9665, 1986.

33. Pääbo, S., Bhat, B. M., Wold, W. S. M., and Peterson, P. A., A short sequence in the COOH-terminus makes an adenovirus membrane glycoprotein a resident of the endoplasmic reticulum, *Cell*, 50, 311, 1987.

34. Townsend, A. and Bodmer, H., Antigen recognition by class I-restricted T lymphocytes, *Annu. Rev. Immunol.*, 7, 601, 1989.

35. Routes, J. M. and Cook, J. L., Resistance of human cells to the adenovirus E3 effect on class I MHC antigen expression. Implications for antiviral immunity, *J. Immunol.*, 144, 2763, 1990.

36. Natuk, R. J., Lubeck, M. D., Chanda, P. K., Chengalvala, M., Wade, M. S., Murthy, S. C. S., Wilhelm, J., Vernon, S. K., Dheer, S. K., Mizutani, S., Lee, S-G., Murthy, K., Eichberg, J. W., Davis, A. R., and Hung, P. P., Immunogenicity of recombinant human adenovirus-human immunodeficiency virus vaccines in chimpanzees, *AIDS Res. Hum. Retrovir.*, 9, 395, 1993.

37. Berkner, K. L., Expression of heterologous sequences in adenoviral vectors, *Curr. Top. Microbiol.*, 158, 39, 1992.

38. Morin, J. E., Lubeck, M. D., Mason, B. B., Molnar-Kimber, K. L., Dheer, S. K., Bhat, B. M., Chanda, P. K., Natuk, R. J., Chengalvala, M., Mizutani, S., Davis, A. R., and Hung, P. P., Recombinant adenovirus vaccine for hepatitis B virus, *New Generation Vaccines,* Woodrow, G. C. and Levine, M. M., Eds., Marcel Dekker, New York, 1990, 448.

39. Tikchonenko, T. I., Adenovirus as vectors for the transfer of genetic information and for the construction of new type vaccines, *Adv. Exp. Med. Biol.*, 257, 193, 1989.

40. Thummel, C., Tjian, R., Hu, S. H., and Grodzicker, T., Translational control of SV40 T antigen expressed from the adenovirus late promoter, *Cell,* 33, 455, 1983.

41. Gluzman, Y., Reichl, H., and Solnick, D., Helper-free adenovirus type 5 vectors, *Eukaryotic Viral Vectors,* Gluzman, Y., Ed., Cold Spring Harbor Laboratory, Cold Spring Harbor, NY, 1982, 187.

42. Rosenfeld, M. A., Yoshimura, K., Trapnell, B. C., Yoneyama, K., Rosenthal, E. R., Dalemans, W., Fukayama, M., Bargon, J., Stier, L. E., Stratford-Perricaudet, L., Perricaudet, M., Guggino, W. B., Pavirani, A., Lococq, J.-P., and Crystal, R. G., *In vivo* transfer of the human cystic fibrosis transmembrane conductance regulator gene to the airway epithelium, *Cell,* 68, 143, 1991.

43. Levero, M., Barban, V., Manteca, S., Ballay, A., Balsamo, C., Avantaggiati, M. L., Natoli, G., Skellekens, H., Tiollais, P., and Perricaudet, M., Defective and nondefective adenovirus vectors for expressing foreign genes *in vitro* and *in vivo, Gene,* 101, 195, 1991.

44. Saito, I., Oya, Y., Yamamoto, K., Yuasa, T., and Shimojo, H., Construction of nondefective adenovirus type 5 bearing a 2.8 kilobase hepatitis B virus DNA near the right end of its genome, *J. Virol.,* 54, 711, 1985.

45. Mason, B. M., Davis, A. R., Bhat, B. M., Chengalvala, M., Lubeck, M. D., Zandle, G., Kosteck, B., Cholodofsky, S., Dheer, S. K., Molnar-Kimber, K., Mizutani, S., and Hung, P. P., Adenovirus vaccine vectors expressing hepatitis B surface antigen: importance of regulatory elements in the adenovirus major late intron, *Virology,* 177, 452, 1990.

46. Berkner, K. L. and Sharp, P. A., Generation of adenovirus by transfection of plasmids, *Nucleic Acids Res.,* 11, 6003, 1983.

47. Hjorth, R. N., Bonde, G. M., Pierzchala, W. A., Vernon, S. K., Wiener, F. P., Levner, M. H., Lubeck, M. D., and Hung, P. P., A new hamster model for adenoviral vaccination, *Arch. Virol.,* 100, 279, 1988.

48. Pacini, D. L., Dubovi, E. J., and Clyde, W., Jr., A new animal model for human respiratory tract disease due to adenovirus, *J. Infect. Dis.,* 150, 92, 1984.

49. McDermott, M. R., Graham, F. L., Hanke, T., and Johnson, D. C., Protection of mice against lethal challenge with herpes simplex virus by vaccination with an adenovirus vector expressing HSV glycoprotein B, *Virology,* 169, 244, 1989.

50. Chengalvala, M., Lubeck, M. D., Davis, A. R., Mizutani, S., Molnar-Kimber, K., Morin, J., and Hung, P. P., Evaluation of adenovirus type 4 and type 7 recombinant hepatitis B vaccines in dogs, *Vaccine,* 9, 485, 1991.

51. Prevec, L., Schneider, M., Rosenthal, K. L., Belbeck, L. W., Derbyshire, J. B., and Graham, F. L., Use of human adenovirus-based vectors for antigen expression in animals, *J. Gen. Virol.,* 70, 429, 1989.

52. Prevec, L., Christie, B. S., Laurie, K. E., Bailey, M. M., (Smith), Graham, F. L., and Rosenthal, K. L., Immune response to HIV-1 gag antigens induced by recombinant adenovirus vectors in mice and rhesus macaque monkeys, *J. Acq. Immun. Defic. Syndr.,* 4, 568, 1991.

53. Lubeck, M. D., Davis, A. R., Chengalvala, M., Natuk, R. J., Morin, J. E., Molnar-Kimber, K. L., Mason, B. B., Bhat, B. B., Mizutani, S., Hung, P. P., and Purcell, R. H., Immunogenicity and efficacy testing in chimpanzees of an oral hepatitis B vaccine based on live recombinant adenoviruses, *Proc. Natl. Acad. Sci. U.S.A.,* 86, 6763, 1989.

54. Ye, W. W., Mason, B. B., Chengalvala, M., Cheng, S.-M., Zandle, G., Lubeck, M. D., Lee, S.-G., Mizutani, S., Davis, A. R., and Hung, P. P., Co-expression of hepatitis B virus antigens by a non-defective adenovirus vaccine vector, *Arch. Virol.,* 118, 11, 1991.

55. Johnson, D. C., Adenovirus vectors as potential vaccines against herpes simplex virus, *Rev. Infect. Dis.,* 13, S912, 1991.

56. Dewar, R. L., Natarajan, V., Vasudevachari, M. B., and Salzman, N. P., Synthesis and processing of human immunodeficiency virus type 1 envelope proteins encoded by a recombinant human adenovirus, *J. Virol.,* 63, 129, 1989.

57. Natuk, R. J., Chanda, P. K., Lubeck, M. D., Davis, A. R., Wilhelm, J., Hjorth, R., Wade, M. S., Bhat, B. M., Mizutani, S., Lee, S., Eichberg, J., Gallo, R. C., Hung, P. P., and Robert-Guroff, M., Adenovirus-human immunodeficiency virus (HIV) envelope recombinant vaccines elicit high-titered HIV-neutralizing antibodies in the dog model, *Proc. Natl. Acad. Sci. U.S.A.,* 89, 7777, 1992.

58. Ragot, T., Eloit, M., and Perricaudet, M., Recombinant E1A-defective adenoviruses expressing pseudorabies and Epstein-Barr virus glycoproteins induce immunological responses as live vaccines in rabbits and mice, *Human Gene Transfer,* Cohen-Haguenauer, O. and Colloque, M. B., Eds., John Libbey Eurotext Ltd., 1991, 219, 249.

59. Collins, P. L., Prince, G. A., Camargo, E., Prucell, R. H., Chanock, R. M., Murphy, B. R., Davis, A. R., Lubeck, M. D., Mizutani, S., and Hung, P. P., Evaluation of the protective efficiency of recombinant vaccinia viruses and adenoviruses that express respiratory syncytial virus glycoproteins, *Vaccines 90,* Brown, F., Chanock, R. M., Ginsberg, H. S., and Lerner, R. A., Eds., Cold Spring Harbor Press, Cold Spring Harbor, NY, 1990, 79.

60. Hsu, K.-H. L., Lubeck, M. D., Davis, A. R., Bhat, R. A., Selling, B. H., Bhat, B. M., Mizutani, S., Murphy, B. R., Collins, P. L., Chanock, R. M., and Hung, P. P., Immunogenicity of recombinant adenovirus-respiratory syncytial virus vaccines with adenovirus types 4, 5, and 7 vectors in dogs and chimpanzee, *J. Infect. Dis.,* 166, 769, 1992.

61. Ebata, S., Prevec, L., Graham, F. L., and Dimock, K., Function and immunogenicity of human parainfluenza virus 3 glycoproteins expressed by recombinant adenoviruses, *Virus Res.,* 24, 21, 1992.

62. Marshall, G. S., Ricciardi, R. P., Rando, R. F., Puck, J., Ge, R., Plotkin, S. A., and Gönczöl, E., An adenovirus recombinant that expresses the human cytomegalovirus major envelope glycoprotein and induces neutralizing antibodies, *J. Infect. Dis.,* 162, 1177, 1990.

63. Jacobs, S. C., Stephenson, J. R., and Wilkinson, G. W. G., High-level expression of the tick-borne encephalitis virus NS1 protein by using an adenovirus-based vector: Protection elicited in a murine model, *J. Virol.,* 66, 2086, 1992.
64. Eloit, M., Gilardi-Hebenstreit, P., Toma, B., and Perricaudet, M., Construction of a defective adenovirus vector expressing the pseudorabies virus glycoprotein gp50 and its use as a live vaccine, *J. Gen. Virol.,* 71, 2425, 1990.
65. Prevec, L., Campbell, J. B., Christie, B. S., Belbeck, L., and Graham, F. L., A recombinant human adenovirus vaccine against rabies, *J. Infect. Dis.,* 161, 27, 1990.
66. Charlton, K. M., Artois, M., Prevec, L., Campbell, J. B., Casey, G. A., Wandeler, A. I., and Armstrong, J., Oral rabies vaccination of skunks and foxes with a recombinant human adenovirus vaccine, *Arch. Virol.,* 123, 169, 1992.
67. Tacket, C. O., Losonsky, G., Lubeck, M. D., Davis, A. R., Mizutani, S., Horwith, G., Hung, P., Edelman, R., and Levine, M. M., Initial safety and immunogenicity studies of an oral recombinant adenohepatitis B vaccine, *Vaccine,* 10, 673, 1992.

Chapter 5

Antigenic and Dicistronic Poliovirus Hybrids as a Novel Oral Delivery System for Foreign Antigens

Hui-Hua Lu,* Louis Alexander, and Eckard Wimmer

TABLE OF CONTENTS

I. INTRODUCTION

Poliovirus, the causative agent of paralytic poliomyelitis, has been extensively studied since its discovery in 1909 by Landsteiner and Popper, making it one of the more well-defined biological entities. The genetic organization, and to a certain extent, the function of the gene products of the poliovirus genome have been elucidated on the basis of biochemical and sequence analyses.[1-4] In addition, the structure of the icosahedral viral capsid has been resolved by X-ray crystallography.[5] Genetic manipulation of poliovirus has been greatly advanced through the construction of infectious cDNA clones [6] and the generation of infectious RNA in an *in vitro* transcription system.[7] Furthermore, poliovirus has been recently synthesized in a cell-free system, which has facilitated the study of poliovirus replication outside living cells.[8]

One of the great achievements of medical science in this century was the development of two poliovaccines which have proven to be remarkably successful in curtailing the incidence of poliomyelitis.[9,10] The formalin-inactivated Salk vaccine (IPV) and the live, attenuated Sabin vaccine (OPV) have compiled an outstanding record of safety with very few vaccine-related cases of poliomyelitis being reported.[11]

In this chapter, we will describe experiments that have taken advantage of the wealth of knowledge concerning poliovirus as well as the properties of the live, attenuated poliovirus vaccine to discuss strategies for the development of novel, oral delivery systems for foreign antigens. One set of experiments involves the construction of antigenic hybrid viruses carrying foreign epitopes on the poliovirus capsid; another set

---

*Corresponding author.

0-8493-4866-8/94/$0.00+$.50

involves the construction of dicistronic viruses harboring foreign genes. In the case of dicistronic viruses, the viral polyprotein and foreign antigens are independently expressed by internal ribosomal entry sites (IRES) from two different picornaviruses.

II. THE NATURE OF POLIOVIRUS

A. CLASSIFICATION

Poliovirus is the prototype of the picornaviridae, a viral family which is currently divided into the five genera Entero-, Rhino-, Cardio-, Aphtho-, and Hepatovirus. These pathogens cause a bewildering array of disease syndromes in humans and animals.[12] The enterovirus genus consists of poliovirus, coxsackieviruses group A and B, human echoviruses and human enteroviruses 68 to 71. Poliovirus is the causative agent of paralytic poliomyelitis. Coxsackieviruses cause numerous human diseases, including myocarditis. Echoviruses are reported to lead to encephalomyelitis and aseptic meningitis. Enterovirus 70 infection results in predominantly acute hemorrhagic conjunctivitis. In addition, rhinovirus infection causes the common cold, and hepatovirus infection (hepatitis A) causes acute hepatitis. A strain of encephalomyocarditis virus (EMCV), a cardiovirus, induces diabetes-like symptoms in mice and the aphthovirus foot-and-mouth disease virus (FMDV) causes debilitating inflammation of the cartilaginous tissue of the hooves and mouths of domesticated cattle.

B. THE GENOME

Picornaviruses have been grouped together predominantly on the basis of their striking similarities in genome organization, protein processing, and replication pathways.[13] Picornavirus genomes are single-stranded RNAs of plus strand polarity covalently linked at the 5′ end to a small protein, VPg, and polyadenylated at the 3′ end. These genomes are very compact, containing only some 8000 nucleotides (nt). This limiting size is likely in response to the selective pressure exerted by the lack of fidelity of the virally encoded RNA polymerase $3D^{pol}$ (mutation rate is approximately 1 in 10,000 bases), and the absence of proof-reading and editing functions.[4] The genome encodes only a single open reading frame coding for a polyprotein, 220 kDa in the case of the prototype, poliovirus. The N terminus of the poliovirus polyprotein specifies P1, the precursor of the capsid proteins. This region is followed by P2 and P3, the precursors of the nonstructural viral proteins. $2A^{pro}$, mapping to the N terminus of P2, cleaves cotranslationally at a tyrosine-glycine amino acid pair, releasing P1. The capsid precursor is subsequently processed at glutamine-glycine amino acid pairs by the virally encoded proteinase $3CD^{pro}$ to produce the capsid proteins VP0, VP1, and VP3.[14] The nonstructural proteins necessary for viral genome replication are also cleaved by $3CD^{pro}$ or by its cleavage product $3C^{pro}$[15] (Figure 1).

The 5′ terminus of the RNA is covalently linked to a small basic protein of 22 amino acids called VPg by a phosphodiester bond between the hydroxyl group of a tyrosine and the 5′-terminal uridylate residue.[16,17] The first step in RNA replication involves the copying of the genomic RNA to produce a complementary strand of negative polarity. This reaction is believed to be catalyzed by the RNA-dependent RNA polymerase, $3D^{pol}$, which is able to elongate RNA chains in vitro.[18] In the next step, the newly made minus strands serve as templates for the synthesis of product genomic RNAs. In addition to $3D^{pol}$, a number of viral proteins and their precursors (2B, 2C, 2BC, 3C, 3CD, 3D) and possibly some cellular proteins have also been implicated in RNA replication, but their exact roles are not yet understood. Some proteins of the P2 region (2C, 2BC), have been proposed to have a function in the formation of membranous replication complexes.[19] Proteinase 3C and its precursor 3CD were found to bind to the 5′ nontranstated region (NTR) and to be involved in plus strand RNA replication.[20] Finally, VPg and possibly 3AB were proposed to function as a primer in the initiation of RNA replication.[21,22] An alternative mechanism for the initiation of RNA replication was suggested by Tobin and

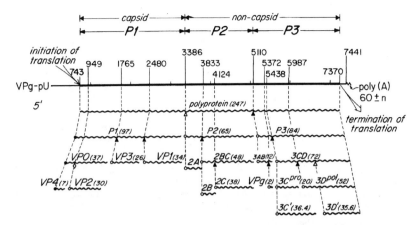

Figure 1 Gene organization and polyprotein processing of poliovirus. Virion RNA, terminated at the 5′ end with the genome-linked protein VPg and at the 3′ end with poly(A), is shown as a solid line, with the translated region more pronounced than the noncoding regions. The numbers above the virion RNA refer to the first nucleotide coden specifying the N-terminal amino acid for the virus specific proteins. The coding region has been divided into three regions (P1, P2, and P3), corresponding to rapid cleavages of the polyprotein. Numbers in parentheses are calculated molecular mass in kDa. Open circles indicate that the terminal amino acid has been experimentally determined. The N terminus is glycine in regions except for VP2, where it is serine. The C-terminal amino acid of protein 3D is phenylalanine. Filled circles indicate that the N termini are known to be blocked. Filled triangles correspond to Gln-Gly pairs that are cleaved during proteolytic processing of a polyprotein by the virally encoded proteinase 3CD (or 3C). Open triangles correspond to Tyr-Gly pairs cleaved by viral proteinase 2A. The open diamond corresponds to an Asn-Ser pair cleaved only during morphogenesis. The polypeptides 3C′ and 3D′ are products of alternative cleavage whose biological significance is unknown. (From Nomoto, A. and Wimmer, E., in *Molecular Basis of Virus Disease,* Russel, M. C. and Almond, J. W., Eds., Soc. Gen. Microbiol. Symp., Vol. 40, Cambridge University Press, 1987, 107. With permission.)

co-workers, in which a hairpin formed at the 3′ end of the RNA is cleaved by VPg, becoming covalently attached to the RNA.[23]

Despite their genetic austerity, all picornavirus genomes contain very long 5′ NTRs, which occupy as much as 10% of the total RNA. Located within this region are highly structured segments of RNA approximately 400 nt in length. These segments, "internal ribosome entry sites" (IRES),[24] are located downstream of the 5′ termini and confer both cap and 5′ end independent translation to the picornaviral RNAs. On the basis of their nucleotide sequences and proposed secondary structures, picornavirus IRES elements have been divided into two types. The entero- and rhinoviruses belong to type I and cardio- and aphthoviruses to group II. Indeed, except for a common Yn-Xm-AUG motif, these types share no structural similarities; yet, surprisingly, they function in an identical fashion.[4,24]

C. THE VIRION

The poliovirion is a small, non-enveloped, icosahedral particle (5:3:2), measuring approximately 30 nm in diameter. Surrounding the genomic RNA core is a isometric protein shell built of 60 protomers, each of which is, in turn, composed of a single copy of the four capsid proteins, VP1-4. The three largest subunits of the protomer, VP1, 2, and 3, are positioned on the surface of the capsid, whereas VP4, the smallest subunit, is located on the interior surface of the capsid.[5] The most striking feature of VP1, 2, and 3, as revealed by X-ray crystallography, is that they have an essentially identical tertiary structure, i.e., they form an eight-stranded, antiparallel beta barrel with a wedge-like shape.[5] This similarity is surprising, considering that the amino acid sequences of these proteins are largely dissimilar. In the virion, wedge-shaped proteins assemble into a tightly bound protein shell. The narrow point of the VP1 wedge is located near the virion's five-fold axes of symmetry, while those of VP2 and VP3 alternate around the three-fold axes. The beta sheets are linked to each other by protruding loops which form much of the surface features of the virion.[5,25] The wedge-shaped folding pattern of poliovirus capsid proteins VP1, 2 and 3 is similar to those of the capsid proteins of many other icosahedral RNA viruses, including those of plant RNA viruses.[26,27] Another well defined feature of the poliovirion is the presence of deep clefts around each of the 12 five-fold axes of symmetry. A similar structure on the surface of rhinovirus, termed the canyon, has been proposed to be the binding site of its cellular receptor, the intercellular adhesion molecule 1 (ICAM-1).[28-30]

D. REPLICATION AND PATHOGENESIS

The early events of the poliovirus life cycle include receptor binding, cellular penetration, and viral uncoating. The poliovirus receptor (PVR) has recently been identified as a member of the immunoglobin superfamily.[31] PVR expression is limited to a small number of tissues in primates such as the Peyer's patches in the ileum, and motor neurons in the brain and spinal cord, although PVR mRNA is detected in a wide range of tissues including kidney.[31,32] The process of receptor binding and subsequent cellular internalization induces an irreversible transition in the viral capsid, giving rise to the formation of altered particles (A-particles).[33,34] A-particles are believed to be intermediates during the penetration of poliovirus through the cell membrane. The viral RNA is then released from the capsid into the cytoplasm by an unknown mechanism. The uncoated viral RNA, which lacks the 5' end cap and possesses an IRES element within the 5' nontranslated region, is then translated in a cap and 5' end independent manner. The newly synthesized viral polyprotein is processed by the virally encoded proteinases, releasing the functional viral proteins. The minus-strand RNA synthesis is carried out by the viral proteins and probably some cellular protein factors, using the viral RNA as template. At this point, a massive process of viral protein synthesis and RNA replication takes place. During the final stage of the virus life cycle, the newly synthesized viral structural proteins and the positive-stranded viral RNA are assembled, producing progeny virion which are released via the virus-induced cell lysis[35] (Figure 2).

Poliovirus enters the host via the enteral route. Uptake into cells of the intestinal mucosa occurs most likely in ileal microfold (M)-cells[36] which could provide a portal of entry for invading virions into adjacent lymphocytic components of intestinal lymphatic structures underlying the mucosal lining. Initial poliovirus replication takes place in pharyngeal lymph nodes and ileal Peyer's patches. Less clear are the pathogenic steps extending viral spread from primary propagation in lymphatic cells to viremia and into the central nervous system (CNS). Viral entry (1) into peripheral motorneuronal axons with following retrograde axonal transport,[37] (2) through the endothelial linings of cerebral capillaries,[38] or (3) across the blood brain barrier via infected macrophages[39] could be possible mechanisms of viral penetration into the CNS. The histopathological hallmarks of polioviral damage in the CNS are selective destruction of motorneuronal elements along the entire neuraxis and reactive lymphocytic infiltration, microglial proliferation, and terminal gliosis in affected areas.

E. THE POLIOVACCINES

The development of both the IPV and OPV vaccines became possible with successful replication of all three serotypes of poliovirus in cultured primate cells of nonneural

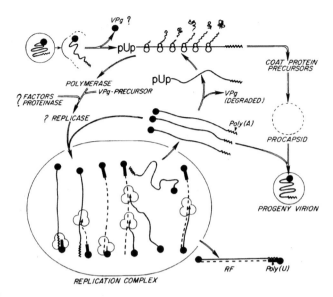

Figure 2 An overview of poliovirus life cycle. Poliovirus binds to its cellular receptor (PVR) and enters the cell probably by receptor-mediated endocytosis. The viral RNA, uncoated and released into the cytoplasm, functions as a messenger RNA for viral polyprotein translation and then as a template for viral RNA replication. The nonstructural viral proteins and possibly some host factors are involved in the RNA replication. The RNA replication complex is membrane bound, and different forms of RNA (RI, RF, and ssRNA) are found associated with this complex. Multicycled protein translation and RNA replication results in an accumulation of viral capsid proteins as well as the genomic RNA, which are assembled into progeny virions during the late stage of poliovirus life cycle, and are released during cell lysis. (Modified after Reference 98.)

origin.[40] The formalin-inactivated vaccine developed by Salk (1954)[9] became available for widespread use slightly before tests of the attenuated virus vaccine were completed.[10]

All three serotypes of attenuated OPV were obtained after multiple passages of the respective virus serotype in simian cell cultures of different origin. Empirical data showed that neurovirulence of the attenuated strains in primates is according to the "neurovirulence score", composed of characteristics of viral replication efficiency and pathogenicity. Neuropathogenetic potential after intraspinal or intracerebral application in cynomolgus monkeys, temperature sensitivity (the RCT marker, reproductive capacity at supraoptimal temperature) and the "d" marker (delayed growth under agar) are valuable parameters to assess neurovirulence of attenuated strains.

Despite its extensive use in the years from 1955 till 1962, the IPV was gradually replaced by the OPV in most countries. The fierce discussion on comparative effectiveness of both vaccines has led to the awareness that both vaccines are highly effective in preventing poliomyelitis. IPV was reported to be less efficient to induce a strong and durable immune response, yet was effective in mass immunization campaigns regarding protection from paralytic poliomyelitis. IPV has the disadvantage of requiring subcutaneous injection, reducing its usefulness in areas with underdeveloped health care systems, due to the limited availability of sterilized, disposable material. However, subcutaneous application reduces the risk of impaired gastrointestinal implantation of the OPV and consequent failing protection in the presence of highly prevalent intercurrent gastrointestinal disease in these countries. The improved thermostability of IPV over OPV facilitates its use in regions with underdeveloped infrastructure. The advantages of OPV are its highly immunogenic potential, due to efficient viral replication in the gut without spread to the CNS, the continuous spread of excreted attenuated virus to nonvaccinated individuals ("herd effect"), and particularly the easy way of oral administration. Of particular importance is the risk of vaccine-related paralytic disease, caused by OPV revertants. Although extremely rare, the possibility of vaccine-induced neuronal damage dictates continuous efforts towards safety improvement of available attenuated vaccines. Reported poliomyelitis in vaccinated patients due to revertants of an attenuated strain was most commonly due to reversal of the type 3/Sabin attenuated phenotype, explainable by the relatively few attenuating changes in the genotype of this strain.[41,42] Administration of the live vaccine to children with hereditary immunodeficiencies has led in very rare instances to induction of paralytic disease. In addition, there are recent cases of poliomyelitis from unvaccinated contact.

Ongoing research efforts have contributed to the elucidation of the determinants of neurovirulence attenuation, although a complete picture of the molecular basis of this complex and multifactorial phenomenon could not be drawn. The determination of the complete nucleotide sequences of the attenuated strains identified differences from their neurovirulent progenitors. Site-directed mutagenesis of potentially attenuating substitutions and following assessment of neurovirulence led to the isolation of mutations conferring the attenuated phenotype.

Attenuated P3/Sabin and neurovirulent P3/Leon differ by 11 base substitutions.[43,44] Mutations, scattered throughout the genome, did not equally contribute to attenuation of neurovirulence. Nucleotide changes at positions 472 and 2034 [45] and 2493[44] proved to cause the major part of phenotypic change.

The neurovirulent parent of P2/Sabin, P712, possessed reduced monkey intraspinal neurovirulence, rendering nucleotide sequence comparisons less revealing. Analysis of a vaccine-associated poliomyelitis field isolate, P2/117, differs from P2/Sabin at 23 bases,[46] two of which, at positions 481 and 2903, respectively, determine neurovirulence attenuation.[47]

The nucleotide sequences of attenuated P1/Sabin indicated that it differed by 55 nucleotide substitutions from its neurovirulent parent P1/Mahoney.[41,48] Reversion to the neurovirulent phenotype could be accomplished by reverting substitutions at positions 480, 6203, and one at the extreme 3' end of the genome.

Neurovirulence-determining mutations in all three serotypes were located in the 5' noncoding region of the genome (position 472 in P3/Sabin, 481 in P2/Sabin, and 480 in P1/Sabin). Clustering of these critical substitutions in a region known to be part of the IRES could affect cap-independent translation by altering the secondary structure of elements in the 5' noncoding region.

Mutation at position 2034 in P3/Sabin maps to the capsid protein VP3. The location of this residue in a protomer interface is responsible for the defective assembly of protomers during morphogenesis of this attenuated strain.[49]

III. ANTIGENIC HYBRIDS OF POLIOVIRUS

A. ANTIGENIC STRUCTURE OF POLIOVIRUS

Poliovirus exists in nature in three distinct serotypes (PV1, 2, and 3). Neutralizing antibodies raised against one serotype are usually incapable of neutralizing the viruses of the other two serotypes. The antigenic structure of these three serotypes of polioviruses is generally identical. It has been defined that regions of the poliovirus capsid capable of inducing and binding neutralizing antibodies were neutralization antigenic (N-Ag) sites. Four such sites (N-AgI, II, IIIA, and IIIB; Figure 3) have been mapped to the virion

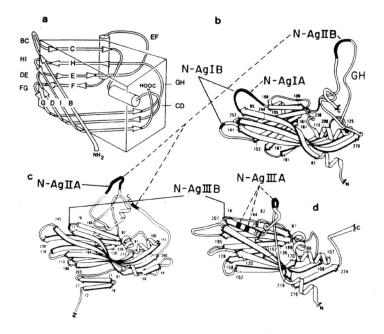

Figure 3 Schematic representation of the tertiary and antigenic structure of the poliovirus capsid proteins. (a) Folding pattern of the polypeptide chain in the core of VP1, 2, and 3. The three viral capsid proteins have a common structure motif, an eight-stranded, antiparallel beta barrel in a wedge-like shape. (b) through (d) Ribbon drawing of the topology of VP1-3. There are four neutralizing antigenic sites (N-Ags), namely, N-AgI, II, IIIA, and IIIB mapped to the beta strands of the capsid proteins on the virion surface. N-AgI and N-AgII can be further divided into N-AgIA, N-AgIB and N-AgIIA, N-AgIIB, respectively. Most of the N-Ags are discontinuous, although some are continuous (e.g., N-Ag IA). N-Ag IA and N-Ag IIA have been targeted for the construction of antigenic hybrids.

surface.[50,51] Most of the N-Ags map to the loops between the beta strands of the capsid proteins. The identification of the N-Ags was largely accomplished by sequence analyses of neutralizing escape mutants selected with various neutralizing monoclonal antibodies.[41] Most neutralization antigenic sites are formed by discontinuous sequences of the capsid proteins although some are continuous (e.g., N-AgIA). In addition, the contributions of linear epitopes were determined through the construction of hybrid polioviruses whose linear epitope(s) were exchanged with those of other serotypes. Finally, the overall antigenic structure of poliovirus was elucidated upon the solution of its three-dimensional structure.[5]

The N-AgI site, which can be divided into N-AgIA and N-AgIB, is a dominant immunogenic determinant for both the type 2 and type 3 viruses.[51] N-AgIA consists of a linear amino acid sequence spanning residues 1091 to 1104 formed by the BC-loop between beta sheets B and C of VP1. (We use a four-digit nomenclature for the amino acids, in which the first digit describes the capsid protein and the next three digits describe the amino acid position within the protein; thus 1091 represents the residue at position 91 of VP1.) N-AgIB includes residues from both the BC and DE loops of VP1. In the case of PV3, residues from the EF and GH loops may participate in N-AgIB also.[51,52] N-AgII is composed of N-AgIIA and IIB. N-AgIIA contains a linear sequence of 2164 to 2172 (the loop connecting beta sheets E and F of VP2) as well as residue 2270.[51,53] N-AgIIB includes sequences 1220 to 1226. N-AgIII is a complex site, being composed of two independent sites, IIIA and IIIB.[51,54] The IIIA site consists of residues 3058 to 3060, 3071 to 3073, and the IIIB site of residues 3076 to 3079 as well as 2072 (Figure 3).

B. INTERTYPIC HYBRIDS

There are three antigenically distinct serotypes of polioviruses. It is of interest to investigate, by the hybrid virus approach, what amino acids in the neutralizing antigenic loops determine type specificity, and to what extent amino acids of the loops can be modified without losing viability of the virus. In addition, the hybrid virus study can also be the basis of the development of multivalent picornavirus vaccines. The linear antigenic determinants, such as N-AgIA, the BC-loop of VP1 (1BC) and N-AgIIA, the EF-loop of VP2 (2EF), have been chosen as the target sequences for the modification, or for the exchange of entire neutralization antigenic sites.[50,55-58]

The successful construction of an antigenic poliovirus hybrid was reported by Murray et al.,[56] who created a mutagenesis cartridge using a naturally occurring as well as an artificially introduced restriction site surrounding N-AgIA in the infectious cDNA clone of PV1, strain Mahoney (PV1[M]). The resultant hybrids virus (W1/3-1D-1), in which N-AgIA (residues 1088 to 1102) of PV1(M) were exchanged with that of PV3, strain Leon (PV3[Le]), was impaired in its growth, but was not temperature sensitive. W1/3-1D-1 was neutralizable by polyclonal anti-PV1 and anti-PV3 antibodies as well as by a neutralizing monoclonal antibody specific for N-AgIA of PV3(Le). In addition, the virus was resistant to a neutralizing monoclonal N-AgIA antibody of PV1(M) as well as polyclonal anti-PV2 antibodies. Furthermore, this virus induced a strong neutralizing response to PV1, and a significant neutralizing response to PV3 in immunized rabbits or monkeys. Thus, in the context of the PV1(M) sequence, the inserted PV3(Le) N-AgIA site is expressed in a conformation which allows for an interaction with neutralizing antibodies as well as for the induction of neutralizing antibodies in rodents or primates.

In an independent study, Burke et al.[57] constructed a similar hybrid (S1/3.10) in which N-AgIA (residues 1095 to 1102) of PV1(S) was replaced with the corresponding sequence of PV3, strain 3.370, via oligonucleotide-directed mutagenesis. The resulting virus interacted with polyclonal antibodies against either PV1 or PV3 as well as panels of anti-PV3 and anti-PV1 monoclonal antibodies. In addition, this virus elicited antibodies against both PV1 and PV3 in immunized rabbits and mice. A similar immune response was observed when the hybrid was orally administered to a cynomolgus monkey.[57] These results demonstrated that the attenuated vaccine strain of poliovirus was able to tolerate significant modification.

A type 1/type 2 hybrid poliovirus was constructed independently by two different groups, using the N-AgIA mutagenesis cartridge.[55,58] The resulting virus (designated W1/2-1D-1 and v510, respectively) in which the 1BC loop of PV1(M) was replaced by that of PV2, strain Lansing (PV2[L]), grew almost as well as the parental strain. In addition, the virus exhibited the expected serological properties. For example, it was neutralizable by PV1- and PV2-specific antisera and it elicited neutralizing antibodies to both PV1 and PV2 in rabbits. This virus was of particular interest with regards to the mouse-neurovirulence phenotype of PV2(L). It is well documented that some strains of PV2 are able to grow in the CNS of mice, causing a paralytic disease resembling poliomyelitis.[59] It is not clear why the mouse is susceptible to certain strains of PV2, but resistant to PV1 and PV3. Most likely PV2(L) can use a receptor to infect the mouse neural cells that PV1 and PV3 polioviruses do not recognize. Using a genetic approach, the mouse neurovirulence phenotype of PV2(L) has been mapped to the capsid protein VP1, with the particular involvement of the N-AgIA loop.[60] Using the type 1/type 2 hybrid previously described,

Martin et al.[58] and Murray et al.[55] identified a short amino acid sequence within the N-AgIA loop responsible for the mouse-adapted phenotype of PV2(L). The crystal structure of hybrid v510, recently determined at 2.6Å resolution, has revealed major structural alterations in this hybrid, when compared to the parental PV1(M).[61] These alterations involve not only the substituted BC loop (residues 1093 to 1104), but also the adjacent HI (residues 1244 to 1252) and DE loop (residues 1141 to 1153) of VP1. Mutational analysis of the mouse-neurovirulence determinants of this hybrid virus has demonstrated that the residues determining the conformation of the 1BC loop were important for the mouse-adapted phenotype of PV2(L).[62]

In further studies, the 1BC loop of PV1(M) was replaced by a combined "1BC loop", which contained either partial or entire sequences of 1BC from both PV2(L) and PV3(Le), thereby generating potentially trivalent poliovirus hybrids.[63] Four such hybrids were constructed, two of which had a normal length 1BC loop originated from 1BC of both PV2(L) and PV3(Le) (designated W1/2/3-1D-23 and -32, respectively), the other two had an extended "1BC loop" which included the entire 1BC loop from both PV2(L) and PV3(Le) (designated W1/2/3-1D-23FL and -32FL, respectively). All four yielded viable viruses, but when tested for their ability to react with, as well as their ability to induce type-specific antibodies, none were serologically trivalent. However, W1/2/3-1D-23, the hybrid containing a normal length 1BC loop with PV2(L) sequences on the left side and the PV3(Le) sequences on the right, did induce a significant anti-PV2 response in immunized rabbits. These data indicated that the immunogenic property of an inserted sequence depends not only on its location on the capsid, but also on its sequence, size, and conformation.

Through peptide mapping and monoclonal antibody selection, it has been found that the EF loop of VP2, a linear sequence containing residues 2164 to 2172, functions as an independent antigenic determinant.[64,65] This sequence, designated N-AgIIA, has been used to construct a second mutagenesis cartridge. Two unique restriction sites flanking the sequences encoding N-AgIIA were introduced, which allowed for the manipulation of part of N-AgIIA (residues 2158 to 2173) by sequence replacement with synthetic oligonucleotides. A type 1/type 2 hybrid virus was constructed in this manner, in which N-AgIIA from PV2(L) was substituted for the corresponding sequence of PV1(M).[50] The resulting virus, W1/2-1B-NII2/2/2, was impaired in its growth characteristics when compared to its wild-type parent PV1(M) and displayed the small plaque phenotype characteristic of most of the poliovirus hybrids. The N-AgIIA site of PV2(L), expressed on the surface of the hybrid, was weakly reactive with rabbit anti-PV2 antisera, an observation consistent with a previous report indicating that N-AgIIA was not a dominant antigenic site in PV2 and PV3 in rodents. However, this same hybrid induced a significant neutralizing immune response when injected into rabbits, which is in contrast to the case of another hybrid which expressed the same 2EF sequence of PV2(L) through replacement of the 1BC loop of PV1(M). The 2EF sequence transplanted to the 1BC position was neither neutralizable by anti-PV2 antibodies, nor able to elicit PV2-specific neutralizing antibodies.[66] Analyses of hybrid W1/2-1B- NII2/2/2 confirmed that the 2EF loop was a neutralization antigenic determinant in its own right. These data demonstrated that the location of a heterologous antigenic determinant on a hybrid poliovirus capsid strongly affects the immunological properties of that determinant.

The construction of the two mutagenesis cartridges, which included N-AgIA and N-AgIIA, makes it possible to construct multivalent hybrids by the simultaneous modification of both sites. Two trivalent hybrids, W1/2/3-1B/1D-3V1 and -3V2, respectively, were generated in this fashion.[63,67] In W1/2/3-1B/1D-3V1, N-AgIA of PV3(Le) and N-AgIIA of PV2(L) replaced the corresponding antigenic sites of PV1(M). In -3V2, N-AgIA was derived from PV2(L) and N-AgIIA from PV3(Le). Both of the viruses were growth impaired when compared to their wild-type parent, but no more so than those hybrids singly modified at either N-AgIA or N-AgIIA. In addition, both viruses are neutralizable by antisera against all three poliovirus serotypes, indicating proper presentation of the inserts on the hybrid virions. Hybrid W1/2/3-1B/1D-3V1 induced neutralizing antibodies to all three serotypes, although the neutralizing activity induced by the PV2(L) determinant in 2EF loop was weak. Hybrid -3V2 induced neutralizing antibodies to PV1(M) and PV2(L), but not PV3(Le), which suggested that the PV3(Le) determinant expressed in the 2EF loop was not immunogenic. Although the overall antigenicity and immunogenicity of the foreign antigens expressed in 2EF of the hybrids were weak, it demonstrated that both N-AgIA and N-AgIIA could be simultaneously manipulated to express independent, heterologous antigenic sequences.

In conclusion, the successful construction of intertypic poliovirus hybrids provides a useful means of testing poliovirus antigenicity and biological properties. However, most intertypic poliovirus hybrids grow poorly and induce insufficient antibody titers against foreign antigens that it is questionable that these agents will replace the existing poliovirus vaccines. In order for this type of hybrid viruses to serve as a vaccine, the growth property of the hybrids as well as the antigen presentation by the hybrids would have to be improved, two parameters of which the molecular biology and cell biology are not understood.

C. HYBRIDS EXPRESSING ANTIGENS FROM OTHER PICORNAVIRUSES

The atomic structures of various representative picornaviruses have been elucidated, including that of human rhinovirus, poliovirus, Mengovirus, and foot-and-mouth disease virus (FMDV).[5,68-70] The capsids of these viruses share extensive structural similarities, differing mainly in the loops linking the conserved beta barrel cores. In the case of poliovirus, rhinovirus, and FMDV, the antigenic sites within the loops have been mapped largely by sequence analyses of neutralization escape mutants selected by neutralizing monoclonal antibodies. The detailed knowledge of virion architecture as well as the antigenic structure of different picornaviruses has allowed for the construction of hybrid polioviruses which expressed antigens of other picornaviruses, such as FMDV, human rhinovirus, and hepatitis A virus.

Kitson et al. have constructed a number of PV1(S) hybrids which expressed different antigenic determinants of FMDV.[71] FMDV, the member of the genus Aphthovirus, causes severe inflammation of the hooves and mouths of cattle and therefore is of great economic importance to the livestock industry. The genus Aphthovirus is divided into seven distinct FMDV serotypes, among which the type O viruses are relatively well defined in terms of their antigenic structure.[42] The antigenic determinants from type O strain O1Kaufbeuren (O1K) of FMDV, which contains four independent antigenic sites, were used to construct PV/FMDV hybrids. Site 1, the major antigenic site of the O1K strain, includes residues 140 to 160 (the large loop connecting the beta strands G and H of VP1) and the C-terminal residues 200 to 213 of VP1, site 2 maps mainly to residues 70 to 77 of VP2 (the loop linking the beta strands B and C of VP2). Site 3 is located at VP1 residues 43 to 45 (the loop between the beta strands B and C of VP1), and site 4 is composed of residues 56 to 58 of VP3. Five PV/FMDV hybrids were constructed using the previously described N-AgIA mutagenesis cartridge.[71] Hybrids O1.1, O1.2, and O1.3, which contain the N-terminal portion (residues 141 to 154), central portion (residues 147 to 156), or the entire 1GH loop (residues 141 to 160) of VP1, respectively, yielded viable viruses that were slightly impaired in their growth characteristics when compared to the parental PV1(S) strain. These hybrids were tested by neutralization and immune diffusion assays, using polyclonal anti-O1K serum, antipeptide (residues 140 to 160) serum, and a panel of mcAbs specific for site 1 of O1K. Hybrid O1.1 was weakly neutralizable by the polyclonal anti-O1K serum, but not by the antipeptide serum or by any of the monoclonal antibodies (mcAbs). Hybrid O1.2 failed to react with any of the mcAbs or antisera. In contrast, hybrid O1.3, which contained the entire 1GH loop of O1K, was efficiently neutralized by mcAbs B2, D7, and 13DB as well as the anti-O1K serum. It was also weakly neutralized by antipeptide serum as well as mcAbs D9 and 13DD. Hybrid O3.1, in which the PV1(S) N-AgIA site was replaced by site 3 (residues 40 to 49 of VP1) of O1K, could not be neutralized by either polyclonal anti-O1K serum or O1k site 3-specific mcAbs. Hybrid A1C.1, in which N-AgIA of PV1(S) was exchanged with the C terminus of VP1 of the type A10 FMDV, was not viable. These data indicated that the entire 1GH loop was required for immunogenicity in the hybrids viruses. The FMDV sequence expressed on the O1.3 capsid retains some, but not all of its reactivity with its mcAbs, which suggested that the conformation of the loop expressed by the hybrid was similar but not identical to that expressed by FMDV. The antigenicity of O3.1 confirmed that FMDV site 3, the equivalent to the N-AgIA site of poliovirus, was not a dominant antigenic site of the O1k strain of FMDV.

The immunogenicity of the PV/FMDV hybrids were examined for their ability to elicit FMDV-specific neutralizing antibodies in guinea pigs. Hybrids O3.1 (containing the entire 1GH loop of O1K) and O3.1 (containing the entire site 3 of O1K) induced site-specific FMDV neutralizing antibodies. Interestingly, when the immunized guinea pigs were challenged with O1K strain of FMDV, the animals with highest level of prechallenge anti-FMDV neutralizing antibodies were protected.

The human rhinovirus genus is composed of more than 100 antigenically distinct serotypes. Human rhinovirus 14 (HRV14), whose crystal structure has been elucidated,[68] displays four independent neutralizing immunogenic (NIm) sites, namely, NImIA, IB, NImII and NImIII. The NImIA site of HRV14 is equivalent to the NAgIA site of poliovirus and, as in poliovirus, is clustered around the five-fold axes of symmetry of the virion. A poliovirus/rhinovirus hybrid has been constructed by replacing the NAgIA of PV1(M) with NImIA of HRV14.[72] This virus, designated W1/HRV14-1D-NImIA (referred here as W1/HRV14), was characterized for its reactivity with neutralizing antibodies against either PV1(M) or HRV14, as well as its ability to induce anti-PV1 and anti-HRV14 neutralizing antibodies in rodents. Both anti-HRV14 and anti-PV1 antisera neutralized W1/HRV14, an observation indicating that the HRV14 NImIA sequence expressed in the hybrid virion retained at least part of the natural conformation usually formed on the HRV14 capsid. Among the five NImIA-specific monoclonal antibodies tested, three (mcAb 1, 20, and 34) were capable of neutralizing W1/HRV14, although the activity was reduced in comparison to their abilities to neutralize HRV14. Two mcAbs (4 and 17) failed to neutralize the hybrid, which suggested a structural divergence existed between the NImIA sequence expressed by W1/HRV14 and that by HRV14. Upon injection into rabbits, W1/HRV14 induced a neutralizing antibody response against both PV1(M) and HRV14, a substantial proportion of which was raised against the HRV14 sequences in W1/HRV14. However, only a small percentage of these antibodies were able to neutralize HRV14, which again suggested that the hybrid had expressed the NImIA sequences in a conformation that differed from that of HRV14. It is possible therefore, that the amino acids surrounding the NImIA site in HRV14 may be necessary for the accurate formation of this antigenic site.

A number of monoclonal antibodies raised against the NImIA site of HRV14 were able to inhibit the binding of the virus to its cellular receptor, ICAM-1, which resulted in neutralization of the virus.[73] These mcAbs were tested for their ability to neutralize W1/HRV14 through the inhibition of the virus interaction with the cellular receptor for poliovirus (PVR). The NImIA-specific mcAbs 1, 20, and 34 did in fact inhibit the binding of W1/HRV14 to PVR. In addition, polyclonal antiserum raised against HRV14, which only recognized the inserted NImIA sequence on W1/HRV14, also blocked the interaction of W1/HRV14 with PVR. Mutagenesis as well as cryoelectron microscopic studies have shown that the rhinovirus canyon, a depressed structure surrounding the five-fold axis of symmetry of the virion, was the binding site for its cellular receptor.[29,30] In the case of poliovirus, however, there is no evidence to suggest that the poliovirus canyon is directly involved in receptor binding. According to the three-dimensional structure of rhinovirus and poliovirus, NImIA and N-AgIA are both located in the BC loop of VP1, close to the canyon of both capsids. In view of the data gained from the study of Altermeyer et al.,[72] namely, that antibodies bound to the NImIA site on W1/HRV14 inhibited the binding of the virus to the cellular receptor for poliovirus and that these antibodies reacted with NImIA to inhibit HRV14 binding to the cellular receptor for HRV14, it was reasonable to conclude that the interaction of poliovirus and rhinovirus with their respective cellular receptors was similar at the molecular level.

Several groups have tried to construct hybrid polioviruses expressing antigenic determinants from hepatitis A virus (HAV). The sole member of the genus Hepatovirus, HAV infection is a serious medical problem in the world due to the lack of an effective anti-HAV vaccine. It was of great interest, therefore, to test whether a vaccine against HAV could be generated through the construction of PV/HAV hybrid viruses. One such construct (W1/HAV-1D-1) was generated in which N-AgIA of PV1(M) was replaced with the corresponding sequence of HAV. The hybrids virus exhibited a small plaque phenotype as well as restricted growth capacity. Unfortunately, this virus could not be neutralized by anti-HAV hyperimmune sera derived from chimpanzees.[74,75] Similarly, negative results were obtained from constructs containing different HAV sequences. Sverdlov et al.[76] reported on the construction of PV1(S)/HAV hybrids generated by means of oligonucleotide-directed mutagenesis. Two presumptive antigenic sites, located at residues 103 through 106 of HAV VP1 and residues 67 through 75 of HAV VP3, respectively, were used separately to substitute for the N-AgIA residues of PV1(S). Both constructs produced viable virus, although their antigenicity and immunogenicity has yet to be tested.[76] Considering that the exact antigenic structure of HAV has not been determined and that HAV antigenic sites appear to be more dependent than those of other picornaviruses on the structural integrity of the virion, it is less likely that HAV vaccine can be generated by this approach at present time.

The hybrid virus strategy has been used to identify a serotype-specific antigenic site of coxsackievirus B4 (CVB4).[77] Belonging to the enterovirus genus of the picornaviridae family, coxsackieviruses are a group of important human pathogens causing a variety of diseases including minor common cold, fatal myocarditis, and neurological disorders. In contrast to the case of poliovirus, little is known about the antigenic structure of coxsackieviruses. Based on the high homology in tertiary structure among the picornaviruses and the degree of sequence identity between coxsackieviruses and polioviruses, it is assumed that the capsid structure of coxsackieviruses is similar to that of polioviruses and that the homologous surface loops contribute to antigenic sites. To test if the hybrid virus strategy can be used to map neutralizing antigenic sites of coxsackieviruses, Kandolf's group constructed a hybrid virus between two different serotypes of coxsackieviruses, i.e., coxsackievirus B3 (CVB3) and CVB4.[77] The hybrid virus was engineered by inserting five amino acids of the putative BC loop of the capsid protein VP1 of CVB4 into the corresponding loop of CVB3 via site-directed mutagenesis of an infectious CVB3 cDNA clone. The resulting hybrid virus, designated CVB3/4, was found to be neutralized and precipitated by both CVB3- and CVB4-specific polyclonal antisera. In addition, CVB3/4 induced antibodies in rabbits which were capable of neutralizing CVB4 as well as CVB3. The hybrid virus exhibited a small-plaque phenotype, an observation indicating that the insertion of the CVB4 specific sequence into the CVB3 capsid protein impaired the viral replication. Interestingly, continued passaging of this hybrid virus resulted in an accumulation of variants with a large plaque phenotype. Sequence analysis of these large plaque variants demonstrated that the inserted sequence is stable and the occurrence of large plaque variants is not due to reversion, an observation suggesting there could be spontaneous mutation(s) in other loci of the viral genome which may improve the growth of the hybrid coxsackievirus.

D. HYBRIDS EXPRESSING ANTIGENS UNRELATED TO PICORNAVIRUSES

A number of hybrid polioviruses have been constructed in which the N-Ag1A site was either interrupted by the insertion of unrelated peptides or was replaced with antigens from pathogens unrelated to picornaviruses.

In an attempt to examine whether the N-Ag1A site of poliovirus was capable of accommodating foreign sequences, Colbere-Garapin and co-workers constructed several insertion mutants through the addition of either tri- or hexapeptides located between residues 1100 and 1101 of PV3(S).[78] Of the three recovered insertion mutants, vFG68 (Asn-Lys-Arg insertion) displayed a plaque phenotype almost identical to that of parental PV3(S) strain. The vFG27 (Leu-Phe-Arg insertion) and vFG13 (Asn-Glu-Arg-Leu-Phe-Arg insertion) mutants on the other hand, produced significantly smaller plaques. None of these enlarged N-Ag1A sites reacted with the PV3(S) N-Ag1A specific-mcAb. vFG68 was highly immunogenic even after the virions were converted from D- to C-particles[79] by brief heat treatment, inducing neutralizing antibodies specific for native vFG68. This observation implied that the enlarged N-Ag1A site functioned as a new neutralization antigenic site that was less rigid than the native site.

Mirzayan et al. reported on the construction of two poliovirus mutants, designated W1-1D-BC1 and -BC2, in which a poliovirus proteinase 3C (3C^{pro}) cleavage site was inserted into the BC loop of VP1.[80] W1-1D-BC1, in which a four-amino acid sequence containing the 3C^{pro} site (Gln*Gly-Pro-Gly; * indicates the cleavage site) substituted for residues 1099 to 1102 of 1BC, was resistant to 3C^{pro} cleavage both *in vivo* and *in vitro*. Considering that W1-1D-BC1 had a 3C^{pro} site (Gln*Gly) located at exactly the same position as the trypsin cleavage site in PV1(S), and that a peptide corresponding to the inserted site could be cleaved by 3C^{pro}, the resistance of W1-1D-BC1 to 3C^{pro} cleavage implied that a structural constraint had been introduced into the mutated 1BC loop. W1-1D-BC2, in which nine amino acids (Gly-Tyr-Ala-Lys-Val-Gln*Gly-Pro-Gly; * is the 3C^{pro} cleavage site) replaced a single threonine residue at position 1099 of the 1BC loop of VP1, was also examined *in vivo* and *in vitro* for its sensitivity to 3C^{pro} cleavage. The 3C^{pro} site in the extended 1BC loop of W1-1D-BC2 was cleaved by 3C^{pro} *in vitro*. In addition, a substantial percentage of the W1-1D-BC2 virus was cleaved at the 1BC loop by either 3C^{pro} or 3CD^{pro} during viral replication *in vivo*. The differential sensitivities of the two mutants to 3C^{Pro} cleavage support the notion that not only the primary but also the tertiary structure of the cleavage sites determine the specific cleavage of the poliovirus polyprotein by the viral proteinases. In contrast to the hybrid virus constructed by Colbere-Garapin and his colleagues,[78] however, C particles of W1-1D-BC2 did not induce antibodies in rabbits capable of neutralizing W1-1D-BC2.[66]

Evans et al.[81] constructed a PV/HIV-1 hybrid virus using the N-AgIA mutagenesis cartridge. These authors chose a defined linear epitope from the transmembrane glycoprotein gp41 (residues 735 to 752) of type 1 human immune deficiency virus (HIV-1) as the substitute for the N-AgIA site (residues 1091 to 1102) of PV1(S). The resulting hybrid virus (S1/env/3), exhibited dual antigenicity and immunogenicity. It retained its reactivity with the polyclonal anti-PV1 serum, as well as with a panel of poliovirus N-AgII- and N-AgIII-specific mcAbs. In addition, the hybrid virus also gained reactivity with group-specific anti-HIV-1 neutralizing antibodies through the expression of the HIV-1 epitope. Preincubation with S1/env/3, but not PV1(S), abolished the anti-HIV-1 (IIIB) neutralizing activity of two antipeptide mcAbs specific for the gp41 epitope. It also reduced the anti-HIV-1 (IIIB) neutralizing activity of a number of HIV-1 positive human sera samples. This same hybrid virus, upon immunization of rabbits, induced antisera specific for HIV-1 gp41 in both peptide binding and immunoblot assays. The antisera was also capable of neutralizing, albeit very weakly, various HIV-1 isolates. McAbs generated against the gp41 epitope on the S1/env/3 capsid also neutralized many of the HIV-1 isolates.[81] The capacity of this PV/HIV-1 hybrid virus to induce anti-HIV-1 neutralizing antibodies in rodents further demonstrated the potential of hybrid polioviruses as vectors for the presentation of a variety of antigens for the production of novel vaccines.

Jenkins et al. reported on the construction of a hybrid poliovirus mutant which contained the antigenic determinant of human papillomavirus type 16 (HPV-16). Using the N-AgIA cartridge, 16 amino acids (residues 269 to 284) of the L1 protein (the major capsid protein) of HPV-16 were exchanged for the N-AgIA site of PV1(S).[82] The growth of this virus (S1/HPV-16/L1) was impaired. In addition, it was neutralizable by mcAb specific for the HPV L1 epitope, as well as by polyclonal and monoclonal anti-PV1(S) antibodies. Antisera raised by the injection of the hybrid into rabbits were capable of interacting with a B-galactosidase/L1 (HPV-16) fusion protein as well as a synthetic peptide corresponding to residues 269-284 of the L1 protein. These antisera also recognized the HPV-16 antigen in infected human tissue.

Another series of PV-1/HIV-1 hybrid viruses was constructed by Dedieu et al.[83] The principal neutralization domain (PND) from either LA1 or RF isolates of HIV-1 replaced the N-AgIA site of PV1(S). The PND of HIV-1 is located in the third variable region (also known as the V3 loop) of the envelope glycoprotein gp120. The V3 loop of HIV-1 induces HIV neutralizing antibodies in both humans and monkeys. A number of hybrid constructs containing various lengths of LA1 or RF V3 sequences, including one containing the entire LA1 V3 loop, failed to produce viable virus, which implied a limited tolerance of the N-AgIA site of poliovirus. Two of the constructs produced viable hybrid viruses, designated vLA1 12B (containing residues 310 to 321 of the LA1 V3 loop) and vRF10B (containing residues 321 to 330 of the V3 loop of RF). vRF10B could be neutralized by an antipeptide serum specific for the V3 loop of HIV-1, strain RF; vLA1 12B was neutralizable by a variety of anti-HIV-1 LA1 sera as well as LA1 V3 loop-specific mcAbs, which indicated that the HIV-1 sequences expressed on the hybrid poliovirions resembled part of the PND structure found in HIV-1. Both hybrids induced high antibody titers in rabbits, which were capable of recognizing the V3 peptides as well as gp120/gp160. However, these antibodies were not effective in neutralizing HIV-1, although antisera from two of the seven rabbits immunized with hybrid vLA1 12B possessed a weak anti-HIV-1 neutralizing activity.[83]

As with the intertypic poliovirus hybrids, the approach to designing novel vaccines by placing foreign antigenic sites into the viral capsid cannot rely as yet on rational design but depends on trial-and-error experiments. So far, no candidate of a hybrid virus with the required properties of efficient growth and antigenicity has been constructed, but chance may provide us one day with a useful agent.

IV. DICISTRONIC POLIOVIRIONS AS EXPRESSION VECTORS FOR FOREIGN GENES

In 1988 and 1989, the internal ribosomal entry sites of encephalomyocarditis virus and poliovirus were discovered independently in two groups.[84-86] Jang and his co-workers engineered a dicistronic messenger RNA (a messenger RNA encodes two different polypeptides) with the following arrangement of genetic elements: poliovirus 5′ nontranslated region, the *sea* oncogene, nucleotide (nt) 260 to 833 of the 5′ NTR of EMCV, and finally the 2A[pro] gene of poliovirus. Significant quantities of the viral proteinase were derived before the appearance of the Sea oncoprotein from this dicistronic mRNA in RRL, which indicated that the translation of the second cistron occurred by a cap and 5′ end independent mechanism. This result was mimicked in COS-1 cells, in which CAT gene translation was promoted by an EMCV IRES element located in the second cistron of transfected, dicistronic mRNA. Simultaneously, the Sonenberg laboratory[87] obtained similar results with dicistronic constructs in which the synthesis of CAT, both *in vivo* and *in vitro*, was driven by the IRES element of poliovirus. In 1992, Molla et al. presented further, convincing evidence for the function of the IRES elements *in vivo* by inserting the IRES of EMCV into the single open reading frame (ORF) of poliovirus RNA between the regions encoding P1 and P2, thereby creating a viable, dicistronic poliovirus.[88] These experiments demonstrate that the IRES elements of picornaviruses are the first genetic elements in a eukaryotic system yet described that are capable of supporting translation initiation of the second ORF in the dicistronic mRNA. In addition, these elements facilitate a novel mechanism of protein synthesis that does not involve ribosome scanning[89] from the 5′ end of the RNA. Furthermore, IRES elements are useful tools in the construction of high-yield expression vectors, or for tagging cellular genetic elements.

Encouraged by the success of the dicistronic expression vectors both *in vitro* and *in vivo*, Alexander and his co-workers have set about developing a dicistronic expression system capable of producing foreign antigens within replicating, infectious poliovirions.[90] To this end, the expression vector pPNENPO was created. In the construction of pPNENPO, the first 630 nt of the poliovirus 5′ NTR (nt 631 to 742 was shown to be extraneous to the viral life cycle[91]) were fused to a segment of the EMCV 5′ NTR (nt 260 to 840) which harbors an IRES element.[85] This foreign (EMCV) IRES was in turn fused directly to the poliovirus ORF, in such a manner that the AUG normally initiating the EMCV polyprotein served as the initiating codon for the PV1(M) polyprotein. This was an important consideration since it allowed a myristoyl acid moiety necessary for viral viability[92] to be posttranslationally linked to the N terminus of VP4. The resulting plasmid, with the genetic arrangement, [PV] 5′ NTR-[EMCV] IRES-[PV] P1, 2,3,-3′ NTR, allowed for the promotion of translation initiation from an elongated 5′NTR, 1233 nt in length as opposed to the 743 nt of wildtype poliovirus (Figure 4).

A T7 promoter engineered immediately upstream of the PV 5′NTR of pPNENPO allowed for the production of pPNENPO RNA *in vitro*. This RNA was used as mRNA in a HeLa cell-free extract, a system also developed by Molla et al. to obtain a translation pattern almost identical to that of wild-type poliovirus.[8] This observation suggested that the tandemly arranged IRES elements functioned to promote normal initiation of protein synthesis as well as proteolysis of the viral polyprotein. This, in fact, was a startling result, considering that the elongated 5′NTR of pPNENPO contained 18 noninitiating AUG triplets, which to our knowledge was the most ever described in a eukaryotic system.

HeLa cell monolayers transfected with PV1(M) RNA displayed a cytopathic effect (CPE), a phenotype indicative of the presence of infectious viral particles spreading through the cell culture. The monolayer cells transfected with pPNENPO RNA displayed CPE 30 h after the introduction of the RNA, a delay of 10 h when compared with transfections with PV1(M) RNA. This result suggested that the mutant RNA was a competent source of infectious poliovirus. This conclusion was confirmed by subsequent plaque assays in which W1-PNENPO infected HeLa cell monolayers were overlaid with agar ensuring viral spread by a cell-to-cell contact mechanism, resulting in a focus of lysed cells, i. e. a plaque. W1-PNENPO expressed a small plaque phenotype when compared to PV1(M), a result consistent with the delayed cytopathic effects observed in transfections.

As mentioned before, two IRES elements can function within a replicating genome when separated by an ORF.[88] Using this system as a model, the possibility was explored as to whether a foreign gene could be inserted between the tandemly arranged IRES elements. The bacterially derived CAT gene had proven to be quite amenable to the study

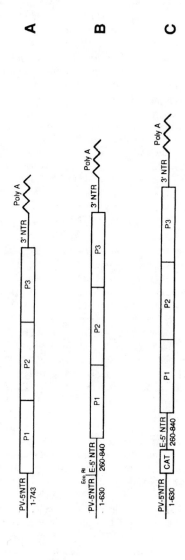

Figure 4

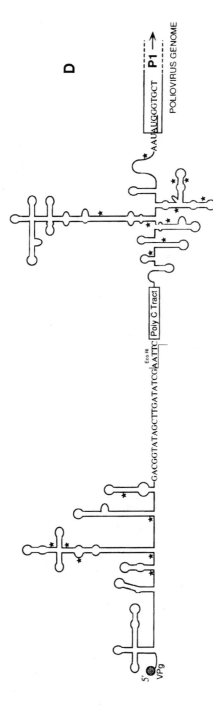

Figure 4 The genotypes of (A) wild-type poliovirus; (B) the dicistronic poliovirus expression vector, pNENPO; and (C) the di-CAT virus, which expresses the bacterially derived CAT gene. (D) A diagram showing the secondary structure of the 5′ NTR of pNENPO, which contains tandemly arranged IRES elements from PV and EMCV. The stars indicate the noninitiating AUG triplets within this elongated 5′ NTR.

of dicistronic RNAs in the past[84,85] and was therefore chosen as the gene to be inserted. This new dicistronic construct, termed DICAT,[90] contained the following arrangement of genetic elements, [PV] 5′ NTR-[bact] CAT- [EMCV] IRES- [PV] P1,2,3- 3′ NTR. DICAT cDNA was transcribed *in vitro* and the resulting RNA was translated in a HeLa cell-free extract. The protein pattern obtained from these reactions confirmed that both ORFs were expressed *in vitro*. Transfection of HeLa cell monolayers with DICAT RNA produced CPE after 45 h, which implied synthesis of infectious poliovirus, a conclusion later confirmed by plaque assay.

Standard CAT assays as well as Western blot analyses[93] were performed on W1-DICAT-infected HeLa cell lysates in order to assess the ability of the dicistronic virus to express the foreign gene. CAT assays indicated the presence of active enzyme in the infected lysates. This activity increased with time, corresponding temporally with an increase in virus titer of a single infectious viral cycle. Moreover, CAT-specific antigen was readily apparent after infection with W1-DICAT. Together, these results indicated that a dicistronic poliovirus containing 17% more RNA than wild-type poliovirus could replicate to produce significant quantities of a foreign gene.

The size of its enlarged genome or the expression of its foreign gene could be responsible for the impaired proliferation of W1-DICAT. In order to relieve itself of the burden inflicted by these foreign sequences, the dicistronic RNA could be rendered genetically unstable. In order to test this hypothesis, W1-DICAT was serially passaged five times into HeLa cells and the resulting lysates were subjected to CAT assay. The production of functional CAT protein decreased with each passage, indicating that the gene was somehow inactivated during viral replication. This result was not surprising, considering the high genetic plasticity of the poliovirus genome,[4] and the strong selection against the larger genomic RNAs. These inherent limitations of self-replicating RNA may have led to the inactivation of the foreign gene either by point mutation or nonhomologous recombination, although the exact mechanism remains to be determined.

V. POTENCY AND LIMITATIONS

The study of antigenic hybrid viruses has produced a great deal of insight into many of the biological functions of poliovirus. For example, the successful exchange of the poliovirus surface loops with a number of foreign antigens demonstrated the extreme flexibility of these protruding surface structures. In fact, the entire 1BC loop can be deleted without effecting the viability of the virus. In addition, the antigenic hybrid strategy has been valuable in the investigation of the viral structure and replication. For example, it has been used to study the antigenic structure of the different serotypes of polioviruses and coxsackieviruses,[50,55,56,58,77,94] the genetic determinant of host range[55,58] as well as the virus/receptor interaction.[72] The construction of antigenic poliovirus hybrids could aid in the development of novel viral vaccines. A large percentage of these constructs produced viable poliovirions, indicating that the virus capsid was in fact capable of accommodating a variety of heterologous antigens. Antigens of different origins have been used to substitute the 1BC and the 2EF loops of the poliovirion. Most of these viruses, especially those of the intertypic hybrids, displayed dual antigenicity and dual immunogenicity, characteristics which may lead to improvements in the existing type 2 and 3 vaccines through the expression of antigenic sites in a stable type 1 background. In addition, the construction and characterization of the PV/HIV as well as the PV/FMDV hybrids have provided a great deal of useful information in evaluating the application of hybrid polioviruses as novel vaccines against a variety of pathogens. It is of great interest for the development of novel oral delivery system that a hybrid poliovirus derived from the attenuated strain elicited antibodies against foreign antigen in orally administered animals.[57] It is known that the attenuated poliovirus replicate efficiently in the gut but not in the CNS in primates; therefore, hybrid poliovirus is one of the candidates of non-CNS carriers.

Nevertheless, the success of the hybrid poliovirus strategy is severely limited for a number of intrinsic reasons. The inserted foreign antigens must be linear and highly immunogenic, criteria met by very few natural antigens.[95] In addition, the size of the foreign antigens to be inserted is limited (less than 30 amino acids) and the immunogenicity of these inserts is usually poor. This is not as efficient as other eukaryotic expression vectors such as the vaccinia virus expression system which is more efficient in antigen presentation and has a larger carrier capacity.[96,97] Finally, most of the hybrid polioviruses were impaired in their growth characteristics. This inhibition was most dramatic in the cases of hybrids constructed on the background of the type 1 Sabin strain, which could make it difficult to generate sufficient quantities of hybrid poliovirus for large-scale vaccination. The insertion of many foreign sequences, especially those unrelated to poliovirus, failed to produce viable hybrid viruses, which suggested that the tolerance of the poliovirus surface loops was limited. It can be assumed that the inserted sequences frequently assume an altered conformation within the restriction of the poliovirus capsid that is not identical to the original antigenic determinants. Since little is known as to what makes a peptide sequence of protein also an antigenic site, it can currently not be predicted whether an antigenic hybrid virus will also produce a useful immune response.

Dicistronic poliovirions expressing complete or almost complete foreign genes could overcome many of the limitations of the antigenic hybrids described above. These viruses can accommodate at least 240 amino acids of foreign protein, a far greater quantity than can be expressed in the virion capsid. This characteristic will allow for a much greater chance of immunogenic response, since antigenic sites will be presented in their natural state, including those possessing nonlinear epitopes. In addition, preliminary data indicate that dicistronic poliovirions grow at least as well as their antigenic hybrid counterparts in tissue culture, indicating that they may in fact be more amenable to large-scale vaccine production. Moreover, the virus structure is not interfered with by the expression of foreign proteins.

In total, antigenic hybrid and dicistronic polioviruses have proven to be quite valuable as windows for viewing many of the biological peculiarities of this well-documented etiologic agent. In addition, they have broken fertile ground for the adaptation of the highly successful Sabin vaccine strains for use against diseases such as HIV and acute hepatitis, which at the present time go almost unchecked due to the lack of adequate vaccine protection.

ACKNOWLEDGMENTS

We thank Aniko Paul and Matthias Gromeier for assistance with the manuscript. We also thank James Harber, James Bibb, and Kevin Harris for their computer expertise, and Chris Helmke for photography. Work described from the laboratory of the authors was supported by NIH grants AI 15122, CA28146, and 1R01AI32100 to E. W., and support from the World Health Organization to H. H. L.

REFERENCES

1. Kitamura, B., Semler, L., Rothberg, P. G., Larsen, G. R., Adler, C. J., Dorner, A. J., Emini, E. A., Hanecak, R., Lee, J., van der Werf, S., Anderson, C.W., and Wimmer, E., Primary structure, gene organization and polypeptide expression of poliovirus RNA, *Nature,* 291, 547, 1981.

148

2. Racaniello, V. R. and Baltimore, D., Molecular cloning of poliovirus cDNA and determination of the complete nucleotide sequence of the viral genome, *Proc. Natl. Acad. Sci. U.S.A.,* 78, 4887, 1981.
3. Dorner, A. J., Dorner, L. F., Larsen, G. R., Wimmer, E., and Anderson, C. W., Identification of the initiation site of poliovirus polyprotein synthesis, *J. Virol.,* 42, 1017, 1982.
4. Wimmer, E., Hellen, C. U. T., and Cao, X., Genetics of poliovirus, *Annu. Rev. Genetics,* 27, 353, 1993.
5. Hogle, J. M., Chow, M., and Filman, D. J., The three dimensional structure of poliovirus at 2.9 Å resolution, *Science,* 229, 1358, 1985.
6. Racaniello, V. and Baltimore, D., Cloned poliovirus complementary DNA is infectious in mammalian cells, *Science,* 214, 916, 1981.
7. van der Werf, S., Bradley, J., Wimmer, E., Studier, F. W., and Dunn, J. J., Synthesis of infectious poliovirus RNA by purified T7 RNA polymerase, *Proc. Natl. Acad. Sci. U.S.A.,* 83, 2330, 1986.
8. Molla, A., Paul, A. V., and Wimmer, E., Cell-free, de novo synthesis of poliovirus, *Science,* 254, 1647, 1991.
9. Salk, J., Krech, U., Younger, J., Bennett, B., Lewis, L., and Bazeley, P., Formaldehyde treatment and safety testing of experimental poliomyelitis vaccines, *Am. J. Public Health,* 44, 563, 1954.
10. Sabin, A. and Boulger, L., History of Sabin attenuated poliovirus oral live vaccine strains, *J. Biol. Stand.,* 1, 115, 1973.
11. Nkowane, B. M., Wassilak, S. G., Oversteen, W. A., Bart, K. J., Schonberger, L. B., Hinman, A. R., and Kew, O. M., Vaccine-associated paralytic poliomyelitis in the United States: 1973 through 1984, *J. Am. Med. Assoc.,* 257, 1335, 1987.
12. Melnick, J. L., Enteroviruses: Polioviruses, Coxsackieviruses, Ecoviruses, and Newer Enteroviruses, in *Virology,* 1, 2nd ed., Fields, B. N., Knipe, D. M., Chanock, R. M., Hirsch, M. S., Melnick, J. L., Morath, T. P., and Roizman, B., Eds., Raven Press, New York, 1990, 549.
13. Rueckert, R. R., Picornaviridae and their replication, in *Virology,* 1, 2nd ed., Fields, B. N., Knipe, D. M., Chanock, R. M., Hirsch, M. S., Melnick, J. L., Morath, T. P., and Roizman, B., Eds., Raven Press, New York, 1990, 507.
14. Hellen, C. U. T., Fäcke, M., Kräusslich, H.-G., Lee, C.-K., and Wimmer, E., Characterization of poliovirus 2A proteinase by mutational analysis: Residues required for autocatalytic activity are essential for induction of cleavage of eukaryotic initiation factor 4F polypeptide p220, *J. Virol.,* 65, 4226, 1992.
15. Harris, K. S., Hellen, C. U. T., and Wimmer, E., Proteolytic processing in the replication of picornaviruses, *Sem. Virol.,* 1, 323, 1990.
16. Lee, Y., Nomoto, A., Detjen, B., and Wimmer, E., The genome-linked protein of picornaviruses. I. A protein covalently linked to poliovirus genome RNA, *Proc. Natl. Acad. Sci. U.S.A.,* 74, 59, 1977.
17. Rothberg, P., Harris, T., Nomoto, A., and Wimmer, E., The genome-linked protein of picornaviruses V. 04-(5'-Uridylyl)-tyrosine is the bond between the genome-linked protein and the RNA of poliovirus, *Proc. Natl. Acad. Sci. U.S.A.,* 75, 4868, 1978.
18. Flanegan, J. B. and Baltimore, D., Poliovirus-specific primer-dependent RNA polymerase able to copy poly(A), *Proc. Natl. Acad. Sci. U.S.A.,* 74, 3677, 1977.
19. Bienz, K., Egger, D., Troxler, M., and Pasamontes, I., Structural organization of poliovirus RNA replication is mediated by viral proteins of the P2 genomic region, *J. Virol.,* 64, 1156, 1990.
20. Andino, R., Rieckhof, G. E., and Baltimore, D., A functional ribonucleoprotein complex forms around the 5' end of poliovirus RNA, *Cell,* 63, 369, 1990.

21. Takeda, N., Yang, C. F., Kuhn, R. J., and Wimmer, E., Uridylylation of the genome-linked protein of poliovirus in vitro is dependent upon an endogenous RNA template, *Virus Res.,* 8, 193, 1987.
22. Takegami, T., Kuhn, R. J., Anderson, C. W., and Wimmer, E., Membrane-dependent uridylylation of the genome-linked protein VPg of poliovirus, *Proc. Natl. Acad. Sci. U.S.A.,* 80, 7447, 1983.
23. Tobin, G. J., Young, D. C., and Flanegan, J. B., Self-catalyzed linkage of poliovirus terminal protein VPg to poliovirus RNA, *Cell,* 59, 511, 1989.
24. Jang, S. K., Pestova, T., Hellen, C. U. T., Witherell, G. W., and Wimmer, E., Cap-independent translation of picornavirus RNAs: structure and function of the internal ribosomal entry site, *Enzyme,* 44, 292, 1990.
25. Filman, D. J., Syed, R., Chow, M., Macadam, A. J., Minor, P. D., and Hogle, J. M., Structural factors that control conformational transitions and serotype specificity in type 3 poliovirus, *EMBO J.,* 8, 1567, 1989.
26. Rossmann, M. G. and Johnson, J. E., Icosahedral RNA virus structure, *Annu. Rev. Biochem.,* 58, 533, 1989.
27. Harrison, S., Olson, A., Schutt, E., Winkler, F., and Bricogne, G., Tomato bushy stunt virus at 2.8 Å resolution, *Nature,* 276, 368, 1978.
28. Rossmann, M. G., The canyon hypothesis. Hiding the host cell receptor attachment site on a viral surface from immune surveillance, *J. Biol. Chem.,* 264, 14587, 1989.
29. Colonno, R. J., Condra, J. H., Mizutani, S., Callahan, P. L., Davies, M. E., and Murcko, M. A., Evidence for the direct involvement of the rhinovirus canyon in receptor binding, *Proc. Natl. Acad. Sci. U.S.A.,* 85, 5449, 1988.
30. Olson, N. H., Kolatkar, P. R., Oliveira, M. A., Cheng, R. H., Greve, J. M., McCelland, A., Baker, T. S., and Rossmann, M. G., Structure of a human rhinovirus complexed with its receptor molecular, *Proc. Natl. Acad. Sci. U.S.A.,* 90, 507, 1993.
31. Mendelsohn, C. L., Wimmer, E., and Racaniello, V. R., Cellular receptor for poliovirus: molecular cloning, nucleotide sequence, and expression of a new member of the immunoglobulin superfamily, *Cell,* 56, 855, 1989.
32. Holland, J., Receptor affinities as major determinants of enterovirus tissue tropisms in humans, *Virology,* 15, 312, 1961.
33. Lonberg-Holm, K., Gosser, L., and Shimshick, E., Interaction of liposomes with subviral particles of poliovirus type 2 and rhinovirus type 2, *J. Virol.,* 19, 746, 1976.
34. Crowell, R. L. and Landau, B. J., Receptors in the initiation of picornavirus infections, in *Comprehensive Virology,* Vol. 18, Fraenfel-Conrat, H. and Wagnar, R. R., Eds., Plenum Press, New York, 1983, 1.
35. Harber, J. and Wimmer, E., Aspects of the molecular biology of picornaviruses, in *Proc. NATO ASI on Regulation of Gene Expression in Animal Viruses,* Carrasco, L., Sonenberg, N., and Wimmer, E., Eds., Plenum Press, New York, 1993, 189.
36. Sicinski, P., Rowinski, J., Warcho, J. B., Jarzabek, Z., Gut, W., Szczygie, B., Bielecki, K., and Koch, G., Poliovirus type 1 enters the human host through intestinal M cells, *Gastroenterology,* 98, 56, 1990.
37. Ren, R. and Racaniello, V. R., Poliovirus spreads from muscle to the central nervous system by neural pathways, *J. Inf. Dis.,* 166, 747, 1992.
38. Blinzinger, K., Simon, J., Magrath, D., and Boulger, L., Poliovirus crystals within the endoplasmic reticulum of endothelial and mononuclear cells in the monkey spinal cord, *Science,* 163, 1336, 1969.
39. Peluso, R., Haase, A., Stowring, L., Edwards, M., and Ventura, P., A Trojan horse mechanism for the spread of visna virus in monocytes, *Virology,* 147, 231, 1985.
40. Enders, J., Weller, T., and Robbins, F., Cultivation of the Lansing strain of poliomyelitis virus in cultures of various human embryonic tissues, *Science,* 109, 85, 1949.

41. Nomoto, A. and Wimmer, E., Genetic studies of the antigenicity and the attenuation phenotype of poliovirus, in *Molecular Basis of Virus Disease,* Russel, M. C. and Almond, J. W., Eds., Soc. Gen. Microbiol. Symp., Vol. 40, Cambridge University Press, 1987, 107.

42. Minor, P. D., Antigenic structure of picornaviruses, in *Picornaviruses,* Racaniello, V. R., Eds., Springer-Verlag, Berlin, 1990, 121.

43. Stanway, G., Hughes, P. J., Mountford, R. C., Reeves, P., Minor, P. D., Schild, G. C., and Almond, J. W., Comparison of the complete nucleotide sequence of the genomes of the neurovirulent poliovirus P3/Leon/37 and its attenuated Sabin vaccine derivative P3/Leon/12 a,b, *Proc. Natl. Acad. Sci. U.S.A.,* 81, 1539, 1984.

44. Tatem, J. M., Weeks-Levy, C., Georgiu, A., DiMcchele, S. J., Gogaez, E. J., Racaniello, V. R., Cano, F. R., and Mento, S. J., A mutation present in the amino terminus of Sabin 3 poliovirus VP1 protein is attenuating, *J. Virol.,* 66, 3194, 1992.

45. Evans, D. M., Dunn, G., Minor, P. D., Schild, G. C., Cann, A. J., Stanway, G., Almond, J. W., Currey, K., and Maizel, J. V., Increased neurovirulence associated with a single nucleotide change in a noncoding region of the Sabin type 3 poliovaccine genome, *Nature,* 314, 548, 1985.

46. Pollard, S. R., Dunn, G., Cammack, N., Minor, P. D., and Almond, J. W., Nucleotide sequence of a neurovirulent variant of the type 2 oral poliovirus vaccine, *J. Virol.,* 63, 4949, 1989.

47. Minor, P. D., The molecular biology of poliovaccines, *J. Gen. Virol.,* 73, 3065, 1992.

48. Nomoto, A., Omata, T., Toyoda, H., Kuge, S., Horie, H., Kataoka, Y., Genba, Y., Nakano, Y., and Imura, N., Complete nucleotide sequence of the attenuated poliovirus Sabin 1 strain genome., *Proc. Natl. Acad. Sci. U.S.A.,* 79, 5793, 1982.

49. Macadam, A. J., Ferguson, G., Arnold, C., and Minor, P. D., An assembly defect as a result of an attenuating mutation in the capsid protein of the Teh poliovirus type 3 vaccine strain, *J. Virol.,* 72, 2475, 1991.

50. Murdin, A. D. and Wimmer, E., Construction of a poliovirus type 1/type 2 antigenic hybrid by manipulation of neutralization antigenic site II, *J. Virol.,* 63, 5251, 1989.

51. Minor, P. D., Ferguson, M., Evans, D. M. A., Almond, J. W., and Icenogle, J. P., Antigenic structure of polioviruses serotypes 1, 2 and 3, *J. Gen. Virol.,* 68, 1857, 1986.

52. Wiegers, K., Uhlig, H., and Dernick, R., N-AgIB of poliovirus type 1: a discontinuous epitope formed by two loops of VP1 comprising residues 96–104 and 141–152, *Virology,* 170, 583, 1989.

53. Emini, E. A., Wimmer, E., Jameson, B. A., Bonin, J., and Diamond, D., Neutralization antigenic sites of poliovirus and peptide induction of neutralizing antibodies, *Ann. Sclavo Collana Monogr.,* 1, 139, 1984.

54. Page, G. S., Mosser, A. G., Hogle, J. M., Filman, D. J., Rueckert, R. R., and Chow, M., Three-dimensional structure of poliovirus serotype 1 neutralizing determinants, *J. Virol.,* 62, 1781, 1988.

55. Murray, M. G., Bradley, J., Yang, X.-F., Wimmer, E., Moss, E. G., and Racaniello, V. R., Poliovirus host range is determined by a short amino acid sequence in neutralization antigenic site I, *Science,* 241, 213, 1988a.

56. Murray, M. G., Kuhn, R. J., Arita, M., Kawamura, N., Nomoto, A., and Wimmer, E., Poliovirus type1/type3 antigenic hybrid virus constructed in vitro elicits type 1 and type 3 neutralizing antibodies in rabbits and monkeys, *Proc. Natl. Acad. Sci. U.S.A.,* 85, 3203, 1988b.

57. Burke, K. L., Dunn, G., Ferguson, M., Minor, P. D., and Almond, J. W., Antigenic chimeras of poliovirus as potential new vaccines, *Nature,* 332, 81, 1988.

58. Martin, A., Wychowski, C., Couderc, T., Crainic, R., Hogle, J., and Girard, M., Engineering a type 2 antigenic site on a type 1 capsid results in a chimeric virus which is neurovirulent for mice, *EMBO J.,* 7, 2839, 1988.

59. Armstrong, C., Successful transfer of the Lansing strain of poliomyelitis virus from the cotton rat to the white mouse, *Public Health Rep.*, 54, 2302, 1939.
60. La Monica, N., Kupsky, W. J., and Racaniello, V. R., Reduced mouse neurovirulence of poliovirus type 2 Lansing antigenic variants selected with monoclonal antibodies, *Virology*, 161, 429, 1987.
61. Yeates, T. O., Jacobson, D. H., Martin, A., Wychowski, C., Girard, M., Filman, D. J., and Hogle, J. M., Three-dimensional structure of a mouse-adapted type 2/type 1 poliovirus chimera, *EMBO J.*, 10, 2331, 1991.
62. Martin, A., Benichou, D., Couderc, T., Hogle, J. M., Wychowski, C., van der Werf, S., and Girard, M., Use of type 1/type 2 chimeric polioviruses to study determinants of poliovirus type 1 neurovirulence in a mouse model, *Virology*, 180, 648, 1991.
63. Murdin, A. D., Lu, H. H., Murray, M. G., and Wimmer, E., Poliovirus antigenic hybrids simultaneously expressing antigenic determinants from all three serotypes, *J. Gen. Virol.*, 73, 607, 1992.
64. Emini, E. A., Jameson, B. A., and Wimmer, E., Identification of a new neutralization antigenic site on poliovirus coat protein VP2, *J. Virol.*, 52, 719, 1984.
65. Minor, P. D., Evans, D. M. A., Ferguson, M., Schild, G. C., Almond, J. W., and Stanway, G., Molecular basis of antigenicity of poliovirus, in *Positive Strand RNA Viruses*, Brinton, M. A. and Rueckert, R. R., Eds., Alan Liss, New York, 1986, 1857.
66. Murdin, A. D., Mirzayan, C., Kameda, A., and Wimmer, E., The effect of site and mode of expression of a heterologous antigenic determinant on the properties of poliovirus hybrids, *Microb. Pathogen.*, 10, 27, 1991.
67. Lu, H. H., Murdin, A. D., Altmeyer, R., Harber, J., and Wimmer, E., Antigenic hybrids of poliovirus: trivalent polioviruses, and characterization of a poliovirus/rhinovirus hybrid, in *Modern Approaches to New Vaccines Including Prevention of AIDS (Vaccines 92)*, Brown, F., Chanock, R. M., Ginsberg, H. S., and Lerner, R. A., Eds., Cold Spring Harbor Press, Cold Spring Harbor, NY, 1992, 287.
68. Rossmann, M. G., Arnold, E., Erikson, J. W., Frankenberger, E. A., Griflith, J. P., Hecht, H. J., Johnson, J. E., Kamer, G., Luo, M., Mosser, A., Rueckert, R., Sherry, B., and Vriend, G., Structure of a human common cold virus and functional relationship to other picornaviruses, *Nature (London)*, 317, 145, 1985.
69. Luo, M., Vriend, G., Kamer, G., Minor, I., Arnold, E., Rossmann, M. G., Boege, U., Scraba, D. G., Duke, G. M., and Palmenberg, A. C., The atomic structure of mengo virus at 3.0 Å resolution, *Science*, 235, 182, 1987.
70. Acharya, R., Fry, E., Stuart, D., Fox, G., Rowlands, D., and Brown, F., The three-dimensional structure of foot-and-mouth disease virus at 2.9 Å resolution, *Nature*, 337, 709, 1989.
71. Kitson, J. D. A., Burke, K. L., Pullen, L. A., Belsham, G. J., and Almond, J. W., Chimeric polioviruses that include sequences derived from two independent antigenic sites of foot-and-mouth disease virus (FMDV) induce neutralizing antibodies against FMDV in guinea pigs, *J. Virol.*, 65, 3068, 1991.
72. Altmeyer, R., Murdin, A. D., Harber, J. J., and Wimmer, E., Construction and characterization of a poliovirus/rhinovirus antigenic hybrid, *Virology*, 184, 636, 1991.
73. Colonno, R. J., Callahan, P. L., Leippe, D. M., Rueckert, R. R., and Tomassisi, J. E., Inhibition of rhinovirus attachment by neutralizing monoclonal antibodies and their Fab fragments, *J. Virol.*, 63, 36, 1989.
74. Bradley, J., Murray, M. G., Kuhn, R. J., Tada, H., Yang, X. F., Mizayan, C., and Wimmer, E., The use of mutagenesis cartridges in the molecular genetics analysis of poliovirus: mutations in the genome-linked protein, VPg and in the neutralization antigenic site I, in *Molecular Aspects of Picornavirus Infection and Detection*, Semler, B. L. and Ehrenfeld, E., Eds., American Society for Microbiology, Washington DC, 1988, 3.

75. Murray, M., Hybrid polio viruses as potential vaccines and as tools to study biological function, Ph.D. thesis, Dept. of Microbiology, State University of New York at Stonybrook, 1989.

76. Sverdlov, E. D., Tsarev, S. A., Markova, S. V., Rostapshov, V. M., Azhikina, T. L., Chernov, I. P., Gorbalenya, A. E., Kolesnikova, M. S., and Romanova, L. I., Insertion of short hepatitis virus A amino acid sequences into poliovirus antigenic determinants results in viable progeny, *FEBS Lett.*, 257, 354, 1989.

77. Reimann, B.-Y., Zell, R., and Kandolf, R., Mapping of a neutralizing antigenic site of coxsackievirus B4 by construction of an antigenic chimera, *J. Virol.*, 65, 3475, 1991.

78. Colbere-Garapin, F., Christodoulou, C., Crainic, R., Garapin, A.-C., and Candrea, A., Addition of a forgien oligopeptide to the major capsid protein of poliovirus, *Proc. Natl. Acad. Sci. U.S.A.*, 85, 8668, 1988.

79. Emini, E., Jameson, B. A., and Wimmer, E., Antigenic structure of poliovirus, in *Immunochemistry of Viruses — The Basis for Serodiagnosis and Vaccines*, Neurath, A. R. and van Regenmortel, M. H. V., Eds., Elsevier Biomedical Press, New York, 1985, 281.

80. Mirzayan, C. M., Pallai, P., and Wimmer, E., Specificity of the polioviral proteinase 3C towards genetically engineered cleavage sites in the viral capsid, *J. Gen. Virol.*, 137, 1159, 1991.

81. Evans, D. J., McKeating, J., Meredith, J. M., Burke, K. L., Katrak, K., John, A., Ferguson, M., Minor, P. D., Weiss, R. A., and Almond, J. W., An engineered poliovirus chimaera elicits broadly reactive HIV-1 neutralizing antibodies, *Nature*, 339, 385, 1989.

82. Jenkins, O., Cason, J., Burke, K. L., Lunney, D., Gillen, A., Patel, D., McCance, D. J., and Almond, J. W., An antigen chimaera of poliovirus induces antibodies against human papillomavirus type 16, *J. Virol.*, 64, 1201, 1990.

83. Dedieu, J.-F., Ronco, J., van der Werf, S., Hogle, J. M., Henin, Y., and Girard, M., Poliovirus chimeras expressing sequences from the principal neutralization domain of human immunodeficiency virus type 1, *J. Virol.*, 66, 3161, 1992.

84. Jang, S. K., Kräusslich, H.-G., Nicklin, M. J. H., Duke, G. M., Palmenberg, A. C., and Wimmer, E., A segment of the 5' nontranslated region of encephalomyocarditis virus RNA directs internal entry of ribosomes during in vitro translation, *J. Virol.*, 62, 2636, 1988.

85. Jang, S. K., Davies, M. V., Kaufman, R. J., and Wimmer, E., Initiation of protein synthesis by internal entry of ribosomes into the 5' nontranslated region of encephalomyocarditis virus RNA in vitro, *J. Virol.*, 63, 1651, 1989.

86. Pelletier, J. and Sonenberg, N., Internal initiation of translation of eukaryotic mRNA directed by a sequence derived from poliovirus RNA, *Nature*, 334, 320, 1988.

87. Pelletier, J., Kaplan, G., Racaniello, V. R., and Sonenberg, N., Cap-independent translation of poliovirus mRNA is conferred by sequence elements within the 5'-noncoding region, *Mol. Cell. Biol.*, 8, 1103, 1988.

88. Molla, A., Jang, S. K., Paul, A. V., Reuer, Q., and Wimmer, E., Cardioviral internal ribosomal entry site is functional in a genetically engineered dicistronic poliovirus, *Nature*, 356, 255, 1992.

89. Kozak, M. J., The scanning model for translation: an update, *J. Cell Biol.*, 108, 229, 1989.

90. Alexander, L., Lu, H.-H., and Wimmer, E., *Proc. Natl. Acad. Sci. U.S.A.*, in press.

91. Kuge, S. and Nomoto, A., Construction of viable deletion and insertion mutants of the Sabin strain type 1 poliovirus: function of the 5' noncoding sequence in vial replication, *J. Virol.*, 61, 1478, 1987.

92. Kräusslich, H.-G., Hölscher, C., Reuer, Q., Harber, J., and Wimmer, E., Myristoylation of the poliovirus polyprotein is required for proteolytic processing of the capsid and for viral infectivity, *J. Virol.*, 64, 2433, 1990.

93. Sambrook, J., Fritsch, E. F., and Maniatis, T., *Molecular Cloning: a Laboratory Manual,* 2nd ed., Cold Spring Harbor Laboratory Press, Cold Spring Harbor, NY, 1989.

94. Burge, W. D., Cramer, W. N., and Kawata, K., Effect of heat on virus inactivation by ammonia, *Appl. Environ. Microbiol.,* 46, 446, 1983.

95. Ada, G. L., Vaccine antigens, in *Structure of Antigens,* Vol. 1, van Regenmortel, M. H. V., Eds., CRC Press, Boca Raton, FL, 1992, 367.

96. Ansardi, D. C., Porter, D. C., and Morrow, C. D., Complementation of a poliovirus defective genome by a recombinant vaccinia virus which provides poliovirus P1 capsid precursor in *trans, J. Virol.,* 67, 3684, 1993.

97. Moss, B., Elroy-Stein, O., Mizukami, T., Alexander, W. A., and Fuerst, T. R., New mammalian expression vectors, *Nature,* 348, 91, 1990.

98. Wimmer, E. W., Kuhn, R. J., Pincus, S., Yang, C.-F., Toyoda, H., Nciklin, M. J. H., and Takeda, N., Molecular events leading to picornavirus genome replication, *J. Cell Sci. (Suppl.),* 7, 251, 1987.

Part II: Nonreplicating Antigen Delivery Systems

Chapter 1

Cholera Toxin and Cholera B Subunit as Oral-Mucosal Adjuvant and Antigen Carrier Systems

Elisabeth Hörnquist, Nils Lycke, Cecil Czerkinsky, and Jan Holmgren

TABLE OF CONTENTS

I. INTRODUCTION

The mucosal surfaces in, e.g., the gastrointestinal, respiratory, and urogenital tracts represent a very large exposure area to exogenous agents, including potentially harmful microorganisms. Not surprisingly, therefore, these mucosal tissues are defended by a large and apparently interconnected local immune system which in essence operates in anatomical and functional separation from systemic immunity.[1] The gastrointestinal tract, which hosts more immunocytes than any other organ in the body, is the largest component of this important mucosal immune system. The host defense against many infectious agents in the gut and on other mucosal surfaces depends heavily on the local production of secretory IgA (sIgA). It is now widely recognized that in order to be efficacious, vaccines against most enteric infections should be able to stimulate the local gut mucosal sIgA immune system.[2,3] This goal is usually better achieved by administering the vaccines by the oral route rather than parenterally. Several oral vaccines have been shown to induce

0-8493-4866-8/94/$0.00+$.50
© 1994 by CRC Press Inc.

sIgA antibody responses also in remote secretions including saliva, tears, nasal-respiratory washings, and breast milk. These and other observations support the possibility that the oral route of vaccination may be used to induce immunity not only against intestinal infection but also against infections in, e.g., the respiratory and urogenital tracts.[2-4]

Several particulate antigens, including both live and killed microorganisms, have proved to be effective oral immunogens.[2-4] Some soluble antigens with specific properties including, for example, stability to intestinal proteases and ability to bind to intestinal epithelium have also been able to stimulate good sIgA antibody responses in mucosal tissue after oral immunization.[2-4] However, the mucosal immune response to most soluble antigens administered by the oral route has been weak and required large and frequently administered oral doses of antigen. Hence, in order to utilize the superior practicality of oral immunization and the specific ability of this route to induce immune responses at mucosal surfaces, there is a great need to find powerful mucosal adjuvants that can improve immunogenicity and thus facilitate the construction of effective oral vaccines. As reviewed by Bienenstock,[5] a number of different compounds have been found to have adjuvant properties when given orally together with antigen. Ox bile was used by many early investigators as a vehicle and adjuvant for orally administered immunogens including early (and apparently effective) killed oral vaccines against dysentery. Other examples of adjuvant-active substances in experimental systems include various polycations such as DEAE-4 dextran and polyornithine, sodium dodecyl benzene sulfate, lipid-conjugated materials, streptomycin, and possibly other agents which alter the intestinal flora, and vitamin A. These agents have in common that they can influence the structural and/or functional integrity of the mucosal surface to which they are applied.

Other substances reported to have mucosal adjuvant activity, however, probably act through different mechanisms. Among these are muramyl dipeptide (MDP), avridine, and cimetidine (for additional discussion of these various adjuvant-active agents and specific references, see Reference 5). The most potent mucosal adjuvant so far identified is, however, cholera toxin (CT). Defining the adjuvant mechanisms of CT could eventually lead to the development of medically more readily acceptable adjuvants for augmenting the immunizing effect of orally administered vaccines.

II. *IN VIVO* ADJUVANT ACTION OF CHOLERA TOXIN

CT is the primary (though not necessarily the only) enterotoxin produced by *Vibrio cholerae* bacteria. The bacterium colonizes the small intestine and binds to the epithelial cells in the mucosa. The CT molecule is well characterized with regard to its structure and function: it consists of five binding (B) subunits assembled into a ring into which a toxic-active (A) subunit is inserted. The B subunits bind the toxin with high affinity to receptors on the epithelial cells, identified as the ganglioside GM1, and the A subunit is then translocated into the cell where it can ADP-ribosylate the G_s subunit of adenylate cyclase which, in turn, converts ATP to cyclic AMP (cAMP) in the affected cell.[6,7] The resulting increase in cAMP then causes diarrhea and fluid loss by inhibiting uptake of sodium chloride and stimulating the secretion of Cl^-. This excessive secretion of electrolytes and fluid leads to the severe, often life-threatening diarrheal disease known as cholera.[6] In addition to its significance as an enterotoxin, CT has recently attracted much interest among immunologists as being an exceptionally powerful oral-mucosal immunogen,[8,9] as well as, at the same time, a potent adjuvant for mucosal IgA responses.[10-12]

Extending the early findings of potent immunomodulatory effects of CT on systemic humoral as well as cell-mediated immune responses,[13] we and others have shown that in mice, CT can strongly augment the mucosal IgA immune response to both admixed and covalently linked, related as well as unrelated antigens.[10,11] From these studies it can be summarized that CT potentiates immune responses to protein antigens administered perorally by up to 50-fold as determined by the increase in numbers of antigen-specific antibody-secreting cells (ASC) in the lamina propria.[11] The dose required for adjuvanticity was 10- to 20-fold lower than the immunogenic dose of CT.[11] The adjuvant action of CT was dose dependent and was only achieved when CT was given PO together with the antigen: both priming (memory induction) and boosting of the gut mucosal immune system by the oral route were greatly potentiated by CT.[11] Although less extensively studied, the heat-labile enterotoxin of *Escherichia coli* (LT) appears to have very similar immunomodulating properties to CT: LT is structurally and antigenically closely related to cholera toxin — anti-CT antibodies can, in fact, neutralize LT. The mode of pathogenic action is also identical to that described for CT, causing diarrhea by stimulating the activity of adenylate cyclase, which results in increased intracellular cyclic AMP concentrations.[7,14] More important, like CT, LT has also been shown to have potent adjuvant activity.[15]

We have investigated possible mechanisms of the adjuvant action of these enterotoxins in mice, and we have also, with the aid of defined nontoxic CT and LT derivatives, tested the possibility of separating the adjuvant action from the enterotoxic/diarrheogenic effect.

III. EFFECTS ON IMMUNE RESPONSE CELLS *IN VITRO* AND *IN VIVO*

The mechanisms responsible for the potent adjuvant effects of CT on the immune system are not fully understood. The results from *in vitro* and *in vivo* studies with isolated T cells, B cells, and macrophages have shown that CT can affect all of the cells engaged in a normal antigen-specific immune response and that the adjuvant action therefore probably is complex, involving more than one step in the immune response.[16-20]

A. CT ENHANCES ANTIGEN PRESENTATION

We have found that CT strongly potentiates antigen presentation by macrophages and enterocytes and that this stimulation of antigen-presenting cells (APC) could be a possible important mechanism involved in the adjuvant function of CT.

1. Effects on Mouse and Rat APC

Treatment of a clonal macrophage cell line, P388D1 (induced by recombinant interferon gamma, rIFN-γ, to express class II MHC-Ag) with CT strongly enhanced the ability of these cells to trigger an allogeneic T cell proliferative response. This effect, which was associated with up to four-fold increased formation of both soluble and cell-associated IL-1-α but not with increased expression of class II MHC-Ag, appears to be mediated mainly or exclusively through a cell-associated form of IL-1-α. Thus, the enhancement of antigen presentation induced by CT was evident also using metabolically inactivated, formalin-fixed P388D1 cells, and was completely abrogated by a specific antiserum to IL-1-α.[17] CT also strongly potentiated, by 100 to 200%, the capacity of normal peritoneal macrophages to present Conalbumine to the Conalbumine-specific T cell line D10.G4., as shown in Figure 1. Furthermore, PO administration of CT to mice enhanced within 24 hours the antigen-presenting function of freshly isolated cells from the Peyer's patches, mesenteric lymph nodes, and even spleen by three- to six-fold (N. Lycke, unpublished observations).

Epithelial cells have been ascribed an antigen-presenting function in the gut. Indeed, several laboratories have reported that freshly isolated epithelial cells can function as APC *in vitro* in both antigen- and allogen-specific systems.[21,22] We used a rat crypt cell line IEC-17 to analyze whether CT enhanced APC-functions in an allogeneic system. We found that CT-treated gut epithelial cells were 50 to 75% more efficient APC as compared to untreated cells. This enhancement was associated with increased IL-6 production and was not due to increased class II MHC expression.[23]

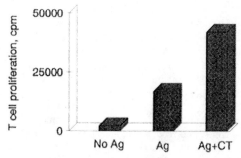

Figure 1 Peritoneal macrophages (H-2^k) were precultured 24 h in medium with or without Conalbumine (100 µg/ml) in the presence or absence of CT (0.1 µg/ml). Thereafter the cells were thoroughly washed and added to cultures of Conalbumine-specific cloned D10.G4.1 T cells and allowed to incubate for 72 h prior to analysis of T cell proliferation by ^{3}H-thymidine-uptake.

2. Effects on Human Monocytes and B Cells as APC

We also recently investigated the effects of CT and of its B subunit (CTB) on cytokine production by highly enriched (>90%) preparations of human peripheral blood monocytes. By analogy with murine studies, we found that CT induced strong intracellular accumulation of IL-1α and IL-1β but did not substantially affect the extracellular export of either cytokine. In fact, CT blocked extracellular export of IL-1β induced by LPS; in contrast, CTB as well as LTB had no effect on either intracellular accumulation or export of IL-1α or β (C. Czerkinsky, I. Nordström, N. Lycke, and J. Holmgren, unpublished observations).

Recent studies have indicated that CT but not CTB increases expression of cell surface-associated HLA-DR molecules on human peripheral blood B cells; this increase was associated with an enhanced ability of these cells to stimulate autologous as well as allogeneic T cells.[18] Since the separated A and B subunits of CT (CTA and CTB) as well as combinations of CTB and pharmacologic cAMP inducers failed to induce similar effects,[18] these studies indicate that the mere binding of the B subunit to GM1 ganglioside or elevations in intracellular cAMP are not sufficient to promote antigen-presentation by human B cells. Nonetheless, the enhanced antigen-presenting ability of peripheral blood B cells may extend to mucosal B cells, a possibility that could underlie at least partly the capacity of CT to potentiate immune responses to orally administered antigens (see below).

B. CT PROMOTES B CELL ISOTYPE DIFFERENTIATION

We have found that CT, at least as studied in mice, directly affects the proliferation as well as differentiation of B cells *in vitro*.[16,20,24,25]

1. Effects on Mouse B Cells

LPS-stimulated B cells exhibited both inhibition and enhancement of proliferation in the presence of CT. At high CT concentrations and early in culture, cell proliferation was inhibited whereas later and/or at physiologically more relevant, lower CT concentrations, B cell proliferation was increased up to 10-fold.[16] Furthermore, a striking increase in the production of IgG and IgA was observed in LPS-stimulated spleen cell cultures in the presence of CT. In contrast, a decrease in IgM content was evident concomitant with the increased production of IgG and IgA.[16]

The enhanced production of IgG and IgA did not result from increased proliferation of membrane IgG$^+$ or IgA$^+$ B cells in culture, but was rather due to greatly increased isotype switch differentiation in the presence of CT. By using cell-sorting technology we could show that CT acted on LPS-stimulated membrane IgM+, IgG/IgA− B cells to undergo isotype differentiation into membrane IgG+ or IgA+ B cells.[20] Subsequent studies revealed that CT also affects B cell responses to regulatory factors released by T cells. We found that CT acted in synergy with the T cell lymphokine IL-4 to induce isotype switch-differentiation in LPS-stimulated B cell cultures.[24] This effect was manifested at the gene level as demonstrated by enhanced expression of germline γ1 RNA transcripts, indicating that CT affects B cell isotype differentiation at an early stage, prior to final gene recombination.[24] An increase in IgG1 differentiation was also observed when CT was replaced by the nontoxic recombinant B subunit (rCTB), which is completely free of contaminating A subunit/whole toxin[25] (Figure 2). CT was, however, at least a thousand-fold (on an equimolar basis) more effective as compared to rCTB in promoting IgG1 differentiation in LPS- and IL-4-stimulated B cell cultures. Moreover, CT but not rCTB stimulated significant increases in IgG1 SFC even in the absence of IL-4.

Analysis of intracellular cAMP-levels in LPS-stimulated spleen B cells in the presence of IL-4, rCTB, or CT revealed that CT but not rCTB nor IL-4 affected the cAMP levels.[25] Thus, the difference in switch-inducing ability between CT and rCTB, together with the fact that whole CT but not rCTB causes increases in intracellular cAMP-levels in murine B cells, suggested a critical role for cAMP in isotype switching. Additional experiments demonstrated that CT could be replaced by dibutyrylcAMP (dBcAMP), a cAMP agonist: optimal concentrations of dBcAMP induced a three-fold increase in IgG1-differentiation, as compared to that seen with an optimal IgG1-inducing concentration of IL-4 alone. In addition, dBcAMP induced enhanced expression of germline γ1-RNA transcripts, a property that was not shared by rCTB, thus indicating that whereas dBcAMP and whole CT affected early events in isotype switching, CTB did not.[25]

These results were further supported by experiments showing that agents capable of inhibiting the cAMP-dependent protein kinase A (Rp-cAMP and H-8) significantly abrogated the synergistic effect of CT on IL-4-stimulated IgG1 differentiation. In contrast, the rCTB-induced IgG1 switch-differentiation was not inhibited by these agents, demonstrating that rCTB enhanced IgG1 differentiation independently of cAMP and the protein kinase A system.[25]

In conclusion, this shows that two different mechanisms are involved in the isotype-switching effect of CT: (1) increased intracellular cAMP levels stimulated by the A subunit potentiates isotype switching early in differentiation by augmenting the formation of sterile germline γ1-RNA transcripts; and (2) the binding of the nontoxic CTB to the membrane GM1-ganglioside receptors promotes later stages of isotype-switch differentiation.[25]

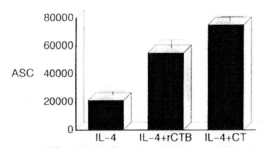

Figure 2 CT and rCTB enhance IL-4 stimulated IgG1 B cell differentiation. Spleen B cells were cultured in LPS (10 µg/ml) and stimulated by an optimal concentration of IL-4 (10,000 U/ml) in the presence or absence of CT (0.1 µg/ml) or rCTB (1.0 µg/ml). Data are shown as IgG1 ASC per 10^7 B cells. (Adapted from Reference 25.)

The existence of dual mechanisms operating together on B cell differentiation may help to explain the strong adjuvant function by CT on IgG and IgA antibody responses following oral and parenteral immunizations.

CT, as well as other cAMP-stimulating agents, have also been found to interact with lymphokines other than IL-4 in enhancing B cell switch differentiation: Stein and Phipps have shown that prostaglandin E_2 together with IFN-γ or IL-4 greatly increases the production of IgG2a and IgG1/IgE, respectively, in LPS-stimulated B cell cultures.[26] In addition, we have demonstrated that while CT alone and IL-5 alone augmented the percent of IgA-producing cells in LPS-stimulated B cell cultures by 3-fold, the combination increased the frequency of IgA cells by 15- to 20-fold,[20,27] again suggesting that CT promotes isotype switching since IL-5 only acts on postswitch IgA B cells (Figure 3). In conclusion, CT seems to have a general switch-promoting effect on B lymphocytes, leading to increased production of, e.g., IgG1, IgG2a, IgE, or IgA, depending on the type of stimulatory agent and the presence or absence of cytokines.

2. Effects on Human B Cells

We investigated the effects of CT and CTB on the proliferation of pure (100%) populations of cloned human B cells. In contrast to findings reported with anti-IgM-stimulated human B cell-rich suspensions, we found that CT as well as CTB had marginal, if any, effects on proliferation of human B cells induced by monoclonal anti-CD40 antibodies and IL-4 (C. Czerkinsky, I. Nordström, and J. Holmgren, unpublished observations). This is a system that has previously been shown to be particularly effective at stimulating the proliferation of broad populations of human B cells (including naive $sIgD^+sIgM^+$ and memory sIgD-isotype committed B cells, $CD5^+$ as well as $CD5^-$ B cells).[28] We are currently studying the effects of CT and its B subunit on the antigen-presenting capacity of purified human B cell subpopulations activated by CD40 and IL-4 and on their differentiation induced by a variety of progression factors such as IL-10, TGF-β, and/or IL-6.

C. CT AFFECTS T CELL PROLIFERATION AND LYMPHOKINE PRODUCTION

Like the effects on B cells, CT had a differential, either stimulatory or inhibitory, effect on T cell functions.

1. Effect on Murine T Cells

CT and CTB have been ascribed mostly inhibitory effects on T cells *in vitro*.[16,29-32] However, we found that CT was not always inhibitory in culture because Con A-stimulated T cells in culture showed enhanced proliferation in the presence of CT at 4 to 6 days of culturing.[16] Earlier in culture, the CT-induced inhibition of T cell proliferation was associated with decreased production of IL-2 and anergy to exogenously added IL-2,

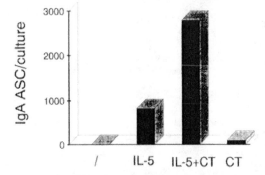

Figure 3 IL-5 plus CT augments the frequency of IgA-producing cells in LPS-stimulated B cell cultures. B cell-enriched spleen cells were stimulated with LPS (10 µg/ml) in the presence or absence of CT (0.1 µg/ml) or IL-5 (1,200 U/ml) or both for 6 days. The frequency of IgA ASC per culture well was determined by the ELISPOT technique. (Adapted from Reference 27.)

despite apparently normal expression of IL-2 receptors.[16] Also, interleukin-4-dependent T cell proliferation was reported to be less sensitive to CT inhibition than IL-2-driven proliferation *in vitro* and, accordingly, murine TH1 cell (producing IL-2 and IFN-γ) function *in vitro* was shown to be impaired, while TH2 cells (producing IL-4, IL-5, IL-6 and IL-10) were not affected by CT in culture.[31]

Furthermore, both CT and CTB have been shown to function as strong immunogens *in vivo*, efficiently stimulating CT-specific T cells.[19,33,34] Elson et al.[34] have shown that CTB-specific T cells could be triggered *in vitro* with denatured but not native CTB after immunization with CT.

Recent work in our laboratory has shown that CT administered together with Keyhole limpet hemocyanin (KLH) *in vivo* greatly promotes priming of KLH-specific T cells in mice.[35] As CT greatly enhances antigen-presentation,[17,23] we used an experimental model which guaranteed that the APC had not been exposed to CT. This was achieved by using peritoneal macrophages from naive syngeneic mice as APC, which were allowed to process antigen prior to adding the *in vivo*-primed T cells. Rechallenge of primed T cells with KLH *in vitro* 1 week after immunization gave several-fold stronger proliferation in KLH-specific spleen, mesenteric lymph node, Peyer's patch, and lamina propria T cells from KLH + CT-treated as opposed to KLH-only-treated mice (Table 1). Moreover, several-fold stronger cytokine production, i.e., IL-2, IL-4, IL-5, IL-6, IL-10, and IFN-γ accompanied the strong proliferative response, indicating that CT promoted priming of both TH1 and TH2 types of precursor cells. Enhanced T cell priming was also achieved after parenteral immunization with KLH admixed with CT adjuvant, demonstrating that the adjuvant effect of CT was not restricted to mucosal immune responses. Accordingly, as CT has a general immunomodulating effect on T cell primimg, the promoting effect on mucosal immune responses cannot be explained merely on the basis of a greater uptake of gut luminal antigens induced by CT.[35]

The increased cell proliferation to recall antigen observed with primed T cells from KLH and CT adjuvant-treated mice is associated with a great increase in the frequencies of KLH-primed antigen-specific T lymphocytes. Limiting dilution analysis gave evidence of a 20- to 40-fold higher frequency of primed antigen-specific T lymphocytes after intravenous immunization in the presence as opposed to the absence of CT adjuvant, as illustrated in Figure 4.[35]

The adjuvant effect of CT has been proposed by Elson and co-workers to result from decreased suppression mediated by CD8+ T cells. They have shown that CD8+ T cells are more susceptible as compared to CD4+ T cells to CT exposure.[34] However, we found that CT induced enhanced antigen responsiveness in CD4+ T cells primarily, suggesting that CT directly affected CD4+ T cell priming rather than regulatory balances between the CD4+ and CD8+ T cell subsets.[35] Also, Clarke et al.[33] have reported on positive effects of

Table 1   Effect of CT on antigen-specific priming of SP, MLN, PP, and LP T lymphocytes

Immunization	SP	MLN	PP	LP
KLH	4376 ± 919	2693 ± 296	2734 ± 246	1277 ± 266
KLH+CT	27112 ± 2772	17489 ± 2449	4583 ± 367	5150 ± 1466

Note: Lymphocytes were isolated from mice immunized once orally with KLH (2.5 mg) alone or together with CT (10 μg). Speen (SP), mesenteric lymph node (MLN), Peyer's patch (PP), and lamina propria (LP) T lymphocytes were cultured with APC which had previously been Mitomycin-treated and pulsed with KLH (100 μg/ml) or incubated in plain medium. Data are shown as incorporation of ³H-thymidine after 72 h of culture. Results are given as mean ± SD cpm for triplicate cultures, with the values obtained from cultures without antigen subtracted.
Adapted from Reference 35.

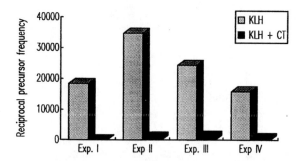

Figure 4 The frequency of KLH-specific T lymphocytes is greatly increased after priming with KLH plus CT. Mice were immunized intravenously with one dose of KLH (100 µg) alone or together with CT (1 µg). The frequencies of KLH-specific T lymphocytes in spleen T cells were determined by limiting dilution analysis 7 days after priming. (Adapted from Reference 35.)

CT on mucosal T cells following oral immunization. They found that after repeated oral immunization with KLH and CT, significant T cell proliferation could be detected *in vitro* on reexposure of primed T cells to KLH .

2. Effects on Human T Cells

We recently investigated the effects of CT on highly purified human polyclonal T cells and cloned T cells and found that CT markedly inhibited T cell proliferation, IL-2 receptor expression, and interferon-γ production induced by immobilized α-CD3 antibodies. In this accessory cell-independent system, the inhibitory effects of CT were seen in both isolated CD4+ and CD8+ T cells with regard to proliferation and IFN-γ production, the former population, however, being more affected (K. Eriksson, C. Czerkinsky, and J. Holmgren, in preparation). In contrast, CTB had, and only at high doses, marginal inhibitory effects on α-CD3-induced proliferation of CD4+ T cells and no effects on IL-2R expression and IFN-γ production. Furthermore, the antiproliferative effects of CT could only be observed when CT had been added at a very early stage in culture, suggesting that its inhibitory activity was exerted by blocking early signal transduction events and/or was counteracted by factors produced by recently activated T cells. Coaddition of IL-2 almost completely reversed the inhibitory effects of CT on α-CD3-induced CD4+ T cell proliferation. Since intracellular levels of cAMP have been shown to interfere with T cell receptor/CD3 signaling and T cell activation,[29] inhibiting IL-2 production[36,37] but inducing IL-2R expression,[38] our observations may suggest that CT affects T cell proliferation through a mechanism independent of cAMP.

Several other studies provide evidence that CT and CTB exert inhibitory actions on T cells by blocking increases in intracellular inositol triphosphate and free calcium.[29,30] Imboden et al. have demonstrated that exposure of the malignant human T cell line Jurkat to CT inhibited T cell receptor-mediated events, i.e., increases in inositol triphosphate and cytoplasmic free calcium.[29] In addition to these inhibitory actions, CT also caused a selective, partial loss of the T cell receptor/CD3 complex from the cell surface. None of these effects were mimicked by the B subunit of cholera toxin or by increasing intracellular cAMP levels with either forskolin or 8-bromo-cAMP.[29] Anderson and Tsoukas demonstrated similar effects on normal human T cells activated by α-CD3 antibodies and rIL-2; treatment of the cells with low concentrations of CT — but not CTB — caused a significant inhibition of the α-CD3-induced rise in cytoplasmic free calcium as well as the α-CD3 plus IL-2-induced proliferation. In contrast, neither the proliferation nor the Ca²⁺ influx were inhibited by CT when the cells were stimulated with PMA and ionomycin, activators that bypass the T cell receptor/CD3 complex.[30] Together these data indicate that CT inhibits T cell activation via a cAMP-independent pathway, perhaps by modification of a G-binding protein associated with triggering of T cells via the T cell receptor/CD3 complex.[29,30]

D. THE ROLE OF CT-ADJUVANT IN THE INDUCTION OF LONG-TERM IMMUNOLOGICAL MEMORY FOLLOWING ORAL VACCINATION

A specific aim of vaccination is clearly to stimulate immunological memory that can confer protective immunity for long periods of time. We have demonstrated both intestinal and extraintestinal long-term immunological memory after oral immunizations with CT.[39] Animals were given four oral priming immunizations with CT, and 2 years later they were boosted perorally with a single dose of CT. A strong α-CT ASC response was evident in the spleen and the lamina propria. The magnitude of the response was comparable to that seen in acutely primed and boosted mice.[39] Moreover, α-CT memory could be transferred to naive syngeneic recipient animals by isolated mesenteric lymph node B cells from memory mice immunized with CT 1 year earlier. A single oral antigen challenge of recipient mice resulted in α-CT antibody secreting cells in lamina propria, mesenteric lymph nodes, and spleen, and the magnitude of the response was similar to that previously found in optimally immunized mice.[40]

Next we investigated whether CT could be used for effective stimulation also of long-term immunological memory to unrelated protein antigens. Mice were given priming immunizations with KLH and CT adjuvant, and 18 months later the memory response to an oral booster with KLH admixed with CT was determined.[41] As shown in Figure 5, even a single priming immunization with KLH and CT adjuvant effectively induced the production of KLH-specific memory cells in the intestinal lamina propria, as demonstrated by high numbers of KLH-specific IgA ASC. In contrast, oral priming immunizations with KLH alone failed to stimulate immunological memory.[41] More important, while CT was found to be a requirement for the generation of memory, reencounter with antigen alone was sufficient to elicit a specific gut mucosal IgA memory response,[41] as shown in Figure 6. This suggests that once immunological memory is established in the

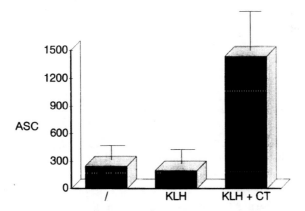

Figure 5 A single oral immunization with CT is sufficient to stimulate the development of long-term memory in the gut. Mice were primed by a single oral immunization with KLH (2.5 mg) alone or together with CT (10 µg) or, as a control, with PBS alone. After 18 months, the mice were challenged with one oral dose of KLH (2.5 mg) plus CT (10 µg). The frequencies of KLH-specific ASC per 10^7 lamina propria mononuclear cells were determined 6 days after challenge. (Adapted from Reference 41.)

166

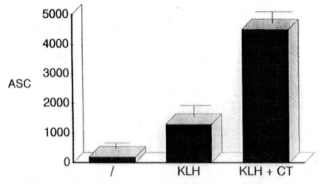

Figure 6 Reencounter with antigen alone is sufficient to elicit a gut mucosal IgA memory response. Mice were given five oral immunizations with KLH (2.5 mg) admixed with CT (10 μg); 22 months later the mice were orally challenged with antigen as indicated. The frequencies of KLH-specific ASC per 10^7 lamina propria mononuclear cells 6 days after oral challenge are shown. (Adapted from Reference 41.)

gut mucosal immune system, e.g., by oral vaccination using CT adjuvant, elicitation of a secondary-type response does not require the presence of CT and could thus result from the reencounter with the specific bacterial or viral pathogen. The ability of CT to induce immunological memory was not achieved by CTB, but required the whole toxin.

In the aforementioned work, we focused on immunological memory in the whole animal after oral vaccination using CT as an adjuvant. The continuation of these studies has addressed immunological memory at the cellular level.[42] An *in vitro* system for stimulation with recall antigen was established in which isolated memory cells were cultured in the presence of specific antigen, and B and T cell responses were recorded. We found that 8 months after oral immunizations with KLH and CT adjuvant, both KLH-specific T and B cells could be isolated from local mucosal (Peyer's patches and lamina propria) as well as systemic (spleen and mesenteric lymph nodes) lymphoid tissues.[42] The memory T lymphocytes responded by proliferation as well as lymphokine production to recall antigen *in vitro*. Moreover, the KLH-specific memory B lymphocytes responded by secretion of anti-KLH antibodies of predominantly IgM isotype. This suggested that at least a proportion of memory B cells following oral vaccination using CT adjuvant had not undergone terminal isotype-switch differentiation to downstream isotypes and thus had not deleted the μ constant heavy-chain gene. These results suggests that CT, incorporated into oral vaccines, may be an effective means to achieve long-term immunological memory and protection not only against pathogenic microorganisms at mucosal surfaces, but also against pathogens that primarily cause systemic infection.

IV. THE ROLE OF LOCAL IGA-PRODUCING B CELLS AND CD4+ T CELLS FOR INTESTINAL PROTECTION AGAINST CHOLERA TOXIN

Knowledge about the factors that confer protection against infection and disease in the gut mucosal immune system is in many respects incomplete. For host resistance against cholera disease, local production of IgA antibodies and mucosal IgA memory are thought to play key roles, in mediating recovery from disease as well as for providing resistance to second attacks of cholera. Animal studies have shown that protection against toxin challenge in intestinal loops after immunization with CT is associated with IgA antitoxin formation in the gut mucosa. However, alternative protective systems such as antisecretory factors (ASFs) have been implicated in resistance to CT.[43] Whether the ASFs function independently of the immune system is as yet not clear. Conceivably the gut T cells may function in immune protection not only by providing B cell help for IgA differentiation, but also for production of factors with a protective function, such as IFN-γ.

We have investigated the role of CD4+ T cells in host defense against cholera enterotoxin-induced diarrhea. Production of CT-specific IgA and protection against toxin challenge in intestinal loops after oral immunizations with CT were evaluated in normal mice and mice that had been depleted of CD4+ T cells by *in vivo* treatment with specific anti-CD4 monoclonal antibodies.[44] Depletion of CD4+ T cells performed prior to oral immunization with CT completely inhibited the ability to respond to CT. No CT-specific IgA-secreting cells were found either in systemic or in local mucosal lymphoid tissues. Nor did we observe serum antitoxin responses in these mice. Anti-CD4 antibody treatment blocked the ability to develop gut protection against CT challenge of ligated intestinal loops after oral CT immunizations. Taken together, these data indicate that CD4+ T cells play a critical role for the development of antitoxin protection and IgA antitoxin production following oral vaccination with CT.[44] Whether IgA antitoxin in the gut is solely and directly responsible for protection against CT is as yet unclear. However, studies in B and T cell-deficient mice are in progress to answer this question.

V. CAN ADJUVANTICITY BE SEPARATED FROM ENTEROTOXICITY?

Since CT is an enterotoxin, which even in amounts as low as 1 to 5 μg in humans can elicit severe cholera diarrhea,[45] it is important to evaluate whether the adjuvant action can be separated from the enterotoxic effect. Nedrud and colleagues have shown that glutaraldehyde treatment of CT leads to a 1000-fold reduction in toxicity but preserves its capacity to enhance mucosal immune responses after oral immunization.[46] Complete blocking of the ADP-ribosylating activity, however, abolished adjuvant properties of CT as well.[46] Currently we are investigating whether it might be possible to dissociate the toxic effect from the adjuvant/immunoenhancing effect. Two types of toxin derivatives have been used to address this problem: the nontoxic B subunit moiety of CT and a mutated *E. coli* LT.

A. CTB IS A STRONG CARRIER VECTOR

The ability of CTB to function as an effective system for mucosal antigen delivery has been evaluated using two different approaches. One system has employed chemical or gene fusion technology to couple foreign antigen to CTB and then use the hybrid molecule for immunization. In several reports, this has led to a marked increase in the ability to stimulate mucosal immunity against the foreign antigen, including specific IgA antibody formation in, for example, the gut,[47] the salivary glands,[47] the respiratory tract,[48] and the genital mucosa[49] after oral and/or topical immunization. We have shown that oral administration of small amounts of streptococcal protein antigen (that is not immunogenic per se when given alone by this route) covalently coupled to the CTB subunit elicits vigorous mucosal as well as extramucosal IgA and IgG antistreptococcal antibody responses in mice.[47] Thus, mice that were fed low doses of CTB-linked streptococcal antigen with free cholera toxin as an adjuvant displayed high frequencies of specific antibody-secreting cells in submandibular salivary glands, mesenteric lymph nodes, and the spleen. In contrast, equivalent or considerably higher doses of streptococcal antigen given alone or conjugated to nonintestinal binding protein (bovine serum albumin) were ineffective or, at best, poor in eliciting antibody responses to the streptococcal antigen.[47] In these instances the enhanced immune responses may primarily, if not exclusively, be attributed to improved antigen uptake and presentation to the mucosal immune system through the ability of CTB to attach to mucosal epithelial GM1 receptors, including those on M cells.[50] Other intestine-binding "lectins" such as certain bacterial fimbriae may also prove useful as vehicles for improved antigen delivery to the mucosal immune tissue in intestinal Peyer's patches and elsewhere.

B. LACK OF TRUE ADJUVANT ACTIVITY OF CTB IN ADMIXED ANTIGENS

An alternative approach has used CTB as an adjuvant admixed to foreign antigens, and not coupled to as described above. This has given conflicting results. We have consistently been unable to observe any adjuvant action of CTB in mice.[11,51] However, Chen and Strober[52] reported increased B cell responses with Peyer's patch B cells after oral administration of influenza virus admixed with CTB. Similar results were reported by Hirabayashi et al.[53] who showed that an intranasal inoculation of influenza vaccine admixed with CTB resulted in enhanced levels of nasal IgA antibodies. We believe that the most likely explanation for the divergent results when reporting adjuvant effects of CTB has been the degree of purity, i.e., the lack of contaminating holotoxin or CTA of the CTB preparation. For example, we have found that B cells exposed to a commercial CTB preparation indeed showed increased intracellular cyclic AMP-levels.[25] This was not found with the recombinant CTB,[25] derived from a genetically CT-deleted *V. cholerae* strain producing plasmid-encoded CTB.[54] At this time we cannot exclude that the adjuvant effect requires the whole toxin. It is conceivable that for oral immunization regimens the whole CT molecule is required, whereas in immunizations by the intranasal route the nontoxic CTB may be sufficient.

Wilson et al.[55] noted a greater adjuvant effect of (a small amount of) CT when given together with (a relatively large amount of) CTB than when given alone. While a true immunomodulating cooperation between CT and CTB cannot be excluded, a simpler explanation would appear to be as follows: CT has an enzymic action on cyclic AMP formation, such that one molecule per cell will suffice to increase cyclic AMP. When a limiting amount of CT is given alone, relatively few cells will bind the toxin molecules, whereas in contrast, when CT is being "diluted" in a much larger amount of CTB many more cells along the intestine will get the chance to bind and respond to CT (and CTB).

Thus it appears that, at least as tested in mice, the *whole toxin molecule is needed for the adjuvant action*. The B subunit moiety in itself seems to lack detectable adjuvant action for admixed antigen although it is able to serve as an efficient oral antigen carrier for CT-adjuvanted mucosal immune responses.

C. SINGLE AMINO ACID SUBSTITUTION IN THE A SUBUNIT ASSOCIATED WITH CONCOMITANT LOSS OF ENTEROTOXIC AND ADJUVANT ACTIVITIES

Recently, it was possible, using chemical mutagenesis with hydroxylamine, to obtain a plasmid encoding a mutated *E. coli* LT molecule (mLT) that bound with similar properties as the native LT protein to cells but was completely devoid of toxicity.[56] Consistent with these findings, the amino acid composition of the mLT-B subunit was identical to that of the normal LT-B subunit. Also the A subunit was identical, with the exception for a single amino acid residue substitution in position 112 (Glu→Lys).[56] This protein provided an excellent tool to address the question whether a discrete, defined single amino acid mutation in the A subunit would concomitantly knock out enterotoxicity and adjuvanticity or whether these properties would be separable.

We confirmed that the oligomeric and receptor-binding properties of purified mLT were identical to those of the parent LT and also that the mLT was devoid of rabbit-loop enterotoxicity as well as ability to induce cyclic AMP formation in different cells including lymphocytes. Furthermore, as tested with a battery of monoclonal antibodies against LT/CT A and B subunits we found no difference in the epitopes between the parent LT and the mutated LT, except for reactivity with a single monoclonal antibody which appears to map directly to an epitope involving the mutated residues 112 in the A subunit. When we then tested the immunogenicity and the adjuvant action of mLT for concomitantly administered KLH antigen after three oral doses, the results were clear-cut.

While the parent LT had similar adjuvant activity to CT on the intestinal lamina propria IgA anti-KLH antibody-forming cell response and also exhibited strong inherent immunogenicity, the mLT failed to give rise to any significant mucosal IgA response against itself and failed completely to stimulate an immune response to KLH,[51] as shown in Figure 7.

VI. PERSPECTIVES: USE IN HUMANS?

It is important to note that most of the studies and findings described above were undertaken in mice and on cells derived from mice (or rats), and that there are substantial differences in the gut mucosal IgA antibody response to CT and CTB between mice and humans. Specifically, in humans both CT and CTB are potent oral immunogens, and the intestinal IgA antibody response to orally administered CTB is fully comparable to that seen against CT in convalescents from severe cholera disease.[57,58] In contrast, in mice only CT is a strong oral immunogen, and, as described, CTB is poorly immunogenic unless added (or contaminated) with a little CT holotoxin. It remains to be determined whether in humans the relative independence of the A subunit for immunogenicity might also extend to an adjuvant action of CTB for admixed foreign antigens. If CTB in itself would prove to be insufficient at least three different strategies are open for experimentation in order to find a strong, yet safe mucosal adjuvant for human use: (1) to see whether defined mutations in the A subunit other than the one so far tested (residue 112) would give a nontoxic, yet adjuvant-active molecule; (2) to see whether the A subunit can be coupled to a different molecule than the B subunit, directing it away from the intestinal epithelial cells while still allowing it to bind to and act on appropriate cells of the immune system; (3) to determine whether a clinically safe adjuvant-active dose of CT (in this case probably admixed with CTB) could be "titrated" out.

Irrespective of the outcome of these efforts, the potential to exploit CTB as an antigen carrier molecule for mucosal immunizations in humans should be explored independently. In addition to the animal data supporting the feasibility of this approach mentioned above, studies in human volunteers have shown that after oral immunization with CTB, a substantial specific IgA antibody-producing cell response was obtained not only in the gut mucosa but also in the blood and, most significantly, in a distant mucosal tissue such as the salivary glands.[58] The documented safety and mucosal immunogenicity of CTB as an oral immunogen in humans, the availability of recombinant systems for large-scale

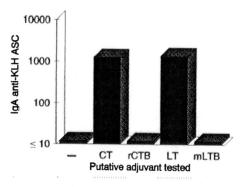

Figure 7 Comparison of the adjuvant effect of cholera toxin (CT), recombinant cholera toxin B subunit (rCTB), *E. coli* heat-labile enterotoxin (LT), and single amino acid residue mLT; (contains a single point mutation changing residue 112 in the A subunit from Glu → Lys) on the local immune response in the lamina propria of the small intestine of mice after three peroral immunizations with KLH (2.5 mg) admixed with the putative adjuvants (10 μg) or given alone (−). The frequencies of specific IgA anti-KLH ASC per million lamina propria mononuclear cells are shown. (Adapted from Reference 51.)

overexpression of CTB or CTB with peptide epitope extensions,[59] and the ability (in animals) of conjugates between CTB and foreign antigen to stimulate mucosal IgA immune responses would appear to lend promise to this approach to stimulate mucosal immunity to an expanded range of antigens.

SUMMARY

Cholera toxin (CT) and the analogous heat-labile enterotoxin (LT) from *Escherichia coli* are both powerful mucosal immunogens and adjuvants. They have several immunomodulating effects that alone or in combination might explain their strong adjuvant action in stimulating mucosal IgA and other immune responses to admixed unrelated antigens after oral immunization. These effects include increased gut permeability and uptake of luminal antigens; enhanced antigen presentation by a variety of cell types, including augmented production of the co-stimulating cytokines IL-1 and IL-6; promotion of isotype differentiation in B cells leading to increased IgA formation; and complex stimulatory as well as inhibitory effects on T cell proliferation and lymphokine production and induction of long-term immunological memory. This adjuvant activity appears to be closely linked to the ADP-ribosylating action of CT and LT associated with enhanced cyclic AMP formation in the affected cells, and thus it may prove difficult to eliminate the enterotoxic activity without loss of adjuvanticity. However, through a separate mechanism, as an antigen-carrier system providing specific binding to intestinal epithelium including the M cells of Peyer's patches, both CT and its nontoxic binding subunit moiety (CTB) have been shown to markedly enhance the mucosal immune response to various foreign antigens or epitopes covalently linked to these molecules. This gives promise for the future use of CTB or related nontoxic binding derivatives as vehicles to facilitate induction of mucosal immune responses to a broad range of antigens for human vaccination purposes.

ACKNOWLEDGMENTS

The experiments summarized here were supported by grants from the Swedish Medical Research Council and the World Health Organization (Transdisease Vaccinology Programme). We gratefully acknowledge collaboration with the laboratories of E. Severinsson, W. Strober, and T. Tsuji in some of the work cited and with A.K. Bromander, L. Ekman, K. Eriksson, U. Karlsson, M. Lindblad, I. Nordström, M. Quiding, and M. Vajdy in our own laboratories. The authors are grateful to S. Bodin for assistance in preparation of this manuscript.

REFERENCES

1. Hanson, L.Å. and Brandtzaeg, P., The mucosal defense system, in *Immunological Disorders in Infants and Children*, Stiehm, E.R., Ed., W.B. Saunders, Philadelphia, 1989, 116.
2. Holmgren, J., Czerkinsky, C., Lycke, N., and Svennerholm, A.-M., Mucosal immunity: implications for vaccine development, *Immunobiology*, 184, 157, 1992.
3. McGhee, J.R., Mestecky, J., Dertzbaugh, T., Eldridge, J.H., Hirasawa, J.H., and Kiyono, H., The mucosal immune system: from fundamental concepts to vaccine development, *Vaccine*, 10, 75, 1992.
4. Mestecky, J. and McGhee, J.R., New strategies for oral immunization, *Curr. Top. Microbiol. Immunol.*, 146, 1, 1989.

5. Bienenstock, J., The nature of immunity at mucosal surfaces — a brief review, in *Bacterial Infections of Respiratory and Gastrointestinal Mucosae,* Doncachie, W., Griffiths, E., and Stephen, J., Eds., IRL Press, Oxford, 1988, 9.

6. Holmgren, J., Actions of cholera toxin and the prevention and treatment of cholera, *Nature,* 292, 413, 1981.

7. Spangler, B.D., Structure and function of cholera toxin and the related *Escherichia coli* heat-labile enterotoxin, *Microbiol. Rev.,* 56, 622, 1992.

8. Pierce, N.S. and Gowans, J.L., Cellular kinetics of the intestinal immune response to cholera toxoid in rats, *J. Exp. Med.,* 142, 1550, 1975.

9. Svennerholm, A.-M., Lange, S., and Holmgren, J., Correlation between intestinal synthesis of specific immunoglobulin A and protection against experimental cholera in mice, *Infect. Immun.,* 21:1, 1978.

10. Elson, C.D. and Ealding, W., Generalized systemic and mucosal immunity in mice after mucosal stimulation with cholera toxin, *J. Immunol.,* 132, 27, 1984.

11. Lycke, N. and Holmgren, J., Strong adjuvant properties of cholera toxin on gut mucosal immune responses to orally presented antigens, *Immunology,* 59, 301, 1986.

12. Dertzbaugh, M.T. and Elson, C.O., Cholera toxin as a mucosal adjuvant, in *Topics in Vaccine Adjuvant Research,* Spriggs, D.R., and Koff, W.C., Eds., CRC Press, Boca Raton, FL, 1991, 119.

13. Holmgren, J. and Lindholm, L., Cholera toxin, ganglioside receptors and the immune response, *Immunol. Commun.,* 5, 737, 1976.

14. Sixma, T.K., Pronk, S.E., Kalk, K.H., Wartna, E.S., van Zanten, B.A.M., Witholt, B., and Hol, W.G.J., Crystal structure of a cholera toxin-related heat-labile enterotoxin from *E. coli, Nature,* 351, 371, 1991.

15. Clements, J.D., Hartzog, N.M., and Lyon, F.L., Adjuvant activity of *Escherichia coli* heat-labile enterotoxin and effect on the induction of oral tolerance in mice to unrelated protein antigens, *Vaccine,* 6, 269, 1988.

16. Lycke, N., Bromander, A.K., Ekman, L., Karlsson, U., and Holmgren, J., Cellular basis of immunomodulation by cholera toxin *in vitro* with possible association to the adjuvant function *in vivo, J. Immunol.,* 142, 20, 1989.

17. Bromander, A.K., Holmgren, J., and Lycke, N., Cholera toxin stimulates IL-1 production and enhances antigen presentation by macrophages *in vitro, J. Immunol.,* 146, 2908, 1991.

18. Anastassiou, E.D., Yamada, H., Francis, M.L., Mond, J.J., and Tsokos, G.C., Effects of cholera toxin on human B cells. Cholera toxin induces surface DR expression while it inhibits anti-IgM antibody-induced B cell proliferation, *J. Immunol.,* 145, 2375, 1990.

19. Wilson, A.D., Bailey, M., Williams, N.A., and Stokes, C.R., The *in vitro* production of cytokines by mucosal lymphocytes immunized by oral administration of keyhole limpet hemocyanin using cholera toxin as an adjuvant, *Eur. J. Immunol.,* 21, 2333, 1991.

20. Lycke, N. and Strober, W., Cholera toxin promotes B cell isotype differentiation, *J. Immunol.,* 142, 3781, 1989.

21. Bland, P.W. and Whiting, C.V., Antigen processing by isolated rat intestinal villus enterocytes, *Immunology,* 68, 497, 1989.

22. Mayer, L., Panja, A., and Li, Y., Antigen recognition in the gastrointestinal tract: death to the dogma, *Immunol. Res.,* 10, 356, 1991.

23. Bromander, A.K., Holmgren, J., and Lycke, N., Cholera toxin enhances alloantigen-presentation by cultured intestinal epithelial cells, *Scand. J. Immunol.,* 37, 452, 1993.

24. Lycke, N., Severinson, E., and Strober, W., Cholera toxin acts synergistically with IL-4 to promote IgG1 switch differentiation, *J. Immunol.,* 145, 3316, 1990.

25. Lycke, N.Y., Cholera toxin promotes B cell isotype-switching by two different mechanisms: cAMP-induction augments germline Ig heavy-chain RNA transcripts while membrane ganglioside GM1-receptor binding enhances later events in differentiation, *J. Immunol.*, 150, 4810, 1993.

26. Stein, S.H. and Phipps, R.P., Anti-class II antibodies potentiate IgG2a production by lipopolysaccharide stimulated B lymphocytes treated with prostaglandin E$_2$ and IFN-γ, *J. Immunol.*, 148, 3943, 1992.

27. Lycke, N., Severinsson, E., and Strober, W., Molecular effects of cholera toxin on isotype differentiation, *Immunol. Res.*, 10, 407, 1991.

28. DeFrance, T., Vanbervielt, B., Durand, I., Briolay, J., and Banchereau, J., Proliferation and differentiation of human CD5+ and CD5– B cell subsets activated through their antigen receptors or CD40 antigens, *Eur. J. Immunol.*, 22, 2831, 1992.

29. Imboden, J.B., Shoback, D.M., Pattison, G., and Stobo, J.D., Cholera toxin inhibits the T-cell antigen receptor-mediated increases in inositol triphosphate and cytoplasmic free calcium, *Proc. Natl. Acad. Sci. U.S.A.*, 83, 5673, 1986.

30. Andersson, D.L. and Tsoukas, C.D., Cholera toxin inhibits resting human T cell activation via a cAMP-independent pathway, *J. Immunol.*, 143, 3647, 1989.

31. Munoz, E., Zubiaga, A.M., Merrow, M., Sauter, N.P., and Huber, B., Cholera toxin discriminates between T helper 1 and 2 cells in T cell receptor-mediated activation: role of cAMP in T cell proliferation, *J. Exp. Med.*, 172, 95, 1990.

32. Elson, C.O., Holland, S., and Woogen, S., Preferential inhibition of the CD8+ T cell subset by cholera toxin (CT) and its B subunit (CT-B), *Faseb J.*, 4, A1864, 1990.

33. Clarke, C.J., Wilson, A.D., Williams, N.A., and Stokes, R., Mucosal priming of T-lymphocyte responses to fed protein antigens using cholera toxin as adjuvant, *Immunology*, 72, 323, 1991.

34. Elson, C.O. and Salomon, S., Activation of cholera toxin-specific T cells in vitro, *Infect. Immun.*, 58, 3711, 1990.

35. Hörnqvist, E. and Lycke, N., Cholera toxin adjuvant greatly promotes antigen-priming of T cells, *Eur. J. Immunol.*, 23, 2136, 1993.

36. Farrar, W.L., Evans, S.W., Rapp, U.R., and Cleveland, J.L., Effects of anti-proliferative cAMP on interleukin 2-stimulated gene expression, *J. Immunol.*, 139, 2075, 1987.

37. Mary, D., Aussel, C., Ferrua, B., and Fehlmann, M., Regulation of IL-2 synthesis by cAMP in human T-cells, *J. Immunol.*, 139, 1179, 1987.

38. Shirikawa, F., Yamashita, U., Chedid, M., and Mizel, S.B., Cyclic AMP: an intracellular second messenger for interleukin 1, *Proc. Natl. Acad. Sci. U.S.A.*, 85, 8201, 1988.

39. Lycke, N. and Holmgren, J., Intestinal mucosal memory and presence of memory cells in lamina propria and Peyer's patches in mice 2 years after oral immunization with cholera toxin, *Scand. J. Immunol.*, 23, 611, 1986.

40. Lycke, N. and Holmgren, J., Adoptive transfer of gut mucosal antitoxin memory by isolated B cells one year after oral immunization with cholera toxin, *Infect. Immun.*, 57, 1137, 1989.

41. Vajdy, M. and Lycke, N.Y., Cholera toxin adjuvant promotes long-term immunological memory in the gut mucosa to unrelated immunogens after oral immunization, *Immunology*, 75, 488, 1992.

42. Vajdy, M. and Lycke, N.Y., Stimulation of antigen-specific T- and B cell memory in local as well as systemic lymphoid tissues following oral immunization with cholera toxin adjuvant, *Immunology*, 80, 197, 1993.

43. Lönnroth, I., Lange, S., and Skadhauge, E., The antisecretory factors: inducible proteins which modulate secretion in the small intestine, *Comp. Biochem. Physiol.*, 90A, 611, 1988.

44. Hörnquist, E., Goldschmidt, T.J., Holmdahl, R., and Lycke, N., Host defense against cholera toxin is strongly CD4+ T cell dependent, *Infect. Immun.*, 59, 3630, 1991.

45. Levine, M.M., Kaper, J.B., Black, R.E., and Clements, M.L., New knowledge on pathogenesis of bacterial enteric infections as applied to vaccine development, *Microbiol. Rev.*, 47, 510, 1983.

46. Liang, X., Lamm, M.E., and Nedrud, J.G., Cholera toxin as a mucosal adjuvant. Glutaraldehyde treatment dissociates adjuvanticity from toxicity, *J. Immunol.*, 143, 484, 1989.

47. Czerkinsky, C., Russell, M.W., Lycke, N., Lindblad, M., and Holmgren, J., Oral administration of a streptococcal antigen coupled to cholera toxin B subunit evokes strong antibody responses in salivary glands and extramucosal tissues, *Infect. Immun.*, 57, 1072, 1989.

48. Liang, X., Lamm, M.E., and Nedrud, J.G., Oral administration of cholera toxin sendai virus conjugate potentiates gut and respiratory immunity against sendai virus, *J. Immunol.*, 141, 3781, 1988.

49. Lehner, T., Bergmeier, L.A., Panagiotidi, C., Tao, L., Brookes, R., Klavinskis, L.S., Walker, P., Walker, J. Ward, R.G., Hussain, L., Gearing, A.J.H., and Adams, S.E., Induction of mucosal and systemic immunity to a recombinant simian immunodeficiency viral protein, *Science*, 258, 1365, 1992.

50. Neutra, M.R., Phillips, T.L., Mayer, E.L., and Fishkind, D.J., Transport of membrane-bound macromolecules by M cells in follicle-associated epithelium of rabbit Peyer's patch, *Cell Tissue Res.*, 247, 537, 1987.

51. Lycke, N., Tsuji, T., and Holmgren, J., The adjuvant effect of *Vibrio cholerae* and *Escherichia coli* heat labile enterotoxins is linked to their ADP-ribosyltransferase activity, *Eur. J. Immunol.*, 22, 2277, 1992.

52. Chen, K.-S. and Strober, W., Cholera holotoxin and its B subunit enhance Peyer's patch B cell responses induced by orally administered influenza virus: disproportionate cholera toxin enhancement of the IgA B cell response, *Eur. J. Immunol.*, 20, 433, 1990.

53. Hirabayashi, Y., Tamura, S.-I., Suzuki, Y., Nagamine, T., Aizawa, C., Shimada, K., and Kurata, T., H-2-unrestricted adjuvant effect of cholera toxin B subunit on murine antibody responses to influenza virus haemagglutinin, *Immunology*, 72, 329, 1991.

54. Sanchez, J. and Holmgren, J., Recombinant system for overexpression of cholera toxin B subunit in *Vibrio cholerae* as a basis for vaccine development, *Proc. Natl. Acad. Sci. U.S.A.*, 86, 481, 1989.

55. Wilson, A.D., Clarke, C.J., and Stokes, C.R., Whole cholera toxin and B subunit act synergistically as an adjuvant for the mucosal immune response of mice to keyhole limpet haemocyanin, *Scand. J. Immunol.*, 31, 443, 1990.

56. Tsuji, T., Inoue, T., Miyama, A., Okamoto, K., Honda, T., and Miwatani, T., A single amino acid substitution in the A subunit of *Escherichia coli* enterotoxin results in loss of its toxic activity, *J. Biol. Chem.*, 265, 22520, 1990.

57. Svennerholm, A.-M., Jertborn, M., Gothefors, L., Karim, A.M.M.M., Sack, D.A., and Holmgren, J., Mucosal antitoxic and antibacterial immunity after cholera disease and after immunization with a combined B subunit-whole cell vaccine, *J. Infect. Dis.*, 149, 884, 1984.

58. Quiding, M., Nordström, I., Kilander, A., Andersson, G., Hanson, L.-Å., Holmgren, J., and Czerkinsky, C., Intestinal immune responses in humans. Oral cholera vaccination induces strong intestinal antibody responses, gamma-interferon production, and evokes local immunological memory, *J. Clin. Invest.*, 88, 143, 1991.

59. Czerkinsky, C., Svennerholm, A.-M., Quiding, M., Jonsson, R., and Holmgren, J., Antibody-producing cells in peripheral blood and salivary glands after oral cholera vaccination of humans, *Infect. Immun.*, 59, 996, 1991.

Chapter 2

Microparticles as Oral Vaccines

Derek T. O'Hagan

TABLE OF CONTENTS

I. INTRODUCTION

The use of microparticles with entrapped antigens as oral vaccines is an exciting area of research, which holds considerable promise for the future development of new and improved vaccines. Because of the characteristics and properties of polymeric microparticles, there is potential both for making currently available vaccines more effective and also for developing new vaccines against infections for which none currently exist. However, the successful exploitation of microparticles as oral vaccines is dependent upon the uptake of particles into the intestinal Peyer's patches following oral administration. This area of investigation is not without controversy, and doubts have been expressed as to whether particle uptake into Peyer's patches occurs at all.

It was concluded by Tomlinson and co-workers in 1987[1] that the transport of intact microparticles across the gastrointestinal tract (GIT) was restricted to exceptional and unusual circumstances. Nevertheless, the extensive and eclectic data describing the uptake of particulates across the GIT were reviewed by O'Hagan in 1990.[2] The data strongly suggested that particle uptake was not nearly so exceptional as had previously been suggested. Although many observations relating to particle uptake remain poorly explained, there has been an interesting debate as to the possible consequences of particulate uptake in humans. Sullivan[3] recently reawakened an older debate[4] and suggested that the uptake of particulates and crystals from toothpaste may be partly responsible for the development of Crohn's disease. Florence et al.[5] provided some support for this hypothesis by demonstrating the uptake of particles (0.5 µm) of titanium oxide into the Peyer's patches of rats. Titanium oxide is a common excipient of tablets and capsules which are routinely administered to humans. The subsequent correspondence in *Lancet* was testimony to the strong feelings aroused. The phenomena of particle uptake and the doubts expressed as to the validity of experimental observations may have historical parallels with related phenomena. For many years, it was generally accepted that proteins and peptides were not absorbed intact across the GIT. However, it is now known that macromolecules may be absorbed intact, and the intestinal absorption of peptides and proteins is a very active area of research.[6] In the 1970s, there was considerable debate as to the possible health risks associated with the intestinal uptake of asbestos and other mineral fibers from drinking water. In a review of the often contradictory data, Cook[7] concluded that a small fraction of fibers was absorbed across the GIT. Interestingly, it was noted that the width of asbestos fibers (0.02 to 0.05 µm) was similar to the diameter of particulates that were reportedly taken up into Peyer's patches following oral administration.

A hypothesis was recently presented by Freedman[8] to suggest that particle uptake in humans may be responsible for pathological consequences. It was suggested that the

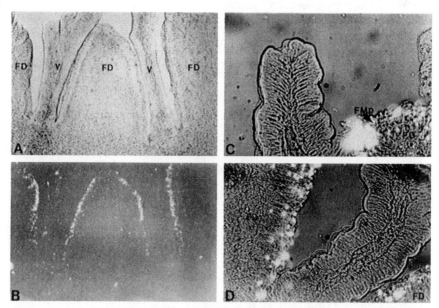

Figure 1 (A) Photomicrograph of a rabbit Peyer's patch showing lymphoid follicle domes (FD) and the surrounding villi (V) (magnification × 25). (B) Micrograph obtained when the image light is turned down to show the presence of polystyrene fluorescent microparticles (0.94 µm), which are almost totally restricted to the dome areas. (C) A follicle dome bordered by two villi, in which fluorescent microparticles (FMp) are present in abundance within the apex of the dome (magnification × 100). (D) Two follicle domes (FD) bordering a villus (V); individual microparticles (FMp, 0.94 µm) are present in the domes, but not in the villus (magnification × 100). (The micrograph was kindly produced by K. Howard and Dr. N.W. Thomas of the Department of Human Morphology, Queen's Medical Centre, Nottingham.)

uptake of starch granule across the GIT may result in embolism of arterioles and capillaries and that embolism of cerebral vessels may be one of the causes of senile dementia. However, it should be noted that within a generally contentious area, the data on the uptake of starch granules are perhaps the least convincing. In a number of publications, reviewed in 1977,[9] Volkheimer described the uptake of large particles (up to 150 μm) across the GIT by a mechanism called "persorption". While the uptake of small particles (<10 μm) appears possible (Figure 1), the uptake of larger particles (70 to 150 μm) seems considerably less likely. Volkheimer[9] reported the presence of particles in blood several hours after oral administration. However, drug targeting studies have shown that particles of a size greater than 7 μm become entrapped in the capillaries of the lung due to mechanical filtration.[10] Volkheimer[9] also described the presence of particles in the cerebrospinal fluid (CSF) and the urine. The apparent ability of particles to penetrate the blood/brain barrier was very surprising, since this is an effective barrier even to small water soluble molecules.[11] Moreover, even if the uptake of large particles is possible, since persorption was described as a passive process occurring at a very low ratio, there is little scope of exploitation for vaccine delivery. Consequently, persorption will not be discussed further. The uptake of particles across the GIT remains an ill-defined phenomenon and many questions remain only partially answered. Doubts remain concerning the mechanisms and sites of uptake, the extent of uptake, the particle size appropriate for optimal uptake, and the fate of particles after uptake. Furthermore, species differences have been identified and the extent to which observations in animal models can be applied to humans is currently unknown.

In this chapter, the term "microparticles" will be used to describe particles in the micrometer (μm) or nanometer (nm) size range (1000 nm = 1 μm). However, when a study has described the use of "nanoparticles" or "nanocapsules", the original term will be used. The term "microspheres" will be used to describe particles >50 μm in size (1000 μm = 1 mm). The two terms, microparticles and microspheres, are used to distinguish between particulate carrier systems that are designed to be taken up into the Peyer's patches and those that are designed to release entrapped antigens within the intestine. It is hoped that this distinction will become clearer as the reader progresses through the chapter.

II. UPTAKE OF PARTICLES INTO PEYER'S PATCHES

While there is now general agreement that particle uptake across the GIT occurs, considerable doubts remain concerning the extent of uptake. Although the majority of studies have suggested that only low levels of uptake are possible,[2] very high levels of uptake have been reported by some.[12,13] Moreover, different groups have emphasized the relative importance of mechanisms and sites of uptake.[2] Nevertheless, it is clear that the Peyer's patches are the predominant site of particle uptake, and recent findings have confirmed this interpretation. Aprahamian et al.[14] initially claimed that nanoparticles were taken up across the intestine through a paracellular mechanism between the enterocytes. However, they subsequently concluded that uptake occurred predominantly into the Peyer's patches.[15] Nevertheless, Jani et al.[16] claimed that microparticles (0.05 and 0.1 μm) may also be taken up by enterocytes, as was originally reported by Sanders and Ashworth.[17]

A. UPTAKE FOLLOWING ORAL ADMINISTRATION

Research into the intestinal uptake of particles was pioneered by Le Fevre and Joel, who demonstrated that carbon and polystyrene (PS) particles accumulated in the Peyer's patches of mice following oral feeding. These studies, reviewed in 1984,[18] showed that the extent of particle uptake was dose dependent. Carbon particles (0.02 to 0.05 μm) in Peyer's patches were detected with difficulty after 2 days, but were detected easily after 2 months of feeding.[18] Long-term feeding studies showed that isolated lymphoid follicles were also able to accumulate orally administered particles.[18] One study was designed to address the important issue of the upper limit of particle size for uptake. It was demonstrated that 5.7-μm PS particles were taken up into the Peyer's patches, but 15.7-μm particles were not.[19] In a later study involving fluorescent PS particles (1.8 μm), it was demonstrated that older animals showed greater uptake of particles than younger animals.[20]

Nevertheless, perhaps the most significant studies are those showing particle uptake after only a single oral dose. Elegant studies were performed by Ebel,[21] who administered fluorescent PS particles to mice and counted the particles in tissue samples using a fluorescence-activated cell sorter (FACS). Ebel showed that particle uptake was both size and dose dependent, with 2.65-μm particles being taken up much more extensively than 9.13-μm particles (Figure 2). In addition, the presence of food was shown to have an effect, and particle uptake occurred more extensively in fed animals (Figure 3). Eldridge et al.[22] also demonstrated that the extent of particle uptake in mice was size dependent and

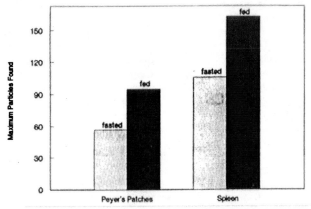

Figure 2 The effect of fed state on the maximum number of PS microparticles found in Peyer's patches and spleen. Mice were dosed 10[8] 2.65 μm particles by a single oral gavage, and fasting began 12 h prior to dosing. Fed mice were allowed to feed ad libitum. (From Ebel, J.P., *Pharm. Res.*, 7, 848, 1990. With permission.)

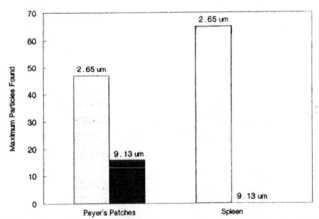

Figure 3 Size dependence of the maximum number of particles found in Peyer's patches and spleen. Mice were dosed 10[7] 2.65 μm or 9.13 μm polystyrene microparticles by a single oral gavage. No 9.13 μm particles were found in the spleen. (From Ebel, J.P., *Pharm. Res.*, 7, 848, 1990. With permission.)

particles >10 μm were not taken up. The nature of the microparticles was also shown to have an effect on the extent of uptake. The most hydrophobic particles, PS microparticles, were taken up to the greatest extent, poly(lactide) (PLA) and poly(lactide-co-glycolide) (PLG) microparticles to a lesser extent, and hydrophilic cellulose microparticles not at all.[22] A recent study in rabbits has confirmed that PS microparticles are taken up more extensively than PLG microparticles.[23] Studies involving the uptake of liposomes into the Peyer's patches of rats have indicated that surface charge may also affect the extent of uptake of particles, since negatively charged liposomes were taken up more extensively.[24] The uptake of microparticles following a single oral dose has been shown in rats.[25]

Additional workers have also described the uptake of microparticles following oral administration. Wells et al.[26] demonstrated the uptake of fluorescent PS microparticles (1 μm) in mice. The same group also described particle uptake in beagle dogs following administration into jejunal loops.[27] However, it was claimed that intestinal macrophages were responsible for particle uptake, rather than the Peyer's patches.[26,27] The uptake of fluorescent PS microparticles (0.1, 0.5, 1.0, and 3.0 μm) into the Peyer's patches of rats was demonstrated by Jani et al.,[28] and the extent of uptake was shown to be dependent both on the size and the nature of the particles. The smaller particles were taken up more extensively and nonionic particles were taken up to a greater extent than carboxylated particles.[28] Jani et al.[16] suggested that the upper size limit for uptake of particles into the Peyer's patches is 1 μm.

Further research on particle uptake has been undertaken using gut loop preparations. The work of Sass et al.[29] indicated that the uptake of PS microparticles (0.5 μm) was very rapid. Within 10 min after intrajejunal administration to rats, the microparticles were visible in the lymphatics, mainly associated with macrophages. The uptake of PS microparticles (0.25 and 0.61 μm) into the Peyer's patches of calves was demonstrated by Landsverk,[30] and the uptake of ferritin by M cells of calves was shown by Paar et al.[31] An earlier study had shown the uptake of resin particles (1 to 5 μm) in calves after administration in milk.[32]

B. UPTAKE BY M CELLS

Accumulated experimental evidence strongly suggests that the Peyer's patches, which are aggregates of lymphoid follicles,[33] are the predominant sites for particle uptake in the intestine.[2] Several studies have shown that a specialized epithelial cell, the M cell, is responsible for uptake (Figure 4). the M cells represent an "antigen-sampling" system and are responsible for the delivery of intestinal antigens into the Peyer's patches.[33]

Although Le Fevre and Joel believed that M cells were responsible for particle uptake,[18] they did not demonstrate this directly. Nevertheless, M cells have been shown to be responsible for the uptake of a wide variety of agents, including macromolecules, bacteria, viruses, and protozoa (Table 1). There are two main implications for the uptake and transport of antigens by M cells: (1) antigens transported through M cells will probably escape degradation and (2) the antigen will be released into an environment rich in immunocompetent cells. Uptake of antigen by M cells allows delivery into the immune inductive environment of the Peyer's patches and restricts access to alternative areas where suppressor T cells predominate.[34]

Jeurissen et al.[35] described the uptake of PS microparticles (0.48 μm) by M cells in mice, and Sass et al.[29] confirmed this observation in rats (Figure 5). Pappo and Ermak[36] demonstrated the uptake of fluorescent PS microparticles (0.6 to 0.75 μm) by M cells in rabbits. The rabbit M cells were identified by a monoclonal antibody, and uptake was shown to be rapid, since the microparticles were internalized within 10 min of their introduction into intestinal loops.[36] Interestingly, this study indicated that uptake into Peyer's patches may occur in synchronous waves, with an initial rapid uptake followed by a "lag" phase of negligible uptake.[36] Additional studies have confirmed the uptake of PS microparticles (0.46 μm) by rabbit M cells, and the extent of uptake was shown to be

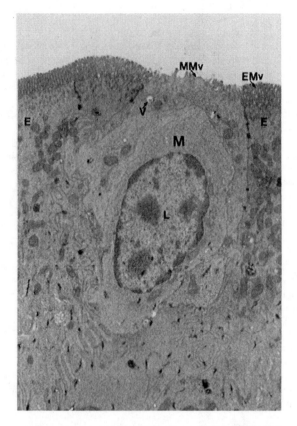

Figure 4 Transmission electron micrograph of a typical intestinal M cell of a rat (magnification × 10,093). The M cell (M) displays short stunted microvilli (MMv) in comparison to the normal "finger-like" microvilli (EMv of the neighboring enterocytes (E). Multivesicular bodies (V) are present in the thin apical cytoplasm of the M cell, and an invading lymphocyte (L) is present in the intercellular pocket. (The electron micrograph was kindly produced by R. Hughes and Dr. N.W. Thomas of the Department of Human Morphology, Queen's Medical Centre, Nottingham.)

dose dependent.[37] The uptake of PLG microparticles by rabbit M cells has been demonstrated by confocal microscopy.[23] The uptake of ingested carbon particles into the M cells of Peyer's patches has also been described in the domestic fowl,[38] indicating that particle uptake occurs in many species.

C. QUANTIFICATION OF PARTICLE UPTAKE

Several attempts were made by Le Fevre et al. to quantify the extent of particle uptake, but this proved difficult, mainly due to the instability of radiolabeled particles.[39] Nevertheless, it was estimated that following oral administration as single doses to mice, 0.01% of PS (0.17 to 0.25 μm)[40] and 0.0055% of carbon (0.027 μm)[41] particles were taken up into the Peyer's patches. Additional studies involving a range of radiolabeled microparticles have subsequently been described.[42-44] Despite problems due to the instability of the radiolabels, these studies confirmed only low levels of particle uptake. For example, De Keyser et al.[44] found only background activity in the organs of mice administered nanoparticles (0.2 μm). Low levels of particle uptake were also reported by Ebel,[21] who

Table 1 Macromolecules and microorganisms known to be transported into Peyer's patches through M cells

Macromolecules	Bacteria	Viruses	Protozoa	Particles
Native ferritin	*Yersinia enterocolitica*	Reovirus	Cryptosporidium	Latex
Cationized ferritin	*Vibrio cholera*	Rotavirus		Carbon
Horseradish peroxidase (HRP)	*Campylobacter jejuni*	Poliovirus		Poly(lactide-co-glycolide)
Ricinus communis agglutinins	*Chlamydia*	Parapox virus		Poly(butyl-cyanoacrylate)
Immunoglobulin A	*Salmonella typhi*	HIV-1		Liposomes
Wheat germ agglutinin	*Shigella flexneri*			HRP on latex
Cholera toxin	*Mycobacterium BCG*			
	Mycobaterium paratuberculosis			
	Brucella arbortus			

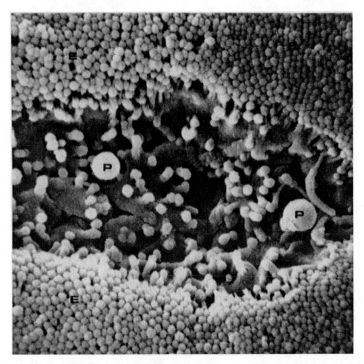

Figure 5 Scanning electron micrograph of two 0.5-μm polystyrene microparticles (P) on the surface of a single M cell (M) displaying typical microfolds. The M cell is surrounded by ordinary enterocytes (E) showing typical "finger-like" microvilli. Rat Peyer's patch epithelium × 14,500. (Micrograph kindly produced by Dr. W. Sass, Department of Experimental Surgery, Christian-Albrechts University, Kiel, Germany.)

calculated that only about 0.01% of doses of between 10^6 and 10^8 fluorescent PS particles (2.65 μm) were taken up into the Peyer's patches.

Nevertheless, Alpar et al.[45] claimed that the extent of particle uptake in rats was several orders of magnitude greater than had previously been reported in mice. These studies involved fluorescent PS microparticles (1.1 μm), which were counted in blood collected from the tail vein. It was calculated that about 39% of a single dose of particles was circulating in the blood 45 min after administration. It was also reported that the formulation vehicle and its volume had an effect on particle uptake.[45,46] Jani et al.[12] also reported high levels of particle uptake following oral administration to rats. The extent of uptake of fluorescent PS microparticles (0.05, 0.1, 0.3, 0.5, 1.0, and 3.0 μm) was determined by quantification of PS in tissues by gel permeation chromatography (GPC). The extent of particle uptake was shown to be size dependent, and 0.05-μm particles were taken up more extensively (34% of the dose) than 1-μm particles (5% of the dose). The distribution of particles was also shown to be size dependent, since the amount of PS found in the liver, spleen, bone marrow, and blood was 6% for 0.05-μm particles, 1% for 1-μm particles, and 0% for 3-μm particles. Studies were also undertaken with radiolabeled PS particles, which confirmed the GPC findings. Nevertheless, studies in rats at Nottingham, involving the direct collection of particles transported in the mesenteric lymph, have shown only low levels of uptake.[47,48] These studies have also indicated that the extent of uptake of particles is greatest at the lower end of the intestine (Jenkins, P., et al., unpublished observations).

Quantitative studies on particle uptake have also been undertaken in gut loop preparations. Under these experimental conditions, the transit of particles along the intestine is prevented. Therefore, uptake might be expected to be enhanced in comparison to feeding studies, in which intestinal transit is unrestricted. However, in feeding studies, the particles may become trapped in the intestinal mucus and delivered more slowly to the Peyer's patches for uptake (see Section VII.B). Delayed delivery of particles to the Peyer's patches through bioadhesion could not operate in gut loop studies because of the shorter duration of these studies. Following the administration of fluorescent PS microparticles (0.6 and 0.75 µm) into jejunal loops in rabbits, it was estimated that about 5% of the total dose of particles was taken up into Peyer's patches.[36] It was noted that the extent of uptake in rabbits was at least one order of magnitude greater than that in murine Peyer's patches, due to the relative abundance of M cells in rabbits.[36] M cells make up about 50% of the Peyer's patch epithelium in rabbits,[49] but only 5 to 10% of cells in murine Peyer's patches.[50] In a similar study, Jepson et al.[37] reported that <1% of florescent PS microparticles (0.46 µm) were taken up into the Peyer's patches of rabbits.

Hence, despite reports to the contrary,[13,45,46] particle uptake across the GIT appears to be an inefficient process. However, this does not necessarily restrict the use of microparticles as oral vaccines. The numbers of particles administered are generally in the order of >10⁶ particles. Even if an uptake efficiency of only 0.01% of the dose is possible, this still represents the delivery of many thousands of particles into the Peyer's patches. Thus, through the use of microencapsulation technology, intact antigen, presented in an immunogenic form and protected against degradation, may be delivered into the sites of the intestine which are responsible for the induction of immune responses.

III. FATE OF PARTICLES AFTER UPTAKE

The potential of microparticles as oral vaccines will be partially dependent on their fate after uptake. If the microparticles stay within the Peyer's patches, the induction of a secretory immune response is likely. However, if the microparticles penetrate to deeper sites, a systemic immune response may also be induced. The development of both secretory and systemic immunity following oral immunization will allow microparticles to be used against a wider range of pathogens.

Le Fevre and Joel reported that small numbers of fluorescent PS microparticles were found in the mesenteric lymph nodes (MLN), but only trace numbers were identified in the liver.[20] Ebel[21] reported the presence of small numbers of particles in the MLN and the spleen. The maximum number of particles in the spleen were found 1 day after administration, but the numbers subsequently declined. Consequently, the findings of Ebel are not inconsistent with those of Le Fevre and Joel, who only looked for particles in the spleen following chronic feeding. The appearance of particles in the spleen was shown to be size dependent, since 2.65-µm particles were present, but 9.13-µm particles were not.[21] The fate of PLG microparticles after uptake into the Peyer's patches has also been shown to be size dependent.[22] Particles <5 µm were found in the MLN and the spleen, but particles >5 µm stayed in the Peyer's patches.

The fate of microparticles following intestinal uptake in rats was shown to be size dependent by Jani et al.[12] Particles of 0.1 µm and less were identified in the MLN, spleen, liver, blood, and bone marrow. However, particles of 0.5 µm and greater were not detected in the blood or the bone marrow, and particles of 3 µm were not detected in the liver or the spleen.[12] A subsequent study confirmed the size-dependent distribution of microparticles following their uptake into Peyer's patches.[27] The rate of distribution of particles after uptake was also shown to be dependent on particle size.[25] Wells et al.[26,27] showed fluorescent microparticles in the MLN following oral administration. Hence, the available evidence suggests that limited numbers of particles may reach the spleen and lymph nodes following intestinal uptake. Undoubtably, the movement of particles through Peyer's patches to deeper sites is facilitated by the porosity of the basement membrane at these sites, where holes as large as 6 µm have been identified.[51,52]

IV. IMMUNOGENICITY OF MICROPARTICLES

It is a long-standing observation that particulate antigens are more immunogenic than soluble antigens. Over the years, this property has been exploited by several groups and there have been many reports describing the adjuvant effect achieved by the association of antigens with microparticles.

A. POLY(METHYL METHACRYLATE) NANOPARTICLES

An early study showed that adsorption of a model protein to PS microparticles (0.05 to 1.3 μm) resulted in enhanced antibody responses in rabbits.[53] Subsequently, Kreuter and colleagues reported the use of poly(methyl methacrylate) (PMMA) nanoparticles (0.05 to 0.3 μm) as adjuvants for whole[54] and split influenza virus vaccines.[55] The immune responses induced in mice and guinea pigs were greater than those induced by the vaccines adsorbed to aluminum hydroxide. It was also demonstrated that the nanoparticles induced protection in a murine model of infection.[56] The adjuvant activity of the nanoparticle was shown to be dependent both on particle size[57,58] and hydrophobicity,[59] with smaller and more hydrophobic particles giving the best responses. PMMA nanoparticles have also been used as adjuvants for adsorbed HIV in mice.[60] The nanoparticles (0.125 μm) induced antibody responses greater than those induced by an aluminum adjuvant.[60]

B. POLYSACCHARIDE MICROPARTICLES

The adjuvant effect resulting from the entrapment of a soluble protein in microparticles was demonstrated by Artursson et al.,[61] using polyacrylstarch microparticles (0.5 to 2.0 μm) with entrapped human serum albumin. The microparticles induced antibody responses in mice which were comparable to those induced by complete Freund's adjuvant (CFA).[61] An alternative approach was described by Schroder and Stahl,[62] who used crystallized dextran nanospheres (1 μm) to induce enhanced antibody responses to entrapped antigens. The predominant mechanism for the adjuvant effect of microparticles is likely to involve the efficient delivery of antigens into antigen-presenting cells (APC) due to particle phagocytosis.[63] In addition, an alternative mechanism may also contribute to the adjuvant effect, the controlled release of antigens.

C. MISCELLANEOUS PARTICULATES

The ability of fungal[64] and viral proteins[65,66] to self-aggregate into particulates has been successfully exploited to present antigens to the immune system. Virus-like particles expressed in yeast cells have recently been shown to be immunogenic following combined oral and rectal immunization in primates.[66a] An alternative way to present antigens to the immune system as particulates is through the construction of "solid-matrix antibody-antigen complexes".[67]

V. CONTROLLED-RELEASE VACCINES

The use of microparticles with entrapped antigens as controlled-release vaccines was first discussed in 1976 by Chang.[68] The overall objective of the current research on microparticles as vaccines is to develop single-dose vaccines.

A. POLYMERIC IMPLANTS

In a preliminary study, model antigens were entrapped within ethylene-vinyl acetate (EVA) copolymer pellets (1000 μm) and implanted subcutaneously into mice. The pellets induced antibody responses for 6 months that were comparable to those induced by CFA.[69] However, the EVA pellets were nondegradable and required surgical removal after completion of the immunization process. Therefore, polymeric implants were developed which degraded *in vivo* to release tyrosine derivatives.[70] Tyrosine had previously been shown to possess adjuvant activity.[71] Following subcutaneous immunization in mice, the biodegradable implants induced antibody responses for 1 year that were comparable to those induced by CFA.[70] An alternative approach to the controlled release of antigens involves the use of cholesterol-lecithin implants.[72] Polymeric implants have also been used for the controlled release of antibodies.[73,74] The use of degradable glasses for controlled delivery of vaccines has also been discussed.[75]

B. POLY(LACTIDE-COGLYCOLIDE) MICROPARTICLES

Recent work on controlled-release vaccines has concentrated on the use of PLG polymers,[76] since these polymers are the primary candidates for the development of vaccines. The PLG polymers and closely related analogues have been used for alternative biomedical applications for many years. They have been used both as resorbable sutures[77] and as bone plates for internal fixation.[78] In addition, PLG polymers have also been used for the preparation of controlled-release drug delivery systems.[79] Long experience with these polymers has shown that they are completely biodegradable and degrade to toxicologically acceptable products, which are eliminated from the body.[80,81] The polymers undergo degradation by random hydrolytic scission of the ester bonds and degrade to lactic and glycolic acids, which are normal metabolites. The biocompatibility of microparticles prepared from PLG polymers has been demonstrated in vivo.[82]

The mechanisms of release of peptides and proteins from PLG microparticles is complex, but appears to be largely controlled by polymer degradation.[76] The rate of degradation for each individual polymer may be controlled, since it is dependent upon variables such as the copolymer composition, molecular weight, molecular weight distribution, and morphology.[81] Hence, controlled-release vaccines prepared from PLG polymers may be designed to release entrapped antigens at predetermined intervals following a single immunization and may obviate the need for booster doses of vaccines.[83]

Following primary and secondary immunization in mice, the immunogenicity of ovalbumin (OVA) in microparticles (5.3 μm) was shown to be comparable to the immunogenicity of OVA emulsified in CFA (Figure 6).[84] Meanwhile, in rats, it was demonstrated that the immunogenicity of microparticles could be enhanced by their dispersion in a water-in-oil emulsion.[85] This finding was confirmed using tetanus toxoid in PLG microparticles.[86] Alonso et al.[86a] recently described the induction of high levels of neutralizing antibodies to TT entrapped in microparticles. The preparation of PLG microparticles with entrapped antigens has been discussed in detail by Jeffery et al.[87,88] The immunogenicity of antigens in PLG microparticles has also been demonstrated by Eldridge et al.[89] Staphylococcal enterotoxin B toxoid (SEB) was entrapped in microparticles (1-10 μm) and induced antibody responses in mice that were comparable to those induced by CFA. The size of the microparticles was shown to have an effect on the immune response, and microparticles <10 μm were shown to be more immunogenic than microparticles >10 μm.[89] Microparticles <10 μm were shown to be taken up by macrophages and transported to the draining lymph nodes, while microparticles >10 μm remained at the injection site.[89] The smaller microparticles (<10 μm) were also shown to induce a more rapid rise in antibody levels, presumably due to their accelerated degradation after uptake into macrophages.[89] Eldridge et al.[90] also demonstrated that different sized microparticles could be administered in combination to provide a biphasic antibody response. The effect of microparticle size on the adjuvant effect of PLG microparticles was also shown by O'Hagan et al.,[91] and microparticles <10 μm (1.5 μm) were significantly more immunogenic than microparticles >10 μm (73 μm). The immunogenicity of PLG microparticles with controlled-release characteristics was also investigated, and the microparticles induced antibody responses that were significantly enhanced for 1 year after a single immunization.[91] The use of microparticles prepared from PLG polymers with controlled release characteristics has also been demonstrated by Gilley et al.[92]

Altman and Dixon[93] described the induction of low levels of antibodies following immunization with a peptide from hepatitis B virus entrapped in PLG microparticles.

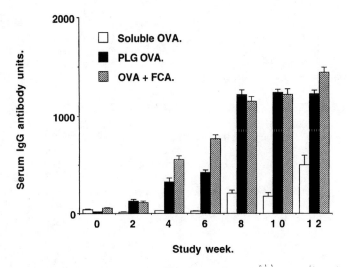

Figure 6 Serum IgG antibody responses (±SE) following subcutaneous immunization in groups of 10 Balb/c mice with 100 µg OVA as a soluble form, entrapped in 2.1 µm PLG microparticles and emulsified in CFA. Identical booster immunizations were administered at study week 6.

Nellore et al.[93a] entrapped hepatitis B surface antigen vaccine in microparticles and showed the induction of enhanced antibody responses. The immunogenicity of diptheria toxoid (DT) entrapped in microparticles was investigated in mice by Singh et al.[94] A single dose of DT in PLA microparticles (30 to 100 µm) gave a response comparable to the normal three-dose schedule. Biodegradable microparticles are also under investigation as vaccines for the control of fertility, and encouraging results have been obtained in animal models.[95] Microparticles have also been shown to be capable of inducing immune responses to entrapped viruses, including influenza virus,[96] parainfluenza virus,[97] and simian immunodeficiency virus.[98] In addition, antibody responses to a protein conjugate of the type 3 capsular polysaccharide of *Streptococcus pneumoniae* have been induced following entrapment in microparticles (<10 µm).[99] O'Hagan et al.[100] showed that microparticles induced proliferative and cytotoxic T lymphocyte (CTL) responses in spleen cells following parenteral immunization. Microparticles also induced CTL activity in spleen cells following oral immunization (Figure 7).[101] Microparticles have also shown potential as delivery systems for use in allergen immunotherapy.[101a]

Alternative polyesters which, unlike PLG and PLA, are water soluble, have also been used for the development of controlled-release vaccines. Bioerodible hydrogels based on polyethylene glycol were used to prepare microspheres (20 to 60 µm) with entrapped luteinizing hormone releasing hormone (LHRH) conjugated to DT. The duration of release of the entrapped LHRH-DT *in vitro* was shown to be dependent on the degree of cross-linking of the polyester, which controlled chain cleavage and polymer swelling.[102] An interesting novel approach to the controlled release of antigens was described by Cohen et al.,[103] who microencapsulated liposomes containing entrapped BSA. The microcapsules (500 µm) were prepared by cross-linking of alginates and gave significantly better antibody responses in mice than CFA. Microencapsulated liposomes were developed because liposomes do not allow for extended antigen release profiles and may not be suitable as single dose vaccines.

Initial studies concerned with the development of a single dose tetanus vaccine have already been completed, and clinical trials with controlled release microparticles are

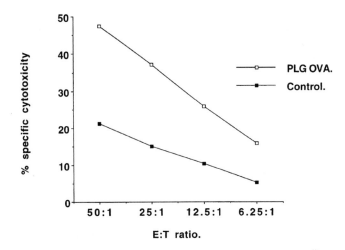

Figure 7 Ovalbumin-specific CTL activity induced in spleen cells of mice (n = 8) following oral immunization with 100 µg OVA on 3 consecutive days, entrapped in 2.3 µm PLG microparticles. Identical booster immunizations were administered 1 week after the primary immunizations, and the spleen cells were removed 7 days after the final dose. The control group (n = 8) shows the level of nonspecific CTL activity against the target cells at the different dilutions of the spleen effector cells. (This study was performed by Dr. A.Mcl. Mowat and K.J. Maloy of the Department of Immunology, Western Infirmary, Glasgow. For further experimental details of the assay system, see Mowat, A.Mcl. et al., *Immunology*, 72, 317, 1991.)

likely in the near future. The controlled release of proteins from PLG microparticles has also been investigated *in vitro*.[104-106]

C. ALBUMIN MICROPARTICLES

An alternative approach to the development of controlled release vaccines was described by Martin et al.,[107] who produced polymerized serum albumin microparticles (100 to 200 µm) with entrapped virus. Following immunization in rabbits, the microparticles induced antibody responses comparable to those induced by Freund's incomplete adjuvant (FIA).[107] Although no adverse effects were reported, the potential immunogenicity of the polymerized albumin remains a cause for concern and may restrict this approach to vaccine development.

VI. PARTICLES AS ORAL DELIVERY SYSTEMS

Research into the use of microparticles as oral drug delivery systems has been underway for considerably longer than research into the use of microparticles as oral vaccines.

A. DRUG DELIVERY SYSTEMS

Early studies showed that linking insulin to PS particles was an effective way to protect the peptide from degradation following oral administration.[108,109] Subsequently, a number of studies have described the use of microparticles to enhance the absorption of drugs. Hexyl(cyanoacrylate) nanoparticles (0.23 μm) were used to enhance the bioavailability of adsorbed vincamine in rabbits.[110] The alkylcyanoacrylates are biodegradable polymers which have been used as tissue adhesives, and a drug delivery system prepared from these polymers has advanced to clinical trials.[111] Poly(butyl cyanoacrylate) (PBC) nanocapsules (0.165 μm) were shown to enhance the intestinal absorption of an entrapped drug in beagles, following administration into isolated gut loops.[112] More interestingly, PBC nanocapsules have also been shown to enhance the absorption of entrapped insulin following oral administration. The nanocapsules (0.22 μm) were administered to diabetic rats and induced a significant decrease in glycemia after 2 days, which was maintained for up to 20 days (Figure 8).[113] An earlier study had shown that alkylcyanoacrylate nanoparticles with adsorbed insulin were not effective following oral administration.[114] The hypoglycemic effect of insulin nanocapsules was confirmed in a second study, in which the effect of site of administration in the GIT was assessed.[115] The hypoglycemic effect from a single dose of nanocapsules (0.3 μm) lasted from 11 to 16 days, depending on the site of administration. The rank order for the potency of nanocapsules was ileum > jejenum > duodenum > colon.[110] *In vitro* studies have confirmed that encapsulated insulin retains the ability to interact with its receptor.[116] However, the efficacy of PBC nanocapsules for oral peptide delivery appears to be confined to insulin, since alternative peptides encapsulated in nanocapsules were not effective.[117]

Nanocapsules (0.23 μm) prepared from PBC have also been used for the oral delivery of indomethacin in rats.[118] The bioavailability was enhanced and the absorption peak was achieved more rapidly.[118] Subsequently, it was demonstrated that indomethacin in PBC

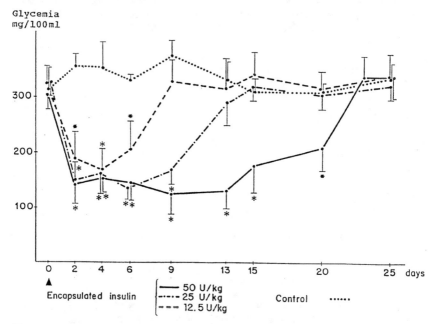

Figure 8 Effect of single intragastric doses of insulin (12.5, 25, and 50 U/kg) entrapped in 0.3-μm poly(isobutyl cyanoacrylate) nanocapsules on glycemia in diabetic rats fasted overnight. Results are the means (±SE) for 7 or 8 animals. * Indicates a statistically significant response. (From Damge, C. et al., *J. Controlled Rel.*, 13, 233, 1990. With permission.)

and PLA (0.29 μm) nanocapsules exerted a biological effect following oral administration.[119] It was also shown that the nanocapsules protected the jejunum from the ulcerating effects of the drug.[120]

B. ANTIGEN DELIVERY SYSTEMS

The success of PBC nanoparticles as oral drug delivery systems encouraged us to assess their potential as antigen delivery systems. Two alternative PBC particle-stabilizing agents were used, and it was possible to produce microparticles with mean sizes of 0.1 μm and 3 μm.[121,122] Following adsorption of OVA to the microparticles, they were orally administered to two groups of rats. Both groups of rats showed enhanced salivary IgA antibody responses in comparison to soluble OVA. However, only the group receiving 0.1-μm particles showed an enhanced response after the animals were boosted (Figure 9). The 0.1-μm group also showed an enhanced serum IgG antibody response.[121,122] Thus, it was shown for the first time that biodegradable microparticles could function as an effective oral antigen delivery system. Furthermore, the results indicated that particle size was an important factor influencing the response.

Nevertheless, the induction of enhanced secretory immunity following oral administration of particulates was not a novel observation. Several years earlier, Cox and co-workers[123,124] had shown that oral immunization with particulate antigens was more effective than soluble antigens. Challacombe[125] also reported that particulate antigens were more effective for oral immunization. O'Hagan et al.[126] confirmed these observations and showed that polyacrylamide (PA) microparticles constituted an effective antigen delivery system for entrapped OVA. The PA microparticles (2.55 μm) were administered orally to rats and induced a significantly enhanced salivary IgA antibody response.[126] The ability of particulates to induce enhanced antibody responses was confirmed by Amerongen et al.,[127] who used microcrystals of hydroxyapatite to present HIV-1 gp120 to M cells for the induction of monoclonal IgA antibodies.

Eldridge et al.[20] described the use of PLG microparticles as an oral antigen delivery system for SEB in mice. The microparticles (4 μm) induced a rise in serum antibody and

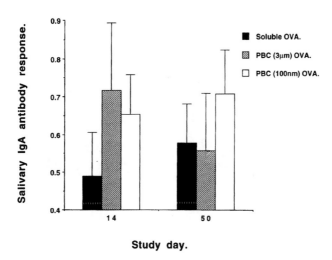

Figure 9 Salivary IgA antibody responses (±S.D.) following oral immunization in groups of 8 Wistar rats with 1 mg ovalbumin on three consecutive days in a soluble form and adsorbed to poly (butylcyanoacrylate) (PBC) microparticles of two different mean sizes. Single booster immunizations were administered to each group at day 46.

secretory IgA.[22] It was also reported that oral immunization with SEB in microparticles induced pulmonary antibody responses[90] and this may have important implications for the development of vaccines against respiratory tract pathogens. Microparticles have also been used as an oral delivery system for entrapped influenza virus,[96] parainfluenza virus,[97] and simian immunodeficiency virus.[98] Following oral immunization in mice, it was demonstrated that OVA in PLG microparticles (3 μm) induced significantly enhanced secretory IgA and systemic IgG antibody responses (Figures 10 and 11).[128] It was also shown that the rate of release of the antigen from the microparticles affected both the serum and secretory antibody responses.[129] Preliminary studies in mice showed that cholera toxin B subunit (CTB) entrapped in microparticles (1.2 μm) induced antibody secreting cells in spleens and MLNs following oral immunization.[100]

Microparticles have been evaluated as an oral delivery system for polysaccharide-based vaccines. The capsular polysaccharide from *S. pneumoniae* was conjugated to SEB, entrapped in microparticles and orally administered to mice. The microparticles enhanced the serum IgM and IgA antibody responses, but not the responses in the saliva, gut wash, or bronchioalveolar lavage fluid (BAL). Intratracheal (IT) immunization with microparticles was more effective than oral immunization, and IT immunization induced a disseminated mucosal IgA response.[99] Intranasal immunization with microparticles has also been shown to induce serum and systemic antibody responses.[97,130,131]

Edelman et al.[132] described the use of PLG microparticles for oral immunization with enterotoxigenic *Escherichia coli* colonization factor 1 (CFA/1) antigen. Following a single immunization in rabbits, a vigorous serum IgG antibody response was induced to the CFA/1. However, only one of three animals in the study showed a secretory IgA response.[132] The microparticles ranged in size from <10 μm to 200 μm (mean size 27 μm),

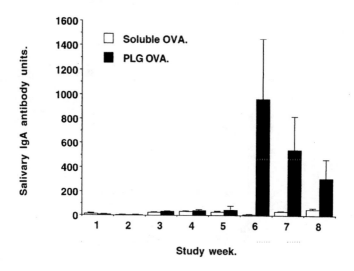

Figure 10 Salivary IgA antibody responses (±SE) following oral immunization in groups of 10 Balb/c mice with 1 mg OVA on 3 consecutive days as a soluble form and entrapped in 3-μm PLG microparticles. Identical booster immunizations were administered at study week 4.

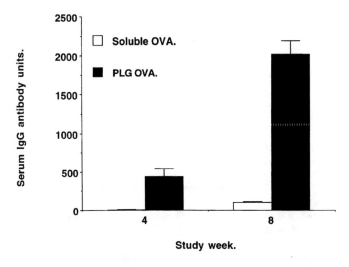

Figure 11 Serum IgG antibody responses (±SE) following oral immunization in groups of 10 Balb/c mice with 1 mg OVA on three consecutive days as a soluble form and entrapped in 3 μm PLG microparticles. Identical booster immunizations were administered at study week 4.

and the majority were too large for uptake into the Peyer's patches. Therefore, the main purpose of microencapsulation was to protect the antigen against degradation, and it was probably released in the intestine prior to uptake into the Peyer's patches. Spenlehauer et al.[133] showed that PLA nanoparticles (0.1 μm) were not degraded in simulated gastric media, but did begin to breakdown after 2 hours in simulated intestinal media. A study by McQueen et al.[134] demonstrated that CFA/1 in microparticles was able to induce protective immunity in rabbits. Moreover, a recent clinical trial in human volunteers has shown limited protective efficacy for a microparticle vaccine containing CFA/11, following challenge with enterotoxigenic *E. coli*.[134a] Hence, particle carrier systems which are too large for uptake into the Peyer's patches may also be exploited for the development of oral vaccines.

C. ENTERIC-COATED MICROSPHERES AS ORAL VACCINES

Klipstein et al.[135] were the first to describe the use of enteric-coated microspheres for oral vaccine development. Heat-labile enterotoxin from *E. coli* (LTB) was encapsulated in microspheres (3000 μm) prepared from starch and cellulose, with hydroxypropyl methylcellulose phthalate as an enteric-coating polymer. After oral administration to rats, the microspheres induced serum and intestinal antibody responses that were comparable to the responses induced by oral immunization after ablation of gastric secretions with the drug cimetidine.[135] Maharaj et al.[136] described a method for the preparation of microspheres (1000 to 3000 μm) with entrapped virus using cellulose acetate phthalate (CAP). CAP has been used extensively for enteric-coating of drugs.[137] The microspheres were stable for 6 h in simulated gastric fluid, but disintegrated rapidly in simulated intestinal fluid. A similar approach to oral vaccine development was described by Lin and co-workers.[138-140] CAP microspheres (500 to 2000 μm) were prepared with entrapped *Mycoplasma hyopneumoniae*,[138] which is an important pathogen in pigs. It was demonstrated that the microspheres showed enhanced stability in the presence of low pH[139] and trypsin.[140] In addition, this vaccine has recently shown protective efficacy in pigs.[140a] In recent years, enteric coatings have been applied to a number of vaccines which were subsequently used in clinical trials, including vaccines against *Haemophilus influenzae*,[141] typhoid fever,[142] tuberculosis,[143] and hepatitis B virus.[144] An alternative polymer, Eudragit L100, has recently been used to produce enteric-coated microspheres (180 to 500 μm) with entrapped insulin.[145,146] Hence, enteric-coated microspheres may find applications in the development of improved oral vaccines. A recent report has described the use of enteric-coated microspheres for oral immunization of salmonid fish.[146a]

VII. OPTIMIZING ORAL DELIVERY SYSTEMS

If microparticles are to achieve widespread use as oral vaccines, then it is clear that the current formulations will need to be improved. Ideally, the dose should be administered as a capsule or a tablet, which should help to protect the antigens from degradation. Furthermore, the formulation should have desirable pharmaceutical characteristics, such as long-term stability on storage under varying conditions. Several formulations which are currently being developed to overcome drug delivery problems may be adapted for the development of improved oral vaccines.

A. MULTIPARTICULATE DELIVERY SYSTEMS

For large-scale human trials, it will probably be necessary to administer microparticles as tablets or capsules. However, the formulation of microparticles into tablets or capsules presents several problems. To allow for successful compression into tablets, it is essential that the microparticles must have good powder flow properties so that they will uniformly fill tablet molds. In addition, the microparticles must be capable of resisting the severe mechanical stress of compression. If not, then the microparticles may rupture and lose important characteristics, such as controlled release properties. Furthermore, fusion of microparticles may occur during compression, resulting in the formation of a nondisintegrating matrix. Jalsenjak et al.[147] reported that the tableting of microcapsules resulted in the production of a nondisintegrating matrix with impaired drug release properties.

Bodmeier et al.[148] described one approach to the development of a dosage form for oral administration of microparticles, in which microparticles were entrapped in beads prepared by gelation of chitosan and sodium alginate. Entrapment in the beads did not change the properties of the microparticles, and high levels of microparticle entrapment were possible. CAP could be used to produce an enteric-coated formulation, although the beads themselves were capable of providing pH-dependent release. The beads displayed good powder flow properties and could be administered as prepared or filled into capsules.

B. BIOADHESIVE DELIVERY SYSTEMS

One of the main factors currently limiting the efficacy of oral drug delivery systems is the rapid transit of dosage forms through the small intestine.[149] In healthy volunteers, small intestinal transit time is normally about 3 to 4 hours[150] and this could conceivably restrict the uptake of particles into Peyer's patches. However, the intestinal transit of microparticles may be delayed through the use of bioadhesive polymers. The polymers may be used to directly prepare microparticles, or alternatively they may be used to "coat" preformed microparticles. Kreuter et al.[43] suggested that PBC nanoparticles were effective orally due to their ability to get trapped between the villi and adsorbed to the mucosa. Studies have confirmed that PBC nanoparticles adsorb to porcine intestinal tissue *in vitro*.[151] In studies undertaken with radiolabeled PBC particles (0.2 to 0.3 μm) in mice, there was an accumulation of radioactivity proximal to the ileocecal junction 90 min after administration.[43] Nevertheless, the levels of radioactivity in the small intestine dropped to 30 to 40% of the 90-min value within 4 to 8 h and to 5%, 24 h after dosing.[43] A study by De Keyser et al.[44] confirmed that nanoparticles (0.2 μm) were almost totally cleared from the GIT of mice after 24 h. Approximately 70% of the particles were cleared from the stomach within 1 h, but the remaining 30% were cleared much more slowly, and 20% of the particles were still in the stomach 8 h after administration. A similar biphasic pattern of gastric emptying of microparticles in mice was described by Povey et al.,[152] using radiolabeled polyethyleneimine microparticles (39 μm). Thus, the evidence suggests that microparticles may show delayed gastric transit, which may be an advantage in the development of microparticles as oral vaccines.

The use of "bioadhesive" polymers as coatings for drug delivery systems is an area of considerable interest.[153] *In vitro* models have been developed to investigate the interaction of particles with mucus,[154] and the effect of coatings on the extent of microparticle adhesion to ileal segments has been studied.[155] However, despite encouraging results *in vitro*, none of the proposed bioadhesive polymers have yet to show improved drug delivery *in vivo*. The attachment sites for the polymers are often unclear, since mucoadhesion is claimed by many and adherence to the enterocytes by others. Moreover, even formulations which have shown encouraging results in animals[156] have not been nearly so effective in humans.[157] One of the major problems limiting the use of bioadhesive polymers for oral delivery is the rapid turnover rate of mucus in the intestine.[158] Even if the polymer attaches firmly to the mucus, the rapid sloughing rate (47 to 270 min in rats)[158] will ensure that the delivery system is soon released. Furthermore, since the delivery system will be attached to the released mucus, its binding sites may be unavailable for reattachment. In addition, since the interaction of polymers with mucus is nonspecific, interactions with food or other components of the gut contents may inactivate the delivery systems.

C. SITE-SPECIFIC DELIVERY SYSTEMS

The potential of lectins and "lectin-like" molecules for the development of oral vaccines will be discussed in detail by Russell-Jones in Chapter II.4. Lectins with site-specific adherence properties may be linked to the surface of microparticles to allow them to be preferentially targeted to selected sites in the intestine. Tomato lectin adsorbed onto the surface of polystyrene (PS) microparticles (0.98 μm) has been shown to enhance the adherence of the particles to enterocytes *in vitro*.[159] An alternative approach used fimbriae from *E. coli* to produce bioadhesive microparticles.[160] More interestingly, the reovirus M cell attachment protein has been incorporated into liposomes and shown to enhance the uptake of the liposomes into Peyer's patches *in vitro*.[161] Thus, targeting ligands may be identified from a variety of sources, including plants and microorganisms and may be exploited to target microparticles to M cells.

An alternative approach to targeting of microparticles to M cells was described by Pappo et al.[162] A monoclonal antibody (MAB) with specificity for rabbit M cells was adsorbed onto the surface of PS microparticles (1 μm) and promoted their uptake into M cells (Table 2).[162] Although MABs may have potential for the targeting of microparticles to the Peyer's patches, it may be necessary to protect the MAB from degradation. The ability of sIgA to enhance the uptake of microparticles (0.5 μm) into M cells has been shown by Porta et al.[163]

The limitations of the currently available drug delivery systems for site-specific delivery in the GIT are discussed in detail elsewhere.[164]

VIII. CONCLUSIONS AND FUTURE PROSPECTS

Although the evidence to demonstrate the uptake of particles into the Peyer's patches of animals is convincing, evidence is lacking in humans. However, this is mainly due to the difficulties associated with undertaking relevant studies in humans. Peyer's patches are certainly abundant in humans; they are present before birth, peak in numbers at about puberty (>200 patches), and thereafter decline gradually.[165] In one patient aged 95 years, 59 patches were clearly visible throughout the intestine.[165] The duodenal patches are small and the largest patches are found near the ileocecal junction. In the terminal ileum, the patches may contain 900 to 1000 individual lymphoid follicles.[166] M cells have been identified on human Peyer's patches,[52,166,167] and it has been demonstrated that poliovirus type 1 adheres specifically to M cells and is subsequently endocytosed.[168] It has also been demonstrated that HIV-1 is transported through rabbit M cells.[169] Therefore, M cells in the rectal epithelium may provide a portal of entry for the virus into humans.[52,166,167,170] It may be significant that the largest Peyer's patches in humans are found where the intestinal transit of oral dosage forms is often delayed, along with the intestinal contents.[149] Thus, the gut contents are static for extended periods where the antigen-sampling M cells are most abundant. In mice and rats, the Peyer's patches consist of 2 to 11 follicles, which are uniform in size, and the mouse intestine contains about 10 Peyer's patches.[50]

There is some clinical evidence to suggest that particulate uptake into Peyer's patches may occur in humans. In one study, a dark brown pigment was identified in the Peyer's patches, submucosal lymphatics, and MLN of all subjects over 6 years of age (34 patients).[171] The pigment, which consisted predominantly of aluminum, silicon, and titanium, was in macrophages and was more abundant in older patients.[171] It was suggested that the pigment was probably derived from minerals in the diet which had been taken up into the Peyer's patches. Pigment resembling atmospheric dust (<1 μm) has also been identified in Peyer's patches and surrounding tissues.[172] In addition, the presence of particles and crystals (2 to 6 μm) in granulomas of the intestine and lymphatics of patients with Crohn's disease has been described.[173] Black pigment has also been identified in the liver and spleens of coal workers, which may be partially of intestinal origin.[173a]

Many problems remain which may ultimately restrict the use of microparticles as oral vaccines. The efficiency of particle uptake may be a problem, although the evidence suggests that even low levels of uptake are sufficient to induce potent immune responses. However, it should be possible to promote particle uptake with targeting agents. Perhaps of greater concern is the potential for inter- and intrasubject variability of particle uptake. Variability in the responses of individual animals have already been observed in small-scale studies.[128,129] The possible effects of preexisting intestinal pathology on particle uptake must also be considered. Particle uptake could be enhanced in subjects with acute gastroenteritis or inflammatory diseases of the intestine. In animal models, intestinal infection has been shown to increase the intestinal absorption of proteins[173-175] and a similar effect on particle uptake might be expected. Alternatively, particle uptake could be restricted or even prevented, due to infection-associated rapid intestinal transit. In the developing world, where oral vaccines are most needed, malnutrition is common. Malnutrition has been shown to promote the uptake of macromolecules in animal models[173,176] and might affect particle uptake. Moreover, mucosal antibody responses have been shown to be impaired by a vitamin A dependent diet.[176a] In the long term, these and other questions

Table 2 Monoclonal antibody (MAB)-dependent localization of green (0.94 μm) and red (1.0 μm) fluorescent polystyrene microparticles in rabbit Peyer's patches

Particle combination	Particle count
MAB–green particles	468 (56)
Green particles	120 (17)
MAB–red particles	364 (77)
Red particles	125 (18)
MAB2–green particles	160 (38)
MAB2–red particles	160 (22)

Note: Particle count is the mean number of particles (±SE) found in the Peyer's patches from three rabbits. The MAB has specificity for rabbit M cells, while MAB2 is a monoclonal antibody of unrelated specificity. Adapted from Pappo, J., Ermak, T.H., and Steger, H.J., *Immunology,* 73, 277, 1991.

Table 3 **Advantages of microparticles for oral immunization**

1. Microparticles are taken up into the Peyer's patches following oral administration.
2. Entrapped antigens are protected from degradation in the gut.
3. Several antigens may be entrapped simultaneously in microparticles.
4. Adjuvants may also be entrapped in microparticles with the antigens.
5. The polymers are nonimmunogenic, so the microparticles can be used for booster immunizations.
6. Controlled or "pulsed" release of antigens from microparticles after uptake is possible.
7. It should be possible to target microparticles to the Peyer's patches to enhance the efficiency of uptake.

must be addressed if microparticles are to achieve widespread use as oral vaccines in humans.

During the microencapsulation process, antigens are subjected to potentially damaging conditions, including exposure to organic solvents and high shear. Therefore, it is crucial that the effects of the formulation process on the integrity of incorporated antigens are assessed. Analysis of OVA entrapped in PLG microparticles by polyacrylamide gel electrophoresis, Western blotting, and isoelectric focusing have indicated that the protein was unaltered.[88] Analysis of bacterial membrane surface proteins after entrapment in microparticles with monoclonal antibodies has also indicated that the proteins are unchanged (O'Hagan et al., unpublished observations). More encouraging, tetanus toxoid and SEB entrapped in microparticles have been shown to retain antigenicity and to induce neutralizing antibodies in mice.[83,86,89] Moreover, antigens entrapped in microparticles have been shown to induce protective immunity in animal models (Jones, T. and O'Hagan, D.T., unpublished observations).[96–98,131] Additional problems which may restrict the use of microparticles as vaccines include, the quality and variability of polymers and the microparticle manufacturing costs. Although microparticles may prove to be more expensive to produce than traditional vaccines, currently only 12% of the total costs for vaccination is for the vaccine.[83] The remainder is for operational costs, including personnel, transportation, refrigeration, etc. Since microparticles may be effective after a single dose and will not require a cold chain, a significant reduction in operational costs for vaccination is possible. These factors are likely to make microparticles affordable worldwide as vaccines. However, it remains to be seen if the exciting potential of microparticles as oral vaccines will be fulfilled. The possible advantages of microparticles in comparison to alternative oral antigen delivery systems are shown in Table 3.

REFERENCES

1. O'Mullane, J.E., Artursson, P., and Tomlinson, E., Biopharmaceutics of microparticulate drug carriers, *Ann. NY. Acad. Sci.,* 507, 120, 1987.
2. O'Hagan, D.T., Intestinal translocation of particulates — implications for drug and antigen delivery, *Adv. Drug Deliv. Rev.,* 5, 265, 1990.
3. Sullivan, S.N., Hypothesis revisited: toothpaste and the cause of Crohn's disease, *Lancet,* 336, 1096, 1990.
4. Chess, S., Chess, D., Olander, G., Benner, W., and Cole, W.H., Production of chronic enteritis and other systemic lesions by ingestion of finely divided foreign materials, *Surgery,* 27, 221, 1950.
5. Florence, A.T., Jani, P.U., and McCarthy, D., Toothpaste and Crohn's disease, *Lancet,* 336, 1580, 1990.

6. Smith, P.L., Wall, D.A., Gochoco, C.H., and Wilson, G., Oral absorption of peptides and proteins, *Adv. Drug. Deliv. Rev.*, 8, 253, 1992.

7. Cook, P.M., Review of published studies on gut penetration by ingested asbestos fibers, *Environ. Health Perspect.*, 53, 121, 1983.

8. Freedman, B.J., Persorption of raw starch: a cause of senile dementia, *Med. Hypotheses*, 35, 87, 1991.

9. Volkheimer, G., Persorption of particles: physiology and pharmacology, *Adv. Pharmacol. Chemother.*, 14, 163, 1977.

10. Douglas, S.J., Davis, S.S., and Illum, L., Nanoparticles in drug delivery, *Crit. Rev. Ther. Drug Carr. Sys.*, 3, 233, 1987.

11. Poznansky, M.J. and Juliano, R.L., Biological approaches to the controlled delivery of drugs: a critical review, *Pharmacol. Rev.*, 36, 277, 1984.

12. Jani, P.U., Halbert, G.W., Langridge, J., and Florence, A.T., Nanoparticle uptake by the rat gastrointestinal mucosal: quantitation and particle size dependence, *J. Pharm. Pharmacol.*, 42, 821, 1990.

13. Lewis, D.A., Field, W.N., Hayes, K., and Alpar, H.O., The use of albumin microspheres in the treatment of carrageenan-induced inflammation in the rat, *J. Pharm. Pharmacol.*, 44, 271, 1992.

14. Aprahamian, M., Michel, C., Humbert, W., Devisaguet, J.-P., and Damge, C., Transmucosal passage of polyalkylcyanoacrylate nanocapsules as a new drug carrier, *Biol. Cell*, 61, 69, 1987.

15. Damge, C., Defontaine, L., Aprahamian, M., Michel, C., Humbert, W., and Devissaguet, J.P., Preferential uptake of nanocapsules through Peyer's patches in the rat, *Proc. Int. Symp. Controlled Rel. Bioact. Mater.*, 18, 349, 1991.

16. Jani, P., Halbert, G.W., Langridge, J., and Florence, A.T., The uptake and translocation of latex nanospheres and microspheres after oral administration to rats, *J. Pharm. Pharmacol.*, 41, 809, 1989.

17. Sanders, E. and Ashworth, C.T., A study of particulate intestinal absorption and hepatocellular uptake, *Exp. Cell Res.*, 22, 137, 1961.

18. Le Fevre, M.E. and Joel, D.D., Peyer's patch epithelium, an imperfect barrier, in *Intestinal Toxicology*, Schiller, C.M., Ed., Raven Press, New York, 1984, 45.

19. Le Fevre, M.E., Hancock, D.C., and Joel, D.D., Intestinal barrier to large particulates in mice, *J. Toxicol. Environ. Health*, 6, 691, 1980.

20. LeFevre, M.E., Boccio, A.M., and Joel, D.D., Intestinal uptake of fluorescent microspheres in young and aged mice (4825), *Proc. Soc. Exp. Biol. Med.*, 190, 23, 1989.

21. Ebel, J.P., A method for quantifying particle absorption from the small intestine of the mouse, *Pharm. Res.*, 7, 848, 1990.

22. Eldridge, J.H., Hammond, C.J., Meulbroeck, J.A., Staas, J.K., Gilley, R.M., and Tice, T.R., Controlled vaccine release in the gut-associated lymphoid tissues. I. Orally administered biodegradable microspheres target the Peyer's patches, *J. Controlled Rel.*, 11, 205, 1990.

23. Jepson, M.A., Simmons, N.L., O'Hagan, D.T., and Hirst, B.H., Comparison of poly (lactide-co-glycolide) and polystyrene microspheres targeting to intestinal M cells, *J. Drug. Target.*, in press.

24. Tomizawa, H., Aramaki, Y., Fujii, Y., Hara, T., Suzuki, N., Yachi, K., Kikuchi, H., and Tsuchiya, S., Uptake of phosphatidylserine liposomes by rat Peyer's patches following intraluminal administration, *Pharm. Res.*, 10, 549, 1993.

25. Jani, P.U., McCarthy, D.E., and Florence, A.T., Nanosphere and microsphere uptake via Peyer's patches: observation of the rate of uptake in the rat after a single oral dose, *Int. J. Pharm.*, 86, 239, 1992.

26. Wells, C.L., Maddaus, M.A., and Simmons, R.L., Role of the macrophage in the translocation of intestinal bacteria, *Arch. Surg.*, 122, 48, 1987.

27. Wells, C.L., Maddaus, M.A., Erlandsen, S.L., and Simmons, R.L., Evidence for the phagocytic transport of intestinal particles in dogs and rats, *Infect. Immun.*, 56, 278, 1988.

28. Jani, P.U., Florence, A.T., and McCarthy, D.E., Further histological evidence of the gastrointestinal absorption of polystyrene nanospheres in the rat, *Int. J. Pharm.*, 84, 245, 1992.

29. Sass, W., Dreyer, H.-P., and Seifert, J., Rapid insorption of small particles in the gut, *Am. J. Gastroenterol.*, 85, 255, 1990.

30. Landsverk, T., Phagocytosis and transcytosis by the follicle associated epithelium of the ileal Peyer's patch in calves, *Immunol. Cell. Biol.*, 66, 261, 1988.

31. Paar, M., Liebler, E.M., and Pohlenz, J.F., Uptake of ferritin by follicle-associated epithelium in the colon of calves, *Vet. Pathol.*, 29, 120, 1992.

32. Payne, J.M., Sansom, B.F., Garner, R.J., Thomson, A.R., and Miles, B.J., *Nature*, 188, 586, 1960.

33. Owen, R.L. and Ermak, T.H., Structural specializations for antigen uptake and processing in the digestive tract, *Springer Semin. Immunopathol.*, 12, 139, 1990.

34. Bland, P.W. and Warren, L.G., Antigen presentation by epithelial cells of the rat small intestine II. Selective induction of suppressor T cells, *Immunology*, 58, 9, 1986.

35. Jeurissen, S.H.M., Kraal, G., and Sminia, T., The role of Peyer's patches in intestinal humoral immune responses is limited to memory formation, *Adv. Exp. Med. Biol.*, 216A, 257, 1987.

36. Pappo, J. and Ermak, T.H., Uptake and translocation of fluorescent latex particles by rabbit Peyer's patch follicle epithelium: a quantitative model for M cell uptake, *Clin. Exp. Immunol.*, 76, 144, 1989.

37. Jepson, M.A., Simmons, N.L., Savidge, T.C., James, P.S., and Hirst, B.H., Selective binding and transcytosis of latex microspheres by rabbit intestinal M cells, *Cell Tissue Res.*, 271, 399, 1993.

38. Burns, R.B., Histology and immunology of Peyer's patches in the domestic fowl *(Gallus domesticus), Res. Vet. Sci.*, 32, 359, 1982.

39. Le Fevre, M.E., Joel, D.D., and Schidlovsky, G., Retention of ingested latex particles in Peyer's patches of germfree and conventional mice (42133), *Proc. Soc. Exp. Biol. Med.*, 179, 522, 1985.

40. Le Fevre, M.E., Joel, D.D., Laissue, J.A., El-Aaser, M.S., and Vanderhoff, J.W., Stability of ^{125}I after intragastric and intravenous administration of radio-iodinated latexes to mice, *J. Reticuloendothel. Soc.*, 22, 189, 1977.

41. Le Fevre, M.E. and Joel, D.D., Distribution of label after intragastric administration of ^{7}Be-labelled carbon to weanling and aged mice (42318), *Proc. Soc. Exp. Biol. Med.*, 182, 112, 1986.

42. Kukan, M., Bezek, S., Koprda, V., Labsky, J., Kalal, J., Ballerova, K., and Trnovec, T., Fate of ^{14}C-terpolymer nanoparticles after peroral administration to rats, *Pharmazie*, 44, 339, 1989.

43. Kreuter, J., Muller, U., and Munz, K., Quantitative and microautoradiographic study on mouse intestinal distribution of polycyanoacrylate nanoparticles, *Int. J. Pharm.*, 55, 39, 1989.

44. De Keyser, J.-L., Poupaert, J.H., and Dumont, P., Poly (diethyl methylidenemalonate) nanoparticles as a potential drug carrier: Preparation, distribution and elimination after intravenous and peroral administration to mice, *J. Pharm. Sci.*, 80, 67, 1991.

45. Alpar, H.O., Field, W.N., Hyde, R., and Lewis, D.A., The transport of microspheres from the gastrointestinal tract to inflammatory air pouches in the rat, *J. Pharm. Pharmacol.*, 41, 194, 1989.

46. Lewis, D.A., Eyles, J., Field, W.N., and Alpar, H.O., Observations on the effect of the volume of water and tonicity in microsphere uptake in rat gut, *J. Pharm. Pharmacol.*, 44 (Suppl.), 1086, 1992.

47. Jenkins, P.G., Howard, K.A., Blackhall, N.W., Thomas, N.W., Davis, S.S., and O'Hagan, D.T., Microparticles absorption from the rat intestine, *J. Controlled Rel.*, in press.

48. Jenkins, P.G., Howard, K.A., Blackhall, N.W., Thomas, N.W., Davis, S.S., and O'Hagan, D.T., The quantitation of the absorption of microparticles into the intestinal lymph of Wistar rats, *Int. J. Pharm.*, in press.

49. Pappo, J., Steger, H.J., and Owen, R.L., Differential adherence of epithelium overlying gut-associated lymphoid tissue, an ultrastructural study, *Lab. Invest.*, 58, 692, 1988.

50. Smith, M.W. and Peacock, M.A., M cell distribution in follicle associated epithelium of mouse Peyer's patches, *Am. J. Anat.*, 159, 167, 1980.

51. McClugage, S.G., Low, F.N., and Zimny, M.L., Porosity of the basement membrane overlying Peyer's patches in rats and monkeys, *Gastroenterology*, 91, 1128, 1986.

52. Fujimura, Y., Hosobe, M., and Kihara, T., Ultrastructural study of M cells from colonic lymphoid nodules obtained by colonic biopsy, *Dig. Dis. Sci.*, 37, 1089, 1992.

53. Litwin, S.D. and Singer, J.M., The adjuvant action of latex particulate carriers, *J. Immunol.*, 95, 1147, 1965.

54. Kreuter, J. and Speiser, P., New adjuvants on a polymethylmethacrylate base, *Infect. Immun.*, 13, 204, 1976.

55. Kreuter, J., Mauler, R., Gruschkau, H., and Speiser, P., The use of new polymethylmethacrylate adjuvants for split influenza vaccines, *Exp. Cell Biol.*, 44, 12, 1976.

56. Kreuter, J. and Liehl, E., Protection induced by inactivated influenza virus vaccines with polymethylmethacrylate adjuvants, *Med. Microbiol. Immunol.*, 165, 111, 1978.

57. Kreuter, J. and Haenzel, I., Mode of action of immunological adjuvants: some physicochemical factors influencing the effectivity of polyacrylic adjuvants, *Infect. Immun.*, 19, 667, 1978.

58. Kreuter, J., Berg, U., Liehl, E., Soliva, M., and Speiser, P.P., Influence of physicochemical properties on the adjuvant effect of particulate polymeric adjuvants, *Vaccine*, 4, 125, 1986.

59. Kreuter, J., Liehl, E., Berg, U., Soliva, M., and Speiser, P.P., Influence of hydrophobicity on the adjuvant effect of particulate polymeric adjuvants, *Vaccine*, 6, 253, 1988.

60. Stieneker, F., Kreuter, J., and Lower, J., High antibody titres in mice with polymethylmethacrylate nanoparticles as adjuvant for HIV vaccines, *AIDS*, 5, 431, 1991.

61. Artursson, P., Martensson, I.L., and Sjoholm, I., Biodegradable microspheres. III. Some immunological properties of polyacryl starch microspheres, *J. Pharm. Sci.*, 75, 697, 1986.

62. Schroder, U. and Stahl, A., Crystallised dextran nanospheres with entrapped antigen and their use as adjuvants, *J. Immunol. Methods*, 70, 127, 1984.

63. Tabata, Y. and Ikada, Y., Phagocytosis of polymer microspheres by macrophages, *Adv. Polym. Sci.*, 94, 107, 1990.

64. Adams, S.E., Dawson, K.M., Gull, K., Kingsman, S.M., and Kingsman, A.J., The expression of hybrid HIV:Ty virus-like particles in yeast, *Nature*, 329, 68, 1987.

65. Clarke, B.E., Newton, S.E., Carroll, A.R., Francis, M.J., Appleyard, G., Syred, A.D., Highfield, P.E., Rowlands, D.J., and Brown, F., Improved immunogenicity of a peptide epitope after fusion to hepatitis B core protein, *Nature*, 330, 381, 1987.

66. Schlienger, K., Mancini, M., Riviere, Y., Dormont, D., Tiollais, P., and Michel, M.L., Human immunodeficiency virus type 1 major neutralizing determinant exposed on hepatitis B surface antigen particles is highly immunogenic in primates, *J. Virol.*, 66, 2570, 1992.

66a. Lehner, T., Brookes, R., Panagiotidi, C., Tao, L., Klavinskis, L.S., Walker, J., Walker, P., Ward, R., Hussain, L., Gearing, A.J.M., Adams, S.E., and Bergmeier, L.A., T- and B-cell functions and epitope expression in nonhuman primates immunized with Simian immunodeficiency virus antigen by the rectal route, *Proc. Natl. Acad. Sci. U.S.A.*, 90, 8638, 1993.

67. Randall, R.E. and Young, D.F., Humoral and cytotoxic T cell immune responses to internal and external structural proteins of simian virus 5 induced by immunization with solid matrix-antibody-antigen complexes, *J. Gen. Virol.*, 69, 2505, 1988.

68. Chang, T.M.S., Biodegradable semipermeable microcapsules containing enzymes, hormones, vaccines and other biologicals, *J. Bioeng.*, 1, 25, 1976.

69. Preis, I. and Langer, R.S., A single step immunization by sustained antigen release, *J. Immunol. Methods,* 28, 193, 1979.

70. Kohn, J., Niemi, S.M., Albert, E.C., Murphy, J.C., Langer, R., and Fox, J.G., Single-step immunisation using a controlled release biodegradable polymer with sustained adjuvant activity, *J. Immunol. Methods,* 95, 31, 1986.

71. Wheeler, A.W., Moran, D.M., Robins, B.E., and Driscol, A., Tyrosine as an immunological adjuvant, *Int. Arch. Allergy Appl. Immunol.,* 69, 113, 1982.

72. Khan, M.Z.I., Tucker, I.G., and Opdebeeck, J.P., Evaluation of cholesterol-lecithin implants for sustained delivery of antigen: Release in vivo and single-step immunisation of mice, *Int. J. Pharm.,* 90, 255, 1993.

73. Radomsky, M.L., Whaley, K.J., Cone, R.A., and Saltzman, W.M., Controlled vaginal delivery of antibodies in the mouse, *Biol. Reprod.,* 47, 133, 1992.

74. Sherwood, J.K., Dause, R.B., and Saltzman, W.M., Controlled antibody delivery system, *Biotechnology,* 10, 1446, 1992.

75. Drake, C.F., Continuous and pulsed delivery of bioactive materials using composite systems based on inorganic glasses, in *Progress towards Better Vaccines,* Bell, R. and Torrigiani, G., Eds., Oxford University Press, London, 1985, 204.

76. Cohen, S., Yoshioka, T., Lucareli, M., Hwang, L.H., and Langer, R., Controlled delivery systems for proteins based on poly (lactic/glycolic acid) microspheres, *Pharm. Res.,* 8, 713, 1991.

77. Reul, G.J., Use of Vicryl (polyglactin 910) sutures in general surgery and cardiothoracic procedures, *Am. J. Surg.,* 134, 297, 1977.

78. Christel, P., Chabot, F., Leray, L.F., Morin, C., and Vert, M., Biodegradable composites for internal fixation, in *Biomaterials,* Winter, G.D., Giobonnes, D.F., and Plenk, H., Eds., John Wiley, New York, 1982, 271.

79. Maulding, H.V., Prolonged delivery of peptides by microcapsules, *J. Controlled Rel.,* 6, 167, 1987.

80. Wise, D.L., Fellman, T.D., Sanderson, J.E., and Wentworth, R.L., Lactic/glycolic acid polymers, in *Drug Carriers in Biology and Medicine,* Gregoriadis, G., Ed., Academic Press, London, 1979, 237.

81. Vert, M., Li, S., and Garreau, H., More about the degradation of LA/GA-derived matrices in aqueous media, *J. Controlled Rel.,* 16, 15, 1991.

82. Visscher, G.E., Robison, R.L., and Argentieri, G.I., Tissue response to biodegradable injectable microcapsules, *J. Biomater. Appl.,* 2, 118, 1987.

83. Aguado, M.T. and Lambert, P.-H., Controlled release vaccines — biodegradable polylactide/polyglycolide (PL/PG) microspheres as antigen vehicles, *Immunobiology,* 184, 113, 1992.

84. O'Hagan, D.T., Rahman, D., McGee, J.P., Jeffery, H., Davies, M.C., Williams, P., Davis, S.S., and Challacombe, S.J., Biodegradable microparticles as controlled release antigen delivery systems, *Immunology,* 73, 239, 1991.

85. O'Hagan, D.T., Jeffery, H., Roberts, M.J.J., McGee, J.P., and Davis, S.S., Controlled release microparticles for vaccine development, *Vaccine,* 9, 768, 1991.

86. Esparza, I. and Kissel, T., Parameters affecting the immunogenicity of microencapsulated tetanus toxoid, *Vaccine,* 10, 714, 1992.

86a. Alonso, M.J., Cohen, S., Park, T.G., Gupta, R.K., Siber, G.R., and Langer, R., Determinants of release tetanus vaccine from polyester microspheres, *Pharm. Res.,* 10, 945, 1993.

87. Jeffery, H., Davis, S.S., and O'Hagan, D.T., The preparation and characterisation of poly (lactide-co-glycolide) microparticles. I. Oil-in-water emulsion solvent evaporation, *Int. J. Pharm.*, 77, 169, 1991.

88. Jeffery, H., Davis, S.S., and O'Hagan, D.T., The preparation and characterisation of poly (lactide-co-glycolide) microparticles. II. Protein entrapment by water-in-oil-in-water emulsion solvent evaporation, *Pharm. Res.*, 10, 362, 1993.

89. Eldridge, J.H., Staas, J.K., Meulbroek, J.A., Tice, T.R., and Gilley, R.M., Biodegradable and biocompatible poly(DL-lactide-co-glycolide) microspheres as an adjuvant for staphylococcal enterotoxin B toxoid which enhances the level of toxin-neutralising antibodies, *Infect. Immun.*, 59, 2978, 1991.

90. Eldridge, J.H., Staas, J.K., Meulbroek, J.A., McGhee, J.R., Tice, T.R., and Gilley, R.M., Biodegradable microspheres as a vaccine delivery system, *Mol. Immunol.*, 28, 287, 1991.

91. O'Hagan, D.T., Jeffery, H., and Davis, S.S., Long term antibody responses in mice following subcutaneous immunization with ovalbumin entrapped in biodegradable microparticles, *Vaccine*, 10, 1993.

92. Gilley, R.M., Staas, J.K., Tice, T.R., Morgan, J.D., and Eldridge, J.H., Microencapsulation and its application to vaccine development, *Proc. Int. Symp. Controlled Rel. Bioact. Mater.*, 19, 110, 1992.

93. Altman, A. and Dixon, F., Immunomodifiers in vaccines, *Adv. Vet. Sci. Comp. Med.*, 33, 301, 1989.

93a. Nellore, R.V., Pande, P.G., Young, D., and Bhagat, H.R., Evaluation of biodegradable microspheres as vaccine adjuvant for hepatitis B surface antigen, *J. Parent. Sci. Technol.*, 46, 176, 1992.

94. Singh, M., Singh, A., and Talwar, G.P., Controlled delivery of Diphtheria toxoid using biodegradable poly (D,L-Lactide) microcapsules, *Pharm. Res.*, 8, 958, 1991.

95. Stevens, V.C., Future perspectives for vaccine development, *Scand. J. Immunol. (Suppl.)*, 11, 137, 1992.

96. Moldoveanu, Z., Novak, M., Huang, W.-Q., Gilley, R.M., Staas, J.K., Schafer, D., Compans, R.W., and Mestecky, J., Oral immunization with influenza virus in biodegradable microspheres, *J. Infect. Dis.*, 167, 84, 1993.

97. Ray, R., Novak, M., Duncan, J.D., Matsuoka, Y., and Compans, R.W., Microencapsulated human parainfluenza virus induces a protective immune response, *J. Infect. Dis.*, 167, 752, 1993.

98. Marx, P.A., Compans, R.W., Gettie, A., Staas, J.K., Gilley, R.M., Mulligan, M.J., Yamshchikov, G.V., Chen, D., and Eldridge, J.H., Protection against vaginal SIV transmission with microencapsulated vaccine, *Science*, 260, 1323, 1993.

99. Meulbroek, J.A., Enhancement of the Antibody Response to a Polysaccharide Based Vaccine by Synthesizing an Artificial Glycoprotein and Using a Novel Microcapsule Delivery System, Ph.D. thesis, University of Alabama at Birmingham, 1990.

100. O'Hagan, D.T., McGee, J.P., Holmgren, J., Mowat, McI.A., Donachie, A.M., Mills, K.H.G., Gaisford, W., Rahman, D., and Challacombe, S.J., Biodegradable microparticles as oral vaccines, *Vaccine*, 11, 149, 1993.

101. O'Hagan, D.T., Jeffery, H., Maloy, K.J., Mowat, McI., Rahman, D., and Challacombe, S.J., Biodegradable microparticles as oral vaccines, *Adv. Exp. Med. Biol.*, in press.

101a. Takagi, I., Nishimura, J., Itoh, H., and Baba, S., Poly(lactic/glycolic) microspheres containing antigen as a novel and potential agent of immunotherapy for allergic disorders, *Jpn. J. Allergol.*, 41, 1388, 1992.

102. Singh, M., Rathi, R., Singh, A., Heller, J., Talwar, G.P., and Kopecek, J., Controlled release of LHRH-DT from bioerodible hydrogel microspheres, *Int., J. Pharm.*, 76, R5, 1991.

103. Cohen, S., Bernstein, H., Hewes, C., Chow, M., and Langer, R., The pharmacokinetics of, and humoral responses to, antigen delivered by microencapsulated liposomes, *Proc. Natl. Acad. Sci. U.S.A.*, 88, 10440, 1992.

104. Marcotte, N. and Goosen, M.F.A., Delayed release of water-soluble macromolecules from polylactide pellets, *J. Controlled Rel.*, 9, 75, 1989.

105. Wang, H.T., Schmitt, E., Flanagan, D.R., and Linhardt, R.J., Influence of formulation methods on the in vitro controlled release of protein from poly (ester) microspheres, *J. Controlled Rel.*, 17, 23, 1991.

106. Park, T.G., Cohen, S., and Langer, R., Controlled protein release from polyethyleneimine-coated poly (L-lactic acid)/pluronic blend matrices, *Pharm. Res.*, 9, 37, 1992.

107. Martin, M.E.D., Dewar, J.B., and Newman, J.F.E., Polymerised serum albumin beads possessing slow release properties for use in vaccines, *Vaccine*, 6, 33-38, 1988.

108. Schichiri, M., Okada, A., Kikkawa, R., Kawamori, R., Shigeta, Y., and Abe, H., B-Naphthyl-azo-polystyrene-insulin as a means of protecting insulin molecule from digestive enzymes, *Biochem. Biophys. Res. Comm.*, 44, 51, 1971.

109. Shigeta, Y., Shichiri, M., Okada, A., and Karasaki, K., Plasma immunoreactive insulin after intestinal administration of B-Naphthyl-azo-polystyrene-insulin to the rabbit, *Endocrinology*, 91, 320, 1972.

110. Maincent, P., Le Verge, R., Sado, P., Couvreur, P., and Devissaguet, J.P., Disposition and oral bioavailability of vincamin loaded polyalkyl cyanoacrylate nanoparticles, *J. Pharm. Sci.*, 75, 955, 1986.

111. Verdun, C., Couvreur, P., Vranckx, H., Lenaerts, V., and Roland, M., Development of a nanoparticle controlled release formulation for human use, *J. Controlled Rel.*, 3, 205, 1986.

112. Damge, C., Aprahamian, M., Balboni, G., Hoeltzel, A., Andrieu, V., and Devissaguet, J.P., Polyalkylcyanoacrylate nanocapsules increase the intestinal absorption of a lipophilic drug, *J. Pharm. Sci.*, 36, 121, 1987.

113. Damge, C., Michel, C., Aprahamian, M., and Couvreur, P., New approach for oral administration of insulin with polyalkylcyanoacrylate nanocapsules as drug carrier, *Diabetes*, 37, 246, 1988.

114. Couvreur, P., Lenaerts, V., Kante, B., Roland, M., and Speiser, P.P., Oral and parenteral administration of insulin associated to hydrolysable nanoparticles, *Acta Pharm. Tech.*, 26, 220, 1980.

115. Michel, C., Aprahamian, M., Defontaine, L., Couvreur, P., and Damge, C., The effect of site of administration in the gastrointestinal tract on the absorption of insulin from nanocapsules in diabetic rats, *J. Pharm. Pharmacol.*, 43, 1, 1991.

116. Roques, M., Damge, C., Michel, C., Staedel, C., Cremel, G., and Hubert, P., Encapsulation of insulin for oral administration preserves interaction of the hormone with its receptor, *Diabetes*, 41, 451, 1992.

117. Damge, C., Michel, C., Aprahamian, M., Couvreur, P., and Devissaguet, J.-P., Nanocapsules as carriers for oral peptide delivery, *J. Controlled Rel.*, 13, 233, 1990.

118. Andrieu, V., Fessi, H., Dubrasquet, M., Devissaguet, J.-P., Puisieux, F., and Benita, S., Pharmacokinetic evaluation of indomethacin nanocapsules, *Drug Des. Deliv.*, 4, 295, 1989.

119. Ammoury, N., Fessi, H., Devissaguet, J.-P., Allix, M., Plotkine, M., and Boulu, R.G., Effect of cerebral blood flow of orally administered indomethacin loaded poly(isobutylcyanoacrylate) and poly(DL-lactide) nanocapsules, *J. Pharm. Pharmacol.*, 42, 558, 1990.

120. Ammoury, N., Fessi, H., Devissaguet, J.-P., Dubrasquet, M., and Benita, S., Jejunal absorption, pharmacological activity and pharmacokinetic evaluation of indomethacin loaded poly(d,I-lactide) and poly(isobutylcyanoacrylate) nanocapsules in rats, *Pharm. Res.*, 8, 101, 1991.

121. O'Hagan, D.T., Pharmaceutical Formulations as Immunological Adjuvants, Ph.D. thesis, University of Nottingham, Nottingham, U.K., 1987.

122. O'Hagan, D.T., Palin, K.J., and Davis, S.S., Poly (butyl-2-cyanoacrylate) particles as adjuvants for oral immunization, *Vaccine,* 7, 213, 1989.

123. Cox, D.S. and Taubman, M.A., Oral induction of the secretory immune response by soluble and particulate antigens, *Int. Arch. Allergy Appl. Immunol.,* 75, 126, 1984.

124. Cox, D.S. and Muench, D., IgA antibody produced by local presentation of antigen in orally primed rats, *Int. Arch. Allergy Appl. Immun.,* 74, 249, 1984.

125. Challacombe, S.J., Systemic tolerance and salivary antibodies after oral immunisation, in *Mucosal Immunity IgA and Polymorphonuclear Neutrophils,* Paris, 1984, 73.

126. O'Hagan, D.T., Palin, K.J., Davis, S.S., Artursson, P., and Sjoholm, I., Microparticles as potentially orally active immunological adjuvants, *Vaccine,* 7, 421, 1989.

127. Amerongen, H.M., Michetti, P., Weltzin, R., Lee, T.H., Kraehenbuhl, J.-P., and Neutra, M.R., Transepithelial delivery of a recombinant HIV protein on hydroxyapitite for production of monoclonal anti-gp120 IgA antibodies, *J. Cell. Biol.,* 115, 237a, 1991.

128. Challacombe, S.J., Rahman, D., Jeffery, H., Davis, S.S., and O'Hagan, D.T., Enhanced secretory IgA and systemic IgG antibody responses after oral immunization with biodegradable microparticles containing antigen, *Immunology,* 76, 164, 1992.

129. O'Hagan, D.T., Rahman, D., Jeffery, H., Sharif, S., and Challacombe, S.J., The rate of release of an antigen from microparticles affects both the serum and the secretory antibody responses following oral immunization, *Int. J. Pharm.,* in press.

130. Almeida, A.J., Alpar, H.O., and Brown, M.R.W., Immune response to nasal delivery of antigenically intact tetanus toxoid associated with poly (L-lactic acid) microspheres in rats, rabbits and guinea pigs, *J. Pharm. Pharmacol.,* 45, 198, 1993.

131. Cahill, E.S., O'Hagan, D.T., Illum, L., Barnard, A., Mills, K.H.G., and Redhead, K., Immune responses in mice following intranasal administration of Bordetella pertussis filamentous haemagglutinin as a solution or entrapped in microparticles, *Vaccine,* submitted.

132. Edelman, R., Russell, R.G., Losonsky, G., Tall, B.D., Tacket, C.O., Levine, M.M., and Lewis, D.H., Immunization of rabbits with enterotoxigenic *E. coli* colonization factor antigen (CFA/1) encapsulated in biodegradable microspheres of poly (lactide-co-glycolide), *Vaccine,* 11, 155, 1993.

133. Spenlehauer, G., Ropert, C., Bazile, D., Brendenbac, J., Marlard, M., and Veillard, M., Fate of ^{14}C radiolabelled poly (D,L-lactic) acid nanoparticles after oral administration to rats, *Proc. Int. Symp. Controlled Rel. Bioact. Mater.,* 18, 684, 1991.

134. McQueen, M.E., Boedeker, E., Reid, R., Jarboe, D., Wolf, M., Le, M., and Brown, W.R., Pili in microspheres protects rabbits from diarrhoea induced by *E. coli* strain RDEC-1, *Vaccine,* 11, 201, 1993.

134a. Boedeker, E., Reid, R., Bhagat, H.R., Dalal, P., Tackett, C., Losonsky, G., Nataro, J., Edelman, R., and Levine, M., Safety, immunogenicity, and efficacy in human volunteers of biodegradable, biocompatible microspheres containing colonization factor antigen/11 (CFA/11) as an enteral vaccine against enterolosigenic *E. coli* (ETEC), *Gastroenterology,* 104, A672, 1993.

135. Klipstein, F.A., Engert, R.F., and Sherman, W.T., Peroral immunization with *Escherichia coli* heat-labile enterotoxin delivered by microspheres, *Infect. Immun.,* 39, 1000, 1983.

136. Maharaj, I., Nairn, J.G., and Campbell, J.B., Simple rapid method for the preparation of enteric-coated microspheres, *J. Pharm. Sci.,* 73, 39, 1984.

137. Healey, J.N.C., Enteric coatings and delayed release, in *Drug Delivery to the Gastrointestinal Tract,* Hardy, J.G., Davis, S.S., and Wilson, C.G., Eds., John Wiley & Sons, New York, 1989, 83.

138. Lin, S.Y., Tzan, Y.L., Lee, C.J., and Weng, C.N., Preparation of enteric-coated microspheres of *Mycoplasma hyopneumoniae* vaccine with cellulose acetate phthalate. I. Formation condition and micromeritic properties, *J. Microencap.,* 8, 317, 1991.

139. Lin, S.Y., Tzan, Y.L., Lee, C.J., and Weng, C.N., Preparation of enteric-coated microspheres of *Mycoplasma hyopneumoniae* vaccine with cellulose acetate phthalate. II. Effect of temperature and pH on the stability and release behaviour of microspheres, *J. Microencap.*, 8, 537, 1991.

140. Lee, C.J. and Tzan, Y.L., Antigenic characteristics and stability of microencapsulated *Mycoplasma hyopneumoniae* vaccine, *Biotechnol. Bioeng.*, 40, 207, 1992.

140a. Weng, C.N., Tzan, Y.L., Liu, S.D., Lin, S.Y., and Lee, C.J., Protective effects of an oral microencapsulated Mycoplasma hyopneumoniae vaccine against experimental infection in pigs, *Res. Vet. Sci.*, 53, 42, 1992.

141. Yeung, S., Pang, G., Cripps, A.W., Clancy, R.L., and Wlodarczyk, J.H., Efficacy of oral immunization against non-typable *Haemophilus influenzae* in man, *Int. J. Immunopharmacol.*, 9, 283, 1987.

142. Levine, M.M., Ferrecio, C., Black, R.E., Germanier, R., and Chilean Typhoid Commitee, Large-scale field trial of Ty21a live oral typhoid vaccine in enteric coated capsule formulation, *Lancet,* i, 1049, 1987.

143. Ishihara, K., Ikeda, S., Arai, E., and Sawada, T., Treatment of malignant skin tumours with oral administration of BCG in enteric-coated capsules, *Dev. Biol. Stand.*, 58, 465, 1986.

144. Lubeck, M.D., Davis, A.R., Chengalvala, M., Natuk, R.J., Morin, J.E., Molnar-Kimber, K., Mason, B.B., Bhat, B.M., Mizutani, S., Hung, P.P., and Purcell, R.H., Immunogenicity and efficacy testing in chimpanzees of an oral hepatitis B vaccine based on live recombinant adenovirus, *Proc. Natl. Acad. Sci. U.S.A.*, 86, 6763, 1989.

145. Morishita, M., Morishita, I., Takayama, K., Machida, Y., and Nagai, T., Novel oral microspheres of insulin with protease inhibitor protecting from enzymatic degradation, *Int. J. Pharm.*, 78, 1, 1992.

146. Morishita, M., Morishita, I., Takayama, K., Machida, Y., and Nagai, T., Hypoglycaemic effect of novel oral microspheres of insulin with protease inhibitor in normal and diabetic rats, *Int. J. Pharm.*, 78, 9, 1992.

146a. Zhang, J.A., Piganelli, J., Christensen, J.M., and Kaatari, S.L., Oral enteric-coated antigen delivery systems in salmonid fish, *Pharm. Res.*, 10, S294, 1993.

147. Jalsenjak, I., Nicolaidou, C.F., and Nixon, J.R., *J. Pharm. Pharmacol.*, 29, 169, 1977.

148. Bodmeier, R., Chen, H., and Paeratakul, O., A novel approach to the oral delivery of micro- or nanoparticles, *Pharm. Res.*, 6, 413, 1989.

149. Davis, S.S., Small intestine transit, in *Drug Delivery to the Gastrointestinal Tract,* Hardy, J.G., Davis, S.S., and Wilson, C.G., Eds., John Wiley & Sons, New York, 1989, 49.

150. Davis, S.S., Fara, J., and Hardy, J.G., The intestinal transit of pharmaceutical dosage forms, *Gut,* 27, 886, 1986.

151. Scherer, D., Mooren, F.C., Kinne, R.K.H., and Kreuter, J., In vitro permeability of PBCA nanoparticles through porcine small intestine, *J. Drug Targ.*, 1, 21, 1993.

152. Povey, A.C., Godeneche, D., and O'Neil, I.K., Time-dependent distribution and excretion of radiolabelled, semipermeable, stable magnetic microcapsules, *J. Pharm. Pharmacol.*, 40, 431, 1988.

153. Gupta, P.K., Leung, S.-H.S., and Robinson, J.R., Bioadhesives/mucoadhesives in drug delivery to the gastrointestinal tract, in *Bioadhesive Drug Delivery Systems,* Lenaerts, V. and Gurny, R., Eds., CRC Press, Boca Raton, FL, 1990, 65.

154. Teng, C.L.C. and Ho, N.F.H., Mechanistic studies in the simultaneous flow and adsorption of polymer-coated latex particles on intestinal mucus. I. Methods and physical model development, *J. Controlled Rel.*, 6, 133, 1987.

155. Pimienta, C., Chouinard, F., Labib, A., and Lenaerts, V., Effect of various poloxamer coatings on an in vitro adhesion of isohexylcyanoacrylate nanospheres to rat ileal segments under liquid flow, *Int. J. Pharm.*, 80, 1, 1992.

156. Harris, D., Fell, J.T., Taylor, D.C., Lynch, J., and Sharma, H.L., GI transit of potential bioadhesive systems in the rat, *J. Controlled Rel.*, 12, 55, 1990.

157. Harris, D., Fell, J.T., Taylor, D.C., Lynch, J., and Sharma, H.L., GI transit of potential bioadhesive systems in man: a scintigraphic study, *J. Controlled Rel.*, 12, 45, 1990.

158. Lehr, C.M., Poelma, F.G.J., Junginger, H.E., and Tukker, J.J., An estimate of turnover time of intestinal mucus gel layer in the rat in situ gut loop, *Int. J. Pharm.*, 70, 235, 1991.

159. Lehr, C.-M., Bouwstra, J.A., Kok, W., Noach, A.B.J., de Boer, A.G., and Junginger, H.E., Bioadhesion by means of specific binding of tomato lectin, *Pharm. Res.*, 9, 547, 1992.

160. Caston, A.J., Davis, S.S., and Williams, P., The potential of fimbrial proteins for delaying intestinal transit of drug delivery systems, *Proc. Int. Symp. Controlled Rel. Bioact. Mater.*, 17, 313, 1990.

161. Rubas, W., Banerjea, A.C., Gallati, H., Speiser, P.P., and Joklik, W.K., Incorporation of the reovirus M cell attachment protein into small unilamellar vesicles: incorporation efficiency and binding capacity to L929 cells in vitro, *J. Microencap.*, 7, 385, 1990.

162. Pappo, J., Ermak, T.H., and Steger, H.J., Monoclonal antibody-directed targeting of fluorescent polystyrene microspheres to Peyer's patch M cells, *Immunology*, 73, 277, 1991.

163. Porta, C., James, P.S., Phillips, A.D., Savidge, T.C., Smith, M.W., and Cremaschi, D., Confocal analysis of fluorescent bead uptake by mouse Peyer's patch follicle-associated M cells, *Exp. Physiol.*, 77, 929, 1992.

164. Wilding, I.R., Davis, S.S., and O'Hagan, D.T., Targeting of drugs and vaccines to the gut, *Pharmacol. Therapeut.*, in press.

165. Cornes, J.S., Number, size and distribution of Peyer's patches in the human small intestine, *Gut*, 6, 225, 1965.

166. Jacob, E., Baker, S.J., and Swaminathan, S.P., M cells in the follicle-associated epithelium of the human colon, *Histopathology*, 11, 941, 1987.

167. Brandtzaeg, P. and Bjerke, K., Human Peyer's patches: lympho-epithelial relationships and characteristics of immunoglobulin-producing cells, *Immunol. Invest.*, 18, 29, 1989.

168. Sicinski, P., Rowinski, J., Warchol, J.B., Jarzabek, Z., Wlodzimierz, G., Szeczygiel, B., Bielecki, K., and Koch, G., Poliovirus type 1 enters the human host through intestinal M cells, *Gastroenterology*, 98, 56, 1990.

169. Amerongen, H.M., Weltzin, R., Farnet, C.M., Michetti, P., Haseltine, W.A., and Neutra, M.R., Transepithelial transport of HIV-1 by intestinal M cells: a mechanism for transmission of AIDS, *J. Acquir. Immun. Defic. Syn.*, 4, 760, 1991.

170. O'Leary, A.D. and Sweeney, E.C., Lymphoglandular complexes of the colon: structure and distribution, *Histopathology*, 10, 267, 1986.

171. Shepherd, N.A., Crocker, P.R., Smith, A.P., and Levison, D.A., Exogenous pigment in Peyer's patches, *Hum. Pathol.*, 18, 50, 1987.

172. Urbanski, S.J., Arsenault, A.L., Green, F.H.Y., and Haber, G., Pigment resembling atmospheric dust in Peyer's patches, *Mod. Pathol.*, 2, 222, 1989.

173. Roge, J., Fabre, M., Levillain, P., and Dubois, P., Unusual particles and crystals in Crohn's disease granulomas, *Lancet*, 337, 502, 1991.

173a. LeFevre, M.E., Green, F.M.Y., Joel, D.D., and Laquer, W., Frequency of black pigment in liver and spleens of coal workers: Correlation with pulmonary pathology and occupational information, *Hum. Pathol.*, 13, 1121, 1982.

174. Uhnoo, I.S., Freihorst, J., Riepenhoff-Talty, M., Fisher, J.E., and Ogra, P.L., Effect of rotavirus infection and malnutrition on uptake of a dietary antigen in the intestine, *Pediatr. Res.*, 27, 153, 1990.

175. Isolauri, E., Gotteland, M., Heyman, M., Pochart, P., and Desjeux, J.F., Antigen absorption in rabbit bacterial diarrhea, *Dig. Dis. Sci.,* 35, 360, 1990.

176. Bloch, K.J., Bloch, D.B., Stearns, M., and Walker, W.A., Intestinal uptake of macromolecules. VI. Uptake of protein antigen in vivo in normal rats and in rats infested with *Nippostrongylus brasiliensis* or subject to mild systemic anaphylaxis, *Gastroenterology,* 77, 1039, 1979.

176a. Wiedermann, U., Hanson, L.A., Holmgren, J., Kahn, H., and Dahlgren, U.I., Impaired mucosal antibody response to cholera toxin in vitamin A deficient rats immunized with oral cholera vaccine, *Infec. Immun.,* 61, 3952, 1993.

177. Worthington, B.S., Boatman, E.S., and Kenny, G.E., Intestinal absorption of intact proteins in normal and protein-deficient rats, *Am. J. Clin. Nutr.,* 27, 276, 1974.

Chapter 3

Immune Stimulating Complexes as Vectors for Oral Immunization

Allan McI. Mowat and Kevin J. Maloy

TABLE OF CONTENTS

I. INTRODUCTION

The wide range of topics covered in this volume testifies to the importance currently given to the development of orally active vaccine vectors, particularly those which might allow immunization with recombinant proteins or peptides. Several strategies have been devised for this purpose, including the use of a number of live carrier organisms. However, for economic, practical, and scientific reasons, synthetic nonliving adjuvant formulations would be preferable as vaccine vehicles under many circumstances. In this chapter, we discuss the possibility that lipophilic immune stimulating complexes (ISCOMS) containing saponin may provide a novel and potent basis for oral immunization.

II. THE "IDEAL" SYNTHETIC ORAL VACCINE VECTOR

Mucosal immunization is essential for stimulating active immunity in a mucosal tissue and can also induce more widespread immune responses in other parts of the body.[1] Synthetic, nonliving oral vaccines would be valuable for provoking protective immunity, not only in the intestine itself, but also in other mucosal tissues including the respiratory and urogenital tracts. In addition, oral immunization is one of the few effective means of inducing immune responses in the breast which would allow passive transfer of immunity from mother to offspring. Finally, the success of the oral polio vaccine highlights the ability of an oral vaccine to protect against systemic infection.

The ideal vaccine must stimulate all forms of the immune response which would normally be provoked by the candidate pathogen itself. In most cases, this will mean that more than one limb of the immune response must be activated, including local and

0-8493-4866-8/94/$0.00+$.50
© 1994 by CRC Press Inc.

systemic antibody responses, cytokine production, and cytotoxic T lymphocytes (CTL). Furthermore, the vaccine must be capable of stimulating these responses in the genetically disparate human population, using a small number of doses of relatively low amounts of antigen. These requirements limit the usefulness of many of the nonliving vectors currently available. The vaccine must also be safe, having no direct toxic effects or ability to sensitize the recipient to develop immunopathology when either the vaccine or the infecting organism itself is encountered in future. Finally, from a practical viewpoint, it would be beneficial if a single vector could be used to incorporate a wide variety of peptide or protein antigens, either separately, or as part of a combined vaccine.

III. PROBLEMS IN DEVELOPING SYNTHETIC ORAL VACCINES

The use of nonliving vaccine vectors containing recombinant antigens presents several immunological difficulties which are greatly increased if the vaccine is to be used by the oral route. Unfortunately, many living and nonliving vectors which are effective by other routes are too susceptible to the hazardous environment of the gut to be considered for use in this tissue.

Purified protein antigens are poorly immunogenic in general and, because they are processed by the exogenous route of antigen presentation, are usually recognized only by class II MHC-restricted T lymphocytes.[2] As a result, such antigens do not stimulate the class I MHC-restricted CTL required for protection against viral and other infections. In the case of orally administered proteins, this problem is compounded by the fact that soluble antigens normally induce a state of profound immunological unresponsiveness when given orally to naive animals.[3] This oral tolerance abrogates any active immune response to the priming antigen itself and prevents secondary responses to subsequent challenge with the antigen, irrespective of its route of administration. The development of oral tolerance is determined by the way in which antigen is processed and presented within the intestinal lymphoid tissues,[3,4] underlining the critical role these functions play in responsiveness to potential vaccines.

Some of these problems can be overcome using the vectors described in other sections of this volume. Nevertheless, many of these strategies are technically complex or require relatively large amounts of antigen, and the majority induce only restricted forms of immune response *in vivo*. In particular, it is exceedingly difficult to stimulate class I MHC-restricted CTL responses by oral administration of purified antigens, even using live vectors such as *Salmonella,* which are potent inducers of most other aspects of local and systemic immunity.[5,6] Furthermore, the ability of adjuvants such as cholera toxin to stimulate strong mucosal antibody and cytokine responses in experimental animals is often genetically restricted, thus limiting its potential usefulness in man.[5,7,8] For the studies reported here, we chose a nonliving vector which had been used for some time to generate strong protective immunity against a number of parenterally administered infectious antigens in a wide range of species. In addition, its chemical properties suggested that it might be effective when given into the intestine.

IV. IMMUNE STIMULATING COMPLEXES (ISCOMS)

Immune stimulating complexes containing the adjuvant mixture of saponins, Quil A, were first described during the early 1980s by Morein and colleagues, as a means of immunizing animals with protein-containing extracts from viral membranes.[9] Since then, a large number of studies have been performed using ISCOMS as vectors for inducing systemic immune responses against antigens from a wide range of pathogens, including viruses, bacteria, and parasites,[10-13] and an ISCOMS-based vaccine is now available commercially for protection against equine influenza. More recently, ISCOMS have been employed with purified antigens, rather than crude membrane preparations, thus extending the applicability of this approach. Furthermore, as we shall discuss, we and others have found that ISCOMS provide a potent means of allowing exogenous antigens to stimulate CTL *in vivo*. Thus, ISCOMS appear to present a novel and potent way of generating a wide range of protective immune responses using purified antigens. Here, we will review the chemical and immunological properties of ISCOMS, before discussing the nature of local and systemic immunity by oral immunization with antigen in ISCOMS.

A. STRUCTURE OF ISCOMS

ISCOMS are rigid, three-dimensional cages of 30 to 70 nm in diameter (Figure 1), with a regular, symmetrical structure which gives them an icosahedral appearance (Figure 2). However, their exact size and shape depends on the type of lipids present, the ratio between lipid, saponin, and cholesterol, and the nature of the antigen which has been incorporated.[14,15] The essential components of the ISCOM particle are saponin (Quil A), cholesterol, and lipid, and these materials alone will form the characteristic structure. However, the immunological importance of ISCOMS lies in the ability of hydrophobic or membrane-associated proteins to incorporate spontaneously if added at this stage. As a result, it is particularly easy to prepare ISCOMS containing even crude extracts of membrane-derived material from pathogenic organisms. Parenteral immunization with such ISCOMS has been successful in raising protective immunity against many viruses and bacteria, as well as several parasites.

It is more difficult to incorporate nonhydrophobic proteins into ISCOMS, but two principal approaches have been used for this purpose. In the first, acid pH has been used to expose hydrophobic regions on proteins such as bovine serum albumin (BSA), HIV gp120, and ovalbumin (OVA). In the presence of additional lipid such as phosphatidyl

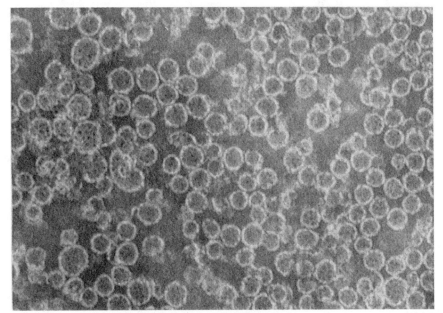

Figure 1 Ultrastructural appearance of ISCOMS. Electron microscopy reveals the cage-like structures formed by the lipophilic micelles. (Magnification × 73,000.)

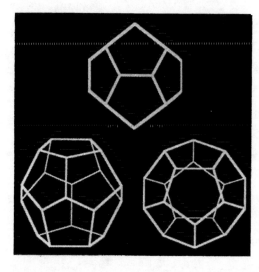

Figure 2 Schematic diagram of the structural symmetry of ISCOMS.

choline (PC) or phosphatidyl ethanolamine (PE), these materials form ISCOMS which are fully immunogenic after parenteral immunization.[16-19] However, as the technique is dependent on the protein containing a sufficient number of hydrophobic residues, it is inefficient and carries the risk of destroying immunogenic epitopes. We have employed an alternative method which should be applicable to most proteins, and which should not interfere with immunological recognition of the antigen. In this approach, palmitic acid residues are attached to the protein using the succinimide esterification reaction and, after addition of PC or PE, the palmitified proteins incorporate with very high efficiency (>95%) into ISCOMS (see References 20 and 21 for details). This technique has been employed successfully with several proteins, including OVA, gp120, hen egg lysozyme, cytochrome c, the C fragment of tetanus toxin, *Bordetella pertussis* toxin p69, FIV p20, and HIV p40 (References 20, 22, and 23 and unpublished observations) and has formed the basis of our studies on oral immunization.

More recently, it has been shown that proteins and/or peptides can also be linked directly to preformed ISCOM matrices (Morein, B., personal communication). Initial results indicate that ISCOMS formed in this way are immunogenic by parenteral routes, but further work is required to determine if this relatively simple technique is applicable to a wide range of antigens and routes of immunization.

B. NATURE OF IMMUNE RESPONSES INDUCED BY PARENTERAL IMMUNIZATION WITH ISCOMS

A full discussion of this aspect of the immunobiology of ISCOMS is beyond the scope of this chapter, and it has been reviewed in detail elsewhere.[10-13] Initial studies showed that ISCOMS-associated antigen stimulated high levels of IgM and IgG antibodies, particularly using multiple immunization regimes. In experimental animals, these responses are equivalent to, or greater than those found using conventional adjuvants such as complete Freund's adjuvant (CFA) and are readily boosted by challenge with antigen whether given alone or in the form of ISCOMS. Importantly, antigen incorporated in ISCOMS induces antibodies which are capable of neutralizing the appropriate pathogens *in vitro* and of mediating protection against challenge infection *in vivo*. Less work has been performed on the ability of ISCOMS to stimulate individual subclasses of IgG, but it has been suggested that ISCOMS containing influenza proteins may share the ability of the virus itself to stimulate high levels of IgG3 antibodies.[24] From the point of view of safety during clinical use, it is of interest that ISCOMS seem to stimulate little or no specific IgE production *in vivo.*

ISCOMS are also very potent stimulators of cell-mediated immunity *in vivo,* generating strong antigen-specific delayed-type hypersensitivity,[22] as well as high proliferative responses and interleukin 2 (IL-2) production by T lymphocytes.[24,25] Indeed, our own results show that ISCOMS are much more efficient than CFA for stimulating DTH and T cell proliferative responses in mice immunized subcutaneously with OVA[22] (Figure 3). Both these responses require very low doses of antigen (<10 μg) and are entirely dependent on CD4+ T cells. Preliminary findings indicate that these cells may belong predominantly to the T_H1 subset, as ISCOMS-immunized lymphocytes produce large amounts of γ-interferon (γIFN), but little or no IL-4 *in vitro* (authors' unpublished observations). ISCOMS also stimulate the production of large amounts of IL-1 *in vivo,* underlining the adjuvant properties of these vectors.[26]

The most novel aspect of ISCOMS is their ability to allow purified protein antigens to prime CTL *in vivo.* Early results indicated that ISCOMS containing influenza membrane extracts primed animals for secondary CTL responses to challenge with the intact virus.[27] More recently, it has been shown that mice immunized subcutaneously or intraperitoneally with purified OVA, β-galactosidase, or HIV gp120 rapidly develop strong CTL responses which are optimal with as little as 5 μg antigen.[17-19,22] The CTL activity is mediated by class I MHC-restricted CD8+ T cells whose antigenic targets comprise the motifs necessary for association with the antigen-binding cleft of appropriate class I MHC molecules.[18,19] These epitopes are generated by endogenous processing of the intact antigen, indicating that the CTL are induced by ISCOMS in a "physiological" manner. Together, these results suggest that this strategy will be of use in protecting against infections in which CTL are of primary importance.

C. ISCOMS AS VECTORS FOR ORAL IMMUNIZATION

The lipid nature of ISCOMS and the general ineffectiveness of liposomes by the oral route initially suggested that ISCOMS would not be suitable for oral immunization.[27] However, the ISCOMS structure is much more stable than that of conventional liposomes and is resistant both to temperature change and acid pH.[8,14] Furthermore, ISCOMS survive treatment with bile salts/acids and are immunogenic if injected directly into the small intestine.[15] For these reasons, we decided to examine directly whether ISCOMS containing OVA would induce systemic and local immunity when given by the oral route.

As we have discussed, feeding normal mice soluble OVA results in tolerance to subsequent systemic challenge with antigen in immunogenic form. The same amount of OVA in ISCOMS given orally does not induce tolerance,[28] but stimulates significant primary systemic immunity in mice, with DTH responses equivalent to those found after conventional parenteral immunization with OVA in CFA. This primary response peaks after 7 to 14 days and persists up to 21 days. There is also a serum IgG antibody response, although this is relatively low in comparison with the cellular response.[22] Low, but consistent CTL responses can also be detected in the spleen of such mice (Figure 4). However, compared with parenteral immunization, larger amounts of antigen are required to produce primary immunity by the oral route, with 100 μg OVA producing optimal DTH responses, and only this dose is effective at generating IgG or CTL responses. In addition, the maximal responses are smaller than those found after a single parenteral immunization. No secretory antibody responses were found in the intestine of mice fed OVA ISCOMS once (see below).

In contrast, repeated oral immunization with ISCOMS stimulates very strong local and systemic immune responses, with optimal immunity occurring after administration of antigen six times over a period of 10 d. Under these circumstances, mice develop good

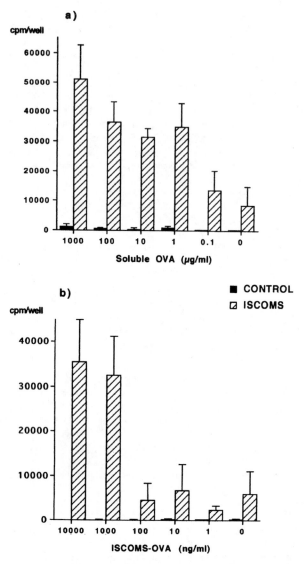

Figure 3 Immunization with ISCOMS containing the protein antigen ovalbumin primes proliferative T cell responses in the draining lymph node of mice which can be recalled with either soluble OVA (a) or with OVA incorporated in ISCOMS (b). Results shown are from 6-day cultures of cells from ISCOMS-immunized mice or unimmunized controls.

serum IgG antibody responses, equivalent to those seen after subcutaneous immunization with OVA in CFA (Figure 5a). The levels of IgG depend on the dose of antigen used on each occasion, with 100 µg OVA producing optimal results. These animals also have high amounts of OVA-specific IgA antibodies in intestinal secretions, and this occurs with as little as 10 µg of OVA per dose (Figure 5b). In more detailed studies, we found that the

% Cytotoxicity

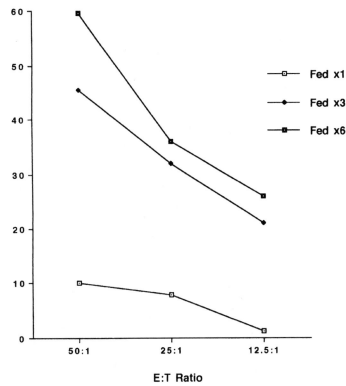

Figure 4 Induction of specific CTL responses by oral immunization with ovalbumin in ISCOMS. Mice were immunized on one, three, or six occasions with ISCOMS containing 100 μg OVA and OVA-specific CTL activity measured against the OVA-transfected EG7.OVA cell line in a ^{51}Cr release assay using spleen cells restimulated with EG7.OVA cells *in vitro*.

induction of intestinal IgA antibodies was dependent on the frequency of immunization, rather than the antigen dose, with at least three feeds being required to stimulate significant local antibody production (Figure 5c). As with many other mucosal immunization regimes, the primary IgA response to OVA ISCOMS is relatively transient, peaking at 7 d and being virtually absent by 14 d.[28] No IgG antibodies can be detected in the intestine, confirming the local origin of these antibodies. The secretory antibody response is OVA specific, but it is interesting to note that mice fed OVA ISCOMS have increased levels of total intestinal IgA, indicating that ISCOMS may have a more generalized adjuvant effect on IgA synthesis (Table 1). No serum or intestinal antibody responses occur in mice fed palmitified OVA as a control, underlining the lack of immunogenicity of protein antigens by the oral route (Figure 5). Despite the strong serum IgG responses and local IgA responses, we were unable to detect any OVA-specific IgA antibody in the serum of mice fed OVA ISCOMS alone. However, significant levels of serum IgA anti-OVA antibody could be induced by priming mice parenterally with a low dose of OVA in ISCOMS, followed by secondary oral challenge with soluble OVA itself (Figure 6). These findings confirm the synergistic effects of combined parenteral and mucosal

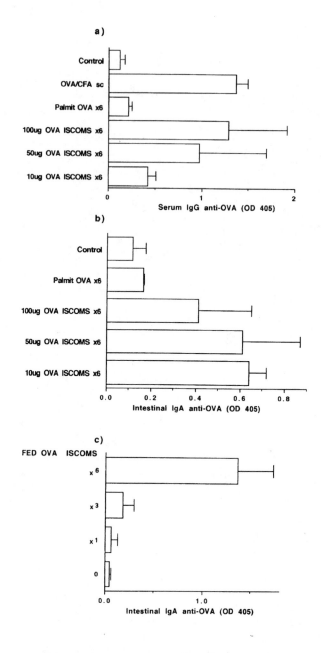

Figure 5 Induction of local and systemic antibody responses by oral immunization with OVA in ISCOMS. (a) Serum OVA-specific IgG antibody levels in mice fed on six occasions with different doses of OVA in ISCOMS, or with palmitified OVA alone. (b) Secretory OVA-specific IgA antibody responses in the small intestine in mice fed OVA ISCOMS six times. (c) Intestinal IgA antibody production requires at least three oral immunizations with ISCOMS.

Table 1   **Adjuvant effects of ISCOMS on intestinal IgA production**

Day after last feed	Fed	Total IgA level (ng/ml)
7	OVA	6.3 ± 1.8
	OVA ISCOMS	$651 \pm 8.3**$
14	OVA	128.6 ± 29.5
	OVA ISCOMS	$245.7 \pm 114*$

Note: Total IgA levels in intestinal washings of mice fed OVA in ISCOMS or in soluble form on six occasions. (** $p < 0.005$; * $p < 0.05$ vs. OVA-fed mice.)

immunization which have been described using other mucosal adjuvants such as cholera toxin[5,29] and suggest the need for further studies of combined immunization regimes using ISCOMS.

Multiple oral immunizations with OVA ISCOMS induce strong CTL responses (Figure 4). These are virtually equivalent when either three or six immunizing doses are used and can be detected in the spleen within 4 d after immunization. Peak responses occur at 7 to 14 d and decline rapidly thereafter. CTL are also generated in the mesenteric lymph node (MLN) of immunized mice, confirming the ability of orally administered ISCOMS to prime local immunity in the intestine itself. However, CTL cannot be detected in the Peyer's patches (PP) of ISCOMS-fed mice, suggesting that the CTL precursors may leave this tissue before fully differentiating (authors' unpublished observations). Alternatively, oral ISCOMS may gain access to the immune system in a manner which does not involve the PP (see below). The CTL induced by feeding OVA ISCOMS are identical to those found in parenterally primed animals. Thus, they are class I MHC-restricted CD8[+] T cells which recognize the physiologically processed immunodominant H-2K[b]-restricted epitope on OVA (Figure 7).

These results are evidence that ISCOMS may provide a novel means of inducing all forms of local and systemic immunity after oral immunization with relatively low amounts of purified protein antigens. Although multiple immunization schedules are necessary and the primary responses which occur are not long-lived, current work indicates that good secondary responses can be recalled for some months after even a single oral dose of OVA ISCOMS. It will now be important to extend our findings to other antigens and to prove the efficacy of oral immunization with ISCOMS-associated antigen in inducing protection against mucosal and systemic pathogens.

D. SAFETY OF ORALLY ADMINISTERED ISCOMS

Systemic administration of ISCOMS is sometimes associated with toxicity, particularly in small animals with ISCOMS containing high concentrations of Quil A. However, in our hands, toxicity is rarely found when ISCOMS are used by the oral route, even in animals receiving very high amounts of Quil A on several occasions. As a result, there is a much wider margin for safety between immunogenic and toxic doses of ISCOMS when oral administration is employed. Recent studies also suggest that the adjuvant component(s) of Quil A can be separated from those responsible for the systemic toxicity,[30,31] indicating it may be possible in the future to synthesize immunogenic ISCOMS containing only nontoxic moieties of Quil A.

Oral immunization with ISCOMS is also not complicated by the intestinal immunopathology which occurs with many other immunomodulatory strategies that prevent the induction of oral tolerance.[3,32-34] Under these circumstances, oral challenge with antigen

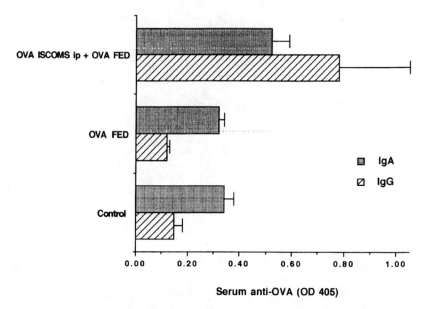

Serum anti-OVA (OD 405)

Figure 6 Induction of systemic IgA antibody responses by combined oral and parenteral immunization with ISCOMS. Serum OVA-specific IgA antibody levels in mice primed once with OVA ISCOMS intraperitoneally and challenged orally with soluble antigen.

produces a local cell-mediated immune response in the intestinal mucosa which is associated with pathological changes such as crypt hyperplasia and lymphocytic infiltration of the epithelium. If allowed to progress, these features may lead to intestinal damage and this phenomenon is a potentially dangerous complication of any immunization regime which stimulates local T cell-mediated immune responses. It is important to note therefore that mice immunized orally with OVA ISCOMS do not develop intestinal pathology when challenged with OVA, despite the high level of local priming which is induced.[28]

E. IMMUNIZATION OF OTHER MUCOSAL SURFACES BY ISCOMS

It is not known whether oral immunization with ISCOMS can induce active immunity in other mucosal tissues, such as the respiratory tract, urogenital tract, or breast. However, it has been known for some time that ISCOMS are highly immunogenic when given directly into the respiratory tract, inducing local and systemic antibody production, as well as local cellular immunity with low doses of antigen.[27,35] Furthermore, mice immunized intranasally with ISCOMS containing influenza membrane antigens are protected from lethal influenza infection and develop virus-specific CTL after challenge.[27,35] Recent studies indicate that ISCOMS containing purified HIV proteins are also immunogenic by the nasal route (Morein, B., personal communication), but the full range of immune responses which can be induced by this route have not yet been established. As yet, there have been no studies of the ability of ISCOMS to be immunogenic in other mucosal tissues.

F. ADJUVANT PROPERTIES OF ISCOMS

Very little is known at present about why ISCOMS are such potent adjuvants. In particular, their ability to stimulate class I MHC-restricted T cells and their mucosal

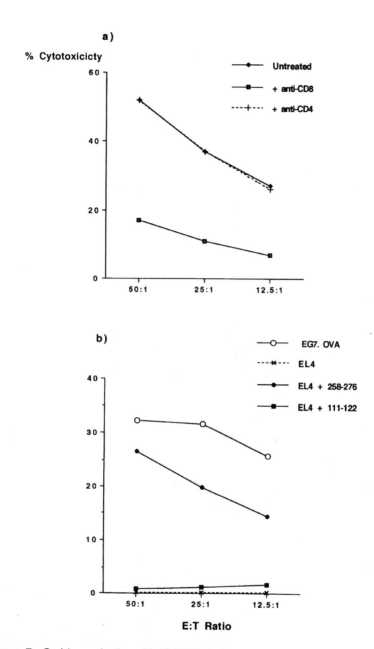

Figure 7 Oral immunization with ISCOMS induces antigen-specific class I MHC-restricted CTL. (a) Splenic CTL responses against EG7.OVA cells are inhibited in the presence of anti-CD8 antibody, but anti-CD4 antibody has no effect. (b) OVA-specific splenic CTL recognize target cells pulsed with the OVA 258-276 peptide which contains the H-2K^b-restricted motif for OVA.[44] There is no recognition of OVA 111-122.

immunogenicity are poorly understood. However, it seems likely that their effects reflect both their chemical composition and their structure.

The adjuvant component of ISCOMS is Quil A, which is a complex mixture of isoterpenoid saponins. Doses of free Quil A similar to those found in ISCOMS enhance antibody and CMI responses to both parenterally and orally administered antigen.[36,37] In addition, feeding Quil A allows protein antigens to stimulate secretory IgA antibody production in the intestine (authors' unpublished observations). These effects appear to be due to a true adjuvant effect on the immune system, since Quil A retains its potentiating activity for antibody and DTH responses even when given by a different route from antigen.[37] The mechanisms underlying this activity remain to be identified, but may involve the nonspecific stimulation of cytokine production. Administration of antigen-free ISCOMS or Quil A produces intense hyperplasia of local lymphoid tissues which involves all subsets of lymphocytes, particularly B cells and CD8+ T cells (unpublished observations). This is associated with the production of several inflammatory cytokines which are likely to stimulate immune responses, including IL-1 and γIFN (Reference 26 and unpublished observations).

This is not the only property of Quil A which contributes to its ability to modulate immune responses. Recently, we and others have found that class I MHC-restricted CTL responses can also be induced *in vivo* by administering soluble antigens together with ISCOMS matrix, intact Quil A, or with the QS21 adjuvant component of Quil A[31] (Figure 8). This phenomenon occurs using both parenteral and oral routes, but much higher amounts of free Quil A are required than the doses which are effective when incorporated in ISCOMS.[31] Unlike its effects on other aspects of the immune response, Quil A only induces CTL when given at the same time and to the same site as antigen (unpublished observations). Recent work indicates that a fraction of Quil A which has no adjuvant effect itself, but which forms ISCOMS, can induce CTL normally *in vivo* (unpublished observations). These results suggest that the ability of Quil A to stimulate CTL responses mainly reflects its physicochemical properties, rather than a modulatory effect on immune function. The basis of this is unclear, but it may be that the detergent activity of Quil A produces pores in the membrane of antigen-presenting cells, allowing those proteins in the vicinity to enter directly into the cytoplasm and thus gain access to the endogenous pathway of antigen processing. Additionally and/or alternatively, this detergent effect may allow the escape into the cytoplasm of materials which have been taken up by endocytosis or phagocytosis (see below). Whatever the mechanism, the induction of CTL by ISCOMS is a complex phenomenon, involving a number of different cell types. Although the CTL themselves are CD8+ T cells, their activation is entirely dependent on the presence of CD4+ T cells *in vivo* (Figure 9a) and requires a population of phagocytic cells (Figure 9b). These findings are consistent with recent data on the induction of CTL in other systems[38-40] and suggest that ISCOMS-associated antigen must be phagocytosed and presented to CD4+ T cells before CTL can be activated. Although this hypothesis would certainly be consistent with the particulate nature of ISCOMS and with their appearance in the phagosomes of macrophages,[41] it is difficult to reconcile with the ability of free Quil A to induce CTL *in vivo*. Resolution of this issue will require detailed studies of the antigen-processing mechanisms utilized by ISCOMS. Very little has been performed in this area, but recent work shows that ISCOMS containing measles virus fusion (MVF) protein can enter both the endogenous and exogenous routes of antigen processing *in vitro*, but the induction of class I MHC-restricted T cells is slow and relatively inefficient.[42] These studies also suggest that ISCOMS-associated MVF can gain access to an unusual, chloroquine-insensitive pathway of class II MHC-restricted processing. Most of these properties of ISCOMS reproduce those of live virus itself, highlighting the potential usefulness of ISCOMS as nonliving adjuvants for vaccination against pathogenic infection.

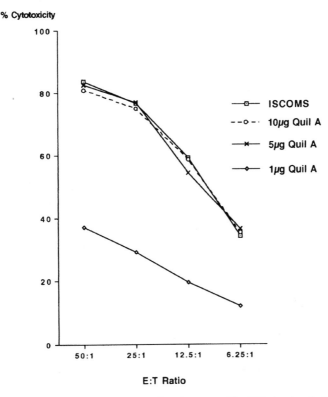

Figure 8 Quil A allows the induction of antigen-specific CTL *in vivo*, but is more effective in the form of an ISCOM. Mice were immunized once intraperitoneally with 10 μg OVA either in ISCOMS (containing 1 μg Quil A), or together with 10 μg, 5 μg, or 1 μg Quil A alone.

G. ADJUVANT ACTIVITY OF ISCOMS IN THE MUCOSA

The unique potency of ISCOMS as orally active vectors must partly reflect the properties of Quil A and ISCOMS discussed above, and it would be interesting to determine how the induction of total and specific IgA responses in the intestine correlate with the production of cytokines such as IL-5 and IL-6. Nevertheless, it seems that additional mechanisms are also involved in the mucosal immunogenicity of ISCOMS. Thus, it has been suggested that ISCOMS particles are taken up preferentially by M cells in the epithelium of PP,[43] the route which is believed to be the most efficient means of stimulating immunity in the gut. Furthermore, we have shown recently that prior administration of ISCOMS enhances the uptake of orally administered protein into the systemic circulation. In parallel, serum from these mice does not contain the tolerogenic material normally found in animals fed soluble proteins (Table 2). These results suggest that ISCOMS influence the absorption of proteins by the intestinal mucosa, both by increasing the amounts absorbed and by altering the immunogenicity of the resulting material. These effects would be more consistent with an action of ISCOMS on the overall barrier function of the intestinal epithelium, rather than a specific effect at the level of the PP. These issues require resolution by following the distribution of ISCOMS-associated antigen after oral administration.

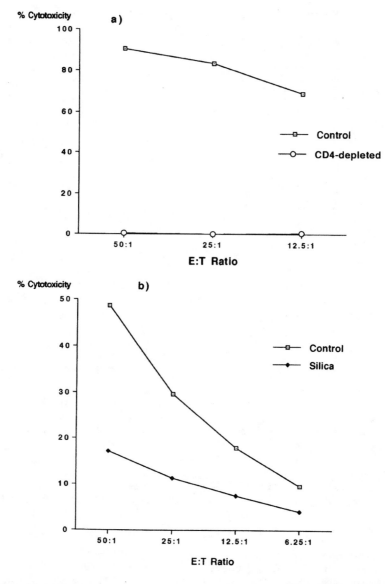

Figure 9 Induction of antigen-specific CTL by ISCOMS requires CD4⁺ T cells and phagocytic cells *in vivo*. The generation of OVA-specific CTL is prevented by treating mice with anti-CD4 antibody (a) or by depleting phagocytic cells by intravenous injection of silica (b) before intraperitoneal immunization with OVA ISCOMS.

V. FUTURE PERSPECTIVES

The information we have presented here suggests that ISCOMS have many novel properties as adjuvants for oral immunization with purified antigens, inducing a unique range of strong local and systemic immune responses. These vectors appear to be highly adaptable, with palmitification providing a potential means of incorporating most chosen antigens. It will now be important to determine whether this strategy is capable of

Table 2 **Effects of ISCOMS on intestinal uptake of antigen**

Fed — 30 min	Fed 0 min	Serum OVA (µg/ml)
Saline	Saline	2.5 ± 15.2
Saline	OVA	281 ± 143
ISCOMS	Saline	5.6 ± 11.1
ISCOMS	OVA	602 ± 202.1*

Note: Mice were fed ISCOMS or saline 30 min before a test feed of 25 mg OVA and serum levels of absorbed protein assessed by an OVA-specific ELISA after a further 30 min. (* $p < 0.02$ vs. OVA-fed controls.)

stimulating protective immunity against pathogens in the intestine and elsewhere and to understand how ISCOMS-associated antigen is processed within both the intestine and the immune system. In the longer term, it would be of interest to explore the feasibility of developing ISCOMS-based vaccines which could be targetted specifically to the intestinal immune system, perhaps by incorporation of epithelial-binding molecules such as cholera toxin, or of antibodies directed at antigen-presenting cells. Finally, it will be necessary to investigate means of incorporating entirely synthetic epitopes into ISCOMS and to examine whether ISCOMS can be used for immunization with nonprotein antigens. By establishing the optimal regimes for oral immunization with ISCOMS, such studies may lead to a new generation of safe and effective oral recombinant vaccines of wide applicability.

ACKNOWLEDGMENTS

The work of the authors described here was supported by the Wellcome Trust and the Scottish Home and Health Department.

REFERENCES

1. Challacombe, S.J., The induction of secretory IgA responses, in *Food Allergy and Intolerance,* Brostoff, J. and Challacombe, S.J., Eds., W.B. Saunders, Eastbourne, U.K., 1987, 269.
2. Cresswell, P., Questions of presentation, *Nature,* 343, 593, 1990.
3. Mowat, A.McI., The regulation of immune responses to dietary protein antigens, *Immunol. Today,* 8, 93, 1987.
4. Mowat, A.McI., Lamont, A.G., and Parrott, D.M.V., Suppressor T cells, antigen-presenting cells and the role of I-J restriction in oral tolerance to ovalbumin, *Immunology,* 64, 141, 1988.
5. McGhee, J.R., Mestecky, J., Dertzbaugh, M.T., Eldridge, J.H., Hirasawa, M., and Kiyono, H., The mucosal immune system: from fundamental concepts to vaccine development, *Vaccine,* 10, 75, 1992.
6. Tite, J.P., Gao, X.-M., Hughes-Jenkins, C.M., Lipscombe, M., O'Callaghan, D., Dougan, G., and Liew, F.Y., Anti-viral immunity induced by recombinant nucleoprotein of influenza A virus. III. Delivery of recombinant nucleoprotein to the immune system using attenuated *Salmonella typhimurium* as a live carrier, *Immunology,* 70, 540, 1990.
7. Elson, C.O. and Ealding, W., Ir gene control of the murine secretory IgA response to cholera toxin, *Eur. J. Immunol.,* 17, 425, 1987.
8. Wilson, A.D., Stokes, C.R., and Bourne, F.J., Adjuvant effect of cholera toxin on the mucosal immune response to soluble proteins. Differences between mouse strains and protein antigens, *Scand. J. Immunol.,* 29, 739, 1989.

9. Morein, B., Sundquist, B., Hoglund, S., Dalsgaard, K., and Osterhaus, A., Iscom, a novel structure for antigenic presentation of membrane proteins from enveloped viruses, *Nature,* 308, 457, 1984.

10. Morein, B., The iscom antigen-presenting system, *Nature,* 332, 287, 1988.

11. Morein, B., Lovgren, K., Hoglund, S., and Sundquist, B., The ISCOM: an immunostimulating complex, *Immunol. Today,* 8, 333, 1987.

12. Morein, B., Fossum, C., Lovgren, K., and Hoglund, S., The iscom — a modern approach to vaccines, *Semin. Virol.,* 1, 49, 1990.

13. Claasen, I. and Osterhaus, A., The iscom structure as an immune-enhancing moiety: experience with viral systems, *Res. Immunol.,* 143, 531, 1992.

14. Ozel, M., Hoglund, S., Gelderblom, H.R., and Morein, B., Quaternary structure of the immunostimulating complex (ISCOM), *J. Ultrastruct. Mol. Struct. Res.,* 102, 240, 1989.

15. Kersten, G.F.A., The Immune Stimulating Complex (ISCOM), Ph.D. thesis, University of Utrecht, 1990.

16. Morein, B., Ekstrom, J., and Lovgren, K., Increased immunogenicity of a non-amphipathic protein (BSA) after inclusion into iscoms, *J. Immunol. Methods,* 128, 177, 1990.

17. Takahashi, H., Takeshita, T., Morein, B., Putney, S., Germain, R.N., and Berzofsky, J.A., Induction of CD8⁺ cytotoxic T cells by immunization with purified HIV-1 envelope protein in ISCOMs, *Nature,* 344, 873, 1990.

18. Heeg, K., Kuon, W., and Wagner, H., Vaccination of class I major histocompatibility complex (MHC)-restricted murine CD8⁺ cytotoxic T lymphocytes toward soluble antigens: immunostaining-ovalbumin complexes enter the class I MHC-restricted antigen pathway and allow sensitization against the immunodominant peptide, *Eur. J. Immunol.,* 21, 152, 1991.

19. Lipford, G.B., Hoffman, M., Wagner, H., and Heeg, K., Primary in vivo responses to ovalbumin. Probing the predictive value of the Kᵇ binding motif, *J. Immunol.,* 150, 1212, 1993.

20. Reid, G., Soluble proteins incorporate into ISCOMS after covalent attachment of fatty acids, *Vaccine,* 10, 597, 1992.

21. Mowat, A.McI. and Reid, G., The preparation of immune stimulating complexes (ISCOMS) as adjuvants for local and systemic immunization with protein antigens, in *Curr. Protocols in Immunology,* Coligan, J.E., Strober, W., Kruisbeek, A.M., and Margulies, D., Eds., in press.

22. Mowat, A.McI., Donachie, A.M., Reid, G., and Jarrett, O., Immune stimulating complexes containing Quil A and protein antigen prime class I MHC-restricted T lymphocytes in vivo and are active by the oral route, *Immunology,* 72, 317, 1991.

23. Browning, M., Reid, G., Osborne, R., and Jarrett, O., Incorporation of soluble antigens into ISCOMS: HIV gp120 ISCOMS induce virus neutralizing antibodies, *Vaccine,* 10, 585, 1992.

24. Villacres-Eriksson, M., Gergstrom-Mollaoglu, M., Kaberg, H., and Morein, B., Involvement of interleukin-2 and interferon-gamma in the immune response induced by influenza virus Iscoms, *Scand. J. Immunol.,* 36, 1992.

25. Fossum, C., Bergstrom, M., Lovgren, K., Watson, D.L., and Morein, B., Effect of ISCOMS and their adjuvant moiety (matrix) on the initial proliferation and IL-2 responses: comparison of spleen cells from mice inoculated with ISCOMS and/or matrix, *Cell. Immunol.,* 129, 414, 1990.

26. Villacres-Eriksson, M., Bergstrom-Mollaoglu, M., Kaberg, H., Lovgren, K., and Morein, B., The induction of cell-associated and secreted interleukin-1 by ISCOMS, matrix or micelles in murine splenic cells, *Scand. J. Immunol.,* in press.

27. Jones, P.D., Tha-Hla, R., Morein, B., Lovgren, K., and Ada, G.L., Cellular immune responses in the murine lung to local immunization with influenza A glycoproteins in micelles and immunostimulatory complexes (ISCOMS), *Scand. J. Immunol.,* 27, 645, 1988.

28. Mowat, A.McI., Maloy, K.J., and Donachie, A.M., Immune stimulating complexes as adjuvants for stimulating local and systemic immunity after oral immunization with protein antigens, *Immunology,* in press.

29. Pierce, N.F., The role of antigen form and function in the primary and secondary intestinal immune responses to cholera toxin, and toxoid in rats, *J. Exp. Med.,* 148, 195, 1978.

30. Kensil, C.R., Patel, U., Lennick, M., and Marciani, D., Separation and characterization of saponins with adjuvant activity from *Quillaja saponaria* Molina cortex, *J. Immunol.,* 146, 431, 1991.

31. Wu, J.-Y., Gardner, B.H., Murphy, C.I., Seals, J.R., Kensil, C.R., Recchia, J., Beltz, G.A., Newman, G.W., and Newman, M.J., Saponin adjuvant enhancement of antigen-specific immune responses to an experimental HIV-1 vaccine, *J. Immunol.,* 148, 1519, 1992.

32. Mowat, A.McI. and Ferguson, A., Hypersensitivity in the small intestinal mucosa. V. Induction of cell mediated immunity to a dietary antigen, *Clin. Exp. Immunol.,* 43, 574, 1981.

33. Mowat, A.McI., Depletion of suppressor T cells by 2'-deoxyguanosine abrogates tolerance in mice fed ovalbumin and permits the induction of intestinal delayed-type hypersensitivity, *Immunology,* 58, 179, 1986.

34. Mowat, A.McI. and Parrott, D.M.V., Immunological responses to fed protein antigens in mice. IV. Effect of reticuloendothelial system stimulation on oral tolerance and intestinal immunity to ovalbumin, *Immunology,* 50, 547, 1983.

35. Lovgren, K., Kabert, H., and Morein, B., An experimental subunit vaccine (iscoms); induction of protective immunity to challenge infection in mice after intranasal or subcutaneous administration, *Clin. Exp. Immunol.,* 82, 435, 1990.

36. Bomford, R., Studies on the cellular site of action of the adjuvant activity of saponin for sheep erythrocytes, *Int. Arch. Allergy Appl. Immunol.,* 67, 127, 1982.

37. Chavali, S.R., Barton, L.D., and Campbell, J.B., Immunopotentiation by orally-administered Quillaja saponins effects in mice vaccinated intraperitoneally against rabies, *Clin. Exp. Immunol.,* 74, 339, 1988.

38. van Rooijen, N., Liposome-mediated elimination of macrophages, *Res. Immunol.,* 143, 215, 1992.

39. Debrick, J.E., Campbell, P.A., and Staerz, U.D., Macrophages as accessory cells for class I MHC-restricted immune responses, *J. Immunol.,* 147, 2846, 1991.

40. Pfeifer, J.D., Wick, M.J., Roberts, R.L., Findlay, K., Normark, S.J., and Harding, C.V., Phagocytic processing of bacterial antigens for class I MHC presentation to T cells, *Nature,* 361, 359, 1993.

41. Watson, D.L., Lovgren, K., Watson, N.A., Fossum, C., Morein, B., and Hoglund, S., Inflammatory response and antigen localization following immunization with influenza virus ISCOMs, *Inflammation,* 13, 641, 1989.

42. Binnendijk, R.S. van, Van Baalen, C.A., Poelen, M.C.M., De Vries, P., Boes, J., Cerundolo, V., Osterhaus, A.D.M.E., and Uytdehaag, F.G.C.M., Measles virus transmembrane fusion protein synthesized de novo or presented in immmunostimulating complexes is endogenously processed for HLA class I and class II-restricted cytotoxic T cell recognition, *J. Exp. Med.,* 176, 119, 1992.

43. Claassen, I., Osterhaus, A., Boersma, W., Schellekens, M., and Claassen, E., Fluorescent labeling of virus, bacteriae and ISCOMs *in vivo:* systemic and mucosal localisation patterns, *Proc. 7th Int. Congr. Mucosal Immunol.,* in press.

44. Falk, K., Rotzschke, O., Stefanovic, S., Jung, G., and Rammensee, H.-G., Allele-specific motifs revealed by sequencing of self-peptides eluted from MHC molecules, *Nature,* 351, 290, 1991.

Chapter 4

Oral Vaccination with Lectins and Lectin-Like Molecules

G. J. Russell-Jones

TABLE OF CONTENTS

I. INTRODUCTION

Attempts to immunize animals orally have generally been hindered by the very small quantities of antigen which survive proteolysis in the gut and which can cross the gut mucosa. In order to overcome these obstacles, it has generally been necessary to repeatedly feed milligram quantities of antigen as many as eight to ten times.[1-7] The immunity induced by this regime has at best been poor, short lasting, and often confined to the mucosal immune system. The small amount of antigen which is actually absorbed is believed to be taken up by "M" cells of the Peyer's patches via a nonspecific, "antigen sampling" mechanism. This presumably explains why only a small quantity of the orally administered antigen is actually absorbed. Following absorption of the antigen it crosses these cells and is presented to the underlying IgA-producing B cells within the dome of the Peyer's patch, or alternatively stimulates the IgG suppressor T cells, resident in the marginal area of the lymphoid follicle,[8,9] which subsequently suppress the production of a systemic IgG response, thereby resulting in systemic tolerance.[3,10-13] The majority of B cells which underlie the intestinal villus epithelium are IgM-, IgE-, or IgG-producing cells, which is in contrast to the predominance of IgA-producing B cells in the area of the

0-8493-4866-8/94/$0.00+$.50
© 1994 by CRC Press Inc.

Peyer's patch and various other subepithelial lymphoid follicles, . These B cells can be stimulated to produce antigen-specific antibody by the many Ia⁺-bearing cells of the villus epithelium.[8,9] There are a number of pathogens which invade the villus epithelial cells of the intestine and stimulate predominantly a serum IgG antibody response rather than the more common secretory IgA (sIgA) response elicited by the majority of soluble antigens. Thus polio virus, cholera toxin, *E. coli* heat-labile toxin (LTB), certain types of rotavirus and reoviruses, and many enterotoxigenic *E. coli* (ETEC) strains all elicit predominantly a serum antibody response following epithelial invasion.[14,15]

The initial event whereby many of these pathogens invade the villus epithelium is by binding to the surface glycolipids and glycoproteins of the villus epithelial cells using a sugar-specific binding protein on the surface of the pathogen. For the purpose of this review, these binding proteins will be referred to as lectin-like molecules (LLMs), due to their functional similarities to the sugar-binding properties of plant lectins.[16] In the case of bacteria, the surface proteins possessing this binding activity are the pili, while the analogous proteins present on the surface of many viruses are hemagglutinins.[17-19] Thus, many of these mucosal pathogens possess various surface appendages which bind in a lectin-like fashion to the mucosal epithelium and play a major role in the pathogenesis of these organisms. Many of the strains of bacteria which cause diarrhea also secrete a toxin which contains a binding subunit (B subunit) which binds in a lectin-like fashion to the intestinal epithelial cell. The toxin is internalized by receptor-mediated endocytosis, after which the toxic A subunit is activated.[20-22] The binding and internalization of these toxin molecules is a remarkably efficient process, as it has been shown that the binding and internalization of a single toxin molecule is enough to kill the cell.[23]

It is the purpose of this review to demonstrate that it is possible to greatly enhance the uptake of orally administered antigen, by utilizing the ability of LLMs to target antigen to the intestinal mucosal cells by binding to their cell surface glycolipids and glycoproteins, and to initiate uptake of the antigens into the cells and thereby present the antigens in a highly efficient manner to the immune system.

II. ORAL VACCINATION WITH LECTINS

A. EXAMINATION OF THE POTENTIAL OF LECTINS OR LECTIN-LIKE MOLECULES TO STIMULATE SYSTEMIC ANTIBODY RESPONSES FOLLOWING ORAL ADMINISTRATION

During preliminary studies on the role of pili in pathogenesis, it was found that several weeks after feeding mice with *E. coli* cells bearing pili of the 987P or K99 serotype, it was possible to detect a serum antibody response to the pili, as well as a concomitant antibody response in the intestinal lumen. Subsequent experiments using purified pili showed that the generation of the antibody response to the pili could be achieved by feeding of pili alone, rather than the whole bacterial cell. Similarly, oral administration of microgram quantities of LTB (the nontoxic, GM1 ganglioside-binding (B) subunit of *E. coli* heat-labile toxin) also stimulated a serum antibody response to this antigen. This was in distinct contrast to the lack of systemic immune response following oral administration of similar doses of BSA to mice. The known functional similarities between pili and LTB (viz., their ability to bind in a lectin-like fashion to glycolipids/glycoproteins on epithelial cells) was postulated[24,25] to account for their ability to elicit a systemic antibody response following oral feeding. Once bound to the epithelial cells, the cells would be triggered to endocytose the antigens, with subsequent paracellular transport and stimulation of a systemic immune response. By analogy, it might be expected that any molecule which was able to bind to the intestinal villus epithelial cells in a similar fashion would be able to elicit a serum antibody response following oral administration.

Oral administration of proteins known to possess lectin-like binding activities to mice stimulated the production of a serum antibody response (Table 1), while feeding of proteins which had no apparent role in pathogenesis or in colonization of the intestine did not.[24,25] Hence, feeding of K99 and 987P pili (bacterial adhesins), LTB, and plant lectins, as well as inactivated influenza vaccine (in which the hemagglutinin activity was still maintained) all elicited comparable serum antibody responses at the doses tested (Table 1). A noticeable exception was seen following feeding of K88ab pili, which did not elicit a serum antibody response, presumably due to the absence of the particular glycoprotein or glycolipid in the mouse intestinal epithelium to which this pilus type binds.[26] Variable stimulation of intestinal antibodies occurred, but was only present upon feeding of the LLMs. None of the other antigens tested was capable of eliciting a substantial serum

Table 1   **Immune response to orally presented antigens**

| Antigen used for immunization (20 µg dose) | Immune response, day 21[a] | | | |
| | Serum | | Intestinal | |
	IgG	IgA	IgG	IgA
K99 pili	968 ± 120	<4	3.0 ± 5.2	3.2 ± 4.9
987P pili	776 ± 64	10.8 ± 8.8	10.9 ± 1.7	4.5 ± 1.88
K88ab pili	<4	<4	<4	<4
LTB	1351 ± 211	<4	<4	12.2 ± 4.4
Influenza vaccine	179 ± 34	<4	<4	<4
Flagella	<4	<4	<4	<4
LPS	12.1 ± 1.0	<4	<4	<4
Polysaccharide	<4	<4	<4	<4
BSA	<4	<4	<4	<4
Con A[b]	666 ± 84	<4	nd	nd
PW mitogen	641 ± 119	<4	nd	nd
L. culinaris	954 ± 48	<4	nd	nd
H. pomatia	591 ± 127	<4	nd	nd
P. vulgaris	1378 ± 110	4.8 ± 2.3	nd	nd
G. max	1529 ± 65	3.1 ± 6.9	nd	nd
A. hypogea	1276 ± 242	<4	nd	nd
U. europaeus	1583 ± 94	<4	nd	nd

Note: Female C57Bl/6J mice (18 to 22 gm) were starved for 3 to 4 h prior to oral administration of antigen at appropriate concentrations in 0.5 ml of 0.1 M carbonate/bicarbonate buffer pH 9.5 on day 0 and day 14. On day 21 mice were bled, sacrificed, and small intestinal washings obtained by washing with 1 ml of 30 mM Tris.HCl pH 8.8, 0.9% NaCl, 50 mM EDTA plus 1.0% Tween 20. Gut washes were stored at –20°C until assayed. Blood samples were allowed to clot at 4°C before removal of the serum and storage at –20°C.[24,25]

[a] The reciprocal of the antiserum dilution that gave an ELISA reading of 0.5 after 45 min at 37°C. Each value represents the mean value obtained from 5 mice ± 1 SD. A titer of one in one thousand corresponds to 1 µg of specific antibody per milliliter of serum.

[b] Each lectin was substituted with 4 DNP molecules per mole lectin using the method of Little and Eisen.[65] The antilectin response could not be measured directly, as sugar specific binding to IgG interfered with the ELISA and so the anti-DNP response is represented. Intestinal antibody titers were not measured for lectin-immunized animals (nd).

response at the doses tested. Intramuscular injection of five of the proteins stimulated very similar antibody titers, regardless of whether the protein was effective orally or not (results not shown).

B. INHIBITION OF THE IMMUNE RESPONSE TO ORAL LECTINS BY COFEEDING SUGARS

The stimulation of an antibody response seen after feeding lectins was a highly specific phenomenon, which appeared to depend upon a specific interaction between the lectin and its ligand. Thus, it was of interest to note that the immune response to LTB and K99 could be completely abolished by cofeeding galactose, lactose, or sorbitol, but not by cofeeding any of the other sugars tested (Table 2). The response to 987P pili was not affected by these sugars. Lactose and sorbitol show considerable structural similarities to galactose, which is claimed to be the specific sugar determinant on both the GM1 ganglioside to which LTB is known to bind,[27-29] and on the GM2 ganglioside to which K99 is thought to bind.[30] The receptor for 987P is yet to be characterized. It is known that binding to the mucosa is a specific, receptor-mediated reaction in which the LLMs bind to specific glycoproteins or glycolipids on the villus epithelium. In this respect, intestinal uptake of these antigens differs significantly from the antigen sampling mechanism suggested for the uptake of orally administered antigens.[1,10,13,31,32]

It must be noted, however, that in order for the LLMs to stimulate an antibody response following oral administration, the specific ligand to which these molecules bind must be present on the intestinal villous epithelial membrane. This presumably explains the restriction of certain ETEC strains of *E. coli* to defined animal species and the inability of K88ab pili to prime mice orally (Table 1). It must also be noted that care must be taken that no glycolipids/glycoproteins with similar structural features to the target ligands are present in the diet of the animal to be orally vaccinated, or otherwise the lectin or LLM will be unable to bind to the intestinal wall.

Pierce and others[31-34] have found similar results following feeding of cholera toxin, a protein with similar binding affinity to LTB, but a slightly different pattern of intestinal binding.[28,35-38] Oral administration of relatively small quantities of this toxin (10 to 100 μg) resulted in the stimulation of relatively good antibody responses in both serum and secretions. However, animals receiving larger doses of this toxin exhibited all the symptoms of

Table 2   Inhibition of the immune response to orally administered antigen by co-feeding certain sugars

Sugar	Immune response to oral antigen (serum IgG)[a]		
	K99 pili	987P pili	LTB
None	968 ± 120	776 ± 64	1351 ± 211
Fructose	1782 ± 966	2046 ± 894	6208 ± 1192
Galactose	65 ± 48	1037 ± 526	4 ± 1.0
Lactose	84 ± 204	1128 ± 662	5 ± 1.0
Mannose	1176 ± 411	4970 ± 2270	4096 ± 658
Melibiose	1840 ± 208	1243 ± 474	412 ± 76
Sorbitol	77 ± 179	1389 ± 307	8 ± 1.2

Note: A 20-μg-dose of LTB or 987P or K99 pili was premixed with 20 μmol of various sugars prior to feeding.

[a] Results represent the mean ELISA titers of serum + 1 SD (n = 5 mice) (see Table 1).[24,25]

a cholera infection.[33] Abolition of binding activity of cholera toxin, by toxoiding, greatly reduced its ability to elicit an antibody response following feeding. Thus, doses of 40 mg of toxoid were required to generate an immune response to the intraduodenal administration of this antigen.[34] It is highly likely that the activity of the holotoxin was due to its ability to cause mucosal damage following activation of adenylate cyclase.[39-41]

C. MODIFICATION OF THE IMMUNE RESPONSE TO ORALLY PRESENTED ANTIGENS BY COFEEDING MUCOSAL ADJUVANTS

A number of molecules (mucosal adjuvants) have been described which, when administered orally, appear to be able to alter the immune response to cofed antigen. DEAE-dextran, for instance, when added to intestinally infused ovalbumin, increased the numbers of antibody-containing cells in the efferent ilial loop.[42] This effect was postulated to result from the ability of DEAE-dextran to increase pinocytosis. Lysozyme has also been shown to possess adjuvant-like properties when administered orally. Lodinova and Jouja[43] added egg white lysozyme to the milk of formula-fed babies and observed an increase in the levels of IgA copro-antibodies. Oral administration of lysozyme and pronase to guinea pigs prior to intrafootpad injection of hep-B antigen significantly enhanced the serum response to this antigen.[44] A similar increase in the humoral response was also seen by these workers when guinea pigs were fed enzymatically digested cell walls of *Bifidobacteria longum*. Parenteral or oral administration of vitamin A has also been shown to increase the serum and intestinal antibody responses to intragastrically administered BSA.[45,46] The mechanism by which lysozyme enhances the immune response is not known; however, it is likely that some small immunostimulatory molecule (similar to muramyl dipeptide, MDP) is released from the wall of *Bifidobacteria longum*. The fat-soluble vitamin A may be acting by a direct affect on the immune system or by causing the release of neuronal mediators from the nerves underlying the mucosal epithelium.

During our studies on oral feeding of lectins, it was noted that it was possible to enhance the immune response to one of these molecules (987P pili) by cofeeding small quantities of the simple monosaccharide, mannose. These observations led us to investigate the possibility that dietary molecules such as simple sugars or vitamins may have the capacity to alter the immune response to orally administered LLMs. The molecules chosen for this study were selected to represent a spectrum of mono- and disaccharides plus a number of water- and fat-soluble vitamins which are normally present in the intestine as the result of digestion of more complex carbohydrates and which are known to be absorbed in the small intestine.

D. IDENTIFICATION OF MOLECULES WHICH ALTER THE IMMUNE RESPONSE TO ORALLY ADMINISTERED LECTINS

Preliminary screening studies using constant dose levels of both dietary molecules and antigen showed that most of the vitamins and sugars had some effect in modulating the size of the immune response to the mucosal immunogens (Table 3) as well as in influencing the type of response (secretory or serum) induced by the various immunogens. Thus, the serum antibody response to K99 pili was significantly increased ($p < 0.05$) by coadministration of vitamin B_{12}, vitamin D, fructose or melibiose; unchanged when given with mannose; decreased to varying extents with vitamin A, vitamin B_1, vitamin B_2, vitamin C, vitamin E, and xylose; and almost completely abolished when fed with vitamin B_6, lactose, or sorbitol. In contrast, the serum antibody response to oral 987P pili was elevated when 987P was coadministered with vitamin B_{12}, vitamin C, vitamin E, fructose or mannose; and was unchanged with vitamin A, vitamin B_1, vitamin B_2, vitamin B_6, vitamin D, lactose, melibiose, sorbitol, and xylose. LTB displayed yet another profile for the effect of cofeeding of dietary molecules on the serum antibody levels. There was an augmented serum response to LTB fed in the presence of vitamin A, vitamin B_2, vitamin

Table 3   Effects of dietary molecules on the immune response to orally administered K99 pili, 987P pili, or LTB[a]

Dietary molecule	Anti-K99[b]		Anti-987P		Anti-LTB	
	Serum IgG	Sec IgA	Serum IgG	Sec IgA	Serum IgG	Sec IgA
None	968 ± 120	3.2 ± 4.9	776 ± 64	48.5 ± 1.8	1351 ± 211	12.2 ± 4.4
Vitamin A	278 ± 184	5.4 ± 3.0	648 ± 40	20.5 ± 24.6	4705 ± 676	21.1 ± 7.6
Vitamin B_1	117 ± 107	2.1 ± 0.9	891 ± 127	14.7 ± 5.5	1782 ± 309	16.0 ± 2.1
Vitamin B_2	604 ± 216	2.0 ± 0.6	1082 ± 271	21.1 ± 11.9	3565 ± 908	16.0 ± 3.7
Vitamin B_6	14 ± 50	3.6 ± 8.2	1782 ± 509	39.9 ± 7.1	9 ± 1.1	—
Vitamin B_{12}	3377 ± 1266	—	3983 ± 1307	91.7 ± 31.9	1024 ± 116	42.2 ± 11.9
Vitamin C	318 ± 255	98 ± 70	4521 ± 1046	84.1 ± 14.3	337 ± 206	16.1 ± 5.0
Vitamin D	1921 ± 640	6.3 ± 2.7	398 ± 89	34.7 ± 8.1	4097 ± 74	13.9 ± 2.2
Vitamin E	512 ± 128	4.4 ± 2.1	3468 ± 776	19.9 ± 3.9	194 ± 64	18.4 ± 3.6
Fructose	1782 ± 966	34.7 ± 14.2	2048 ± 894	23.5 ± 3.2	6208 ± 1192	10.5 ± 3.3
Lactose	84 ± 204	22.9 ± 6.7	1128 ± 662	21.7 ± 6.1	5 ± 1.0	—
Mannose	1176 ± 411	21.1 ± 40.3	4970 ± 2270	16.9 ± 26.4	4096 ± 658	24.2 ± 8.1
Melibiose	1840 ± 208	4.4 ± 3.7	1243 ± 474	124.5 ± 22.6	512 ± 76	8.0 ± 4.0
Sorbitol	77 ± 179	20.5 ± 3.4	1389 ± 307	91.7 ± 18.6	8 ± 1.2	—
Xylose	328 ± 217	2.8 ± 1.3	1024 ± 941	21.4 ± 5.4	5404 ± 2211	21.1 ± 9.2

Note: Pili or LTB were administered after mixing with either 20 μg of vitamin, or 25 μmol of sugar.

[a] See Figure 1.

[b] Each value is the mean antibody titer of 15 mice $\pm$ 1 SD.[25]

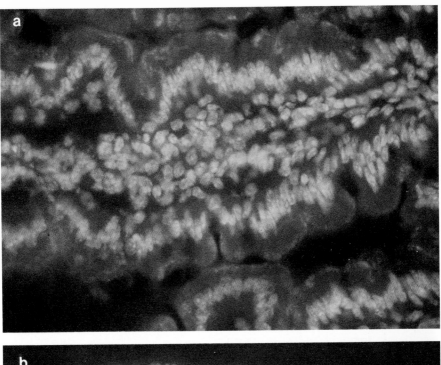

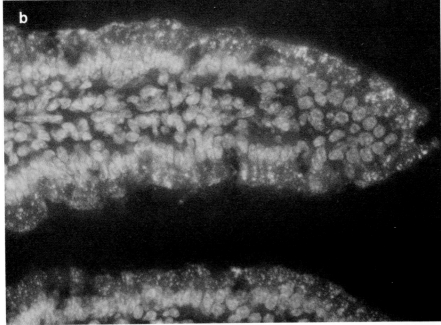

PLATE 1. Histological localization of the site of uptake of the lectin-like molecule, LTB. Mice were fed FITC-labeled LTB in saline and were sacrificed after 30 (1a, 1c) and 120 (1b, 1d) min. The small intestines were removed and sectioned for microscopy. Specificity of uptake was shown by feeding FITC-labeled LTB preincubated with GM1 ganglioside. Controls were fed FITC-BSA (not shown). (1a) Villous cells, 30 min; (1b) villous cells, 120 min; (1c) lymphoid follicles, 30 min; (1d) lymphoid follicles 120 min.[60,64]

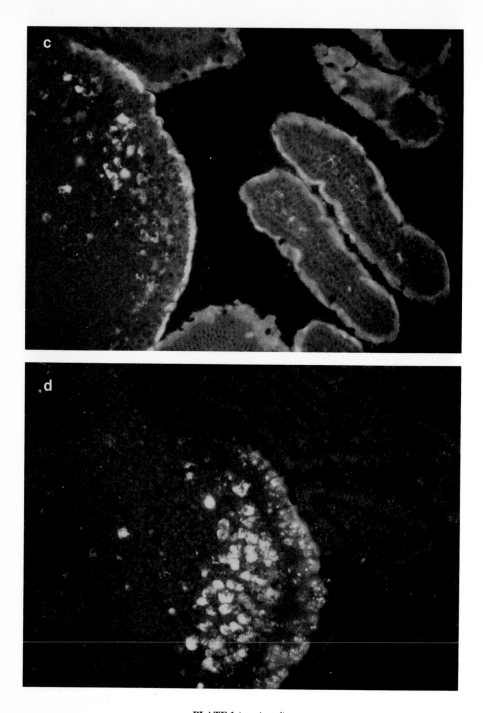

PLATE 1 *(continued).*

D, fructose, mannose, and xylose; but little or no change with vitamin B_1 or vitamin B_{12}; a slight reduction with vitamin C, vitamin E, or melibiose; and almost complete inhibition with vitamin B_6, lactose, and sorbitol. These results are broadly suggestive that K99 and 987P pili and LTB bind to and are internalized by discrete cells of the microvillous epithelium, which express surface ligands specific for each LLM, and which have different absorptive activities.

One possible explanation for the alteration in the immune response seen when mucosal immunogens were cofed with sugars and vitamins was that the mice may have been suffering from a dietary deficiency of the fed substance, or that some of the sugars or vitamins may have been toxic at high doses. When, however, the lectins were injected IM with the sugar or vitamin, there was no change in the immune response in comparison to the lectin injected alone (results not shown). Thus the reason for the change in response due to cofeeding of these molecules with the mucosal immunogens must be due to some event on or near the site of absorption of these molecules rather than by direct interaction with the immune system.

There is a change in the absorptive role of cells from the proximal to distal region of the small intestine. Thus the uptake of fats, vitamins and xylose occurs in the proximal region of the intestine; the uptake of sugars and amino acids occurs lower in the jejunum; while the uptake of bile salts and vitamin B_{12} occurs in the more distal ileum.[47,48] This change in role of the absorptive cells is accompanied by a related change in the various glycolipids which make up the membranes of these cells as well as the membrane-bound glycoproteins, exposed on the lumenal epithelium, which comprise the receptors and enzymes responsible for processing and uptake of the various sugars, vitamins, amino acids, and fats taken up by these cells.[49-52] It is this change in the distribution of the various glycolipids and glycoproteins which will determine where individual lectins or LLMs will bind. Thus different LLMs, which are known to bind to different glycoproteins and glycolipids, will adhere to and be internalized by different villous epithelial cells as they move down the length of the gastrointestinal tract.[50,53-56] The extent to which a particular immunogen interacts with any one cell will depend on the relative number and distribution of the specific ligands on that cell. It is possible that the alteration in response seen when the immunogens were fed with various dietary molecules is due to a change in the receptor-mediated endocytotic activity of specific cells with different uptake potentials for the various lectins and dietary molecules.

Binding of the lectins or LLMs to these absorptive cells somehow stimulates the uptake of the LLMs (presumably by receptor-mediated endocytosis, RME) with subsequent transport of these molecules from the lumenal side of the intestine across the epithelium and into the systemic circulation. Once the LLMs have reached the circulation, they are free to interact with the immune system. Experiments of Gill and others have shown that the enterotoxins of *V. cholera* and of *E. coli* are able to promote RME simply by binding to a number of cell types.[57-59] It is possible that the general mechanism which triggers RME of cholera toxin will also occur following the binding of K99 and 987P pili.

The results depicted in Table 3 suggest that it is possible to increase the uptake of the mucosal immunogens by stimulation of the relevant cells to which they bind by coadministering specific sugars and vitamins. The change in profile of stimulatory molecules for each particular immunogen presumably reflects the variable distribution of receptors for the mucosal immunogens as well as the change in absorptive functions of the cells along the intestine. It can be predicted that the receptors for K99 pili are expressed on the cells responsible for uptake of vitamin B_{12}, vitamin D, fructose, and melibiose; those for 987P pili are on cells responsible for uptake of vitamin B_6, vitamin C, vitamin E, fructose, and mannose; while those for LTB occur on cells responsible for the uptake of vitamin A, vitamin B_2, vitamin D, mannose, and xylose.

The data presented above have two important implications for the generation of immune responses following oral feeding. First, the diet of animals receiving oral vaccination with an antigen may be an important factor in determining the type of immune response generated to the immunogen. The presence of various sugars or vitamins may enhance or completely abolish the immune response to the immunogen, especially if the immunogen is known to possess a lectin-like binding activity. For this reason, experimental animals receiving oral vaccination regimes should preferably be starved. This regime may appear to be impractical in the field; however, in many instances we have observed little difference in the immune response generated to LLMs between fed or starved animals! Second, the data suggest that it may be possible to selectively modify the immune response, both in type and magnitude, by selective coadministration of certain sugars or vitamins with the immunogen. The selection of vitamins or sugars will vary from immunogen to immunogen and from species to species, since the distribution of glycolipids and glycoproteins is known to vary both between organs within a species and from one animal species to another.

E. BIOADHESION TO THE INTESTINE BY MEANS OF SPECIFIC BINDING OF LECTINS

One of the major problems of oral drug delivery has been postulated to be the speed at which the administered drug passes through the gastrointestinal tract. This rapid transit of drugs through the major absorptive regions of the intestine, the jejunum and ileum, is a major barrier to the development of delayed or controlled release drug delivery systems for oral use. In an attempt to slow this passage through the intestine, Robinson and others have used bioadhesive polymers to increase mucin/epithelial adhesion.[60,61,62] An alternative approach using lectins is currently being investigated by the groups of Lehr and Woodley using the tomato lectin (isolated from *Lycopersicum esculentum*).

Lehr and co-workers have found that tomato lectin binds specifically to cultured monolayers of the human colon carcinoma line Caco-2, as well as to isolated fixed pig enterocytes.[63] When the tomato lectin was passively absorbed to 0.98 μm fluorescently labeled polystyrene microspheres, the spheres could be shown to bind to isolated pig enterocytes. Binding to the enterocytes appeared be specific as it was inhibitable by $(GluNAc)_4$. Woodley's group have been studying binding of radiolabeled lectin to everted rings of rat small intestine.[64] In comparative studies with labeled lectin, BSA, and poylvinylpyrollidone (PVP), a four- to eight-fold higher association of label was found following incubation of the intestinal rings with tomato lectin. Binding was greatly reduced in the presence of $(GluNAc)_4$. Oral administration of PVP or lectin showed little difference in intestine-associated counts, 1 or 5 h after administration to rats.

III. LECTINS AS CARRIERS FOR ORAL IMMUNIZATION

A. INTRODUCTION

In the previous sections of this chapter it has been shown that it is possible to administer orally a number of lectins or lectin-like molecules which have the ability to bind to the glycoproteins and glycolipids of the intestinal epithelium and stimulate uptake, presumably by RME, and thereby to induce significant serum IgG titers with or without a parallel rise in sIgA antibody levels. Furthermore, it was shown that the type of immune response so elicited can be tailored by the coadministration of many simple dietary molecules.

Of particular note is the finding that a number of these LLMs were capable of acting as carriers to prime for an anti-DNP response. Thus, the eight plant lectins, Concanavalin A (Con A), pokeweed mitogen (PW mitogen), and the lectins of *L. culinaris, H. pomatia, P. vulgaris, G. max, A. hypogea,* and *U. europaeus* were all able to cotransport the hapten, dinitrophenol (DNP), across the intestinal epithelium following oral administration and thereby to elicit a systemic antibody response to the conjugated hapten (Table 1). This finding suggested that the potential could exist for at least some of these LLMs to act as "carriers" for other antigens and to therefore improve the relatively poor uptake of most antigens across the intestinal epithelium.

The following study was designed to investigate whether this carrier potential of the LLPs could be extended to molecules larger than the simple hapten, DNP (mol wt 168) and to establish some of the various parameters for their successful use as a means of formulating new and more effective oral vaccines.

B. DEMONSTRATION OF THE CARRIER POTENTIAL OF LECTINS

All of the lectins and LLMs tested showed the capacity to effectively transport the co-valently attached hapten DNP across the intestinal mucosa and to elicit a serum anti-DNP antibody response after feeding of the dinitrophenylated lectin. DNP-modified BSA, how-ever was completely ineffective in eliciting an anti-DNP or anti-BSA response when fed at the concentrations tested (Table 4). K99 and 987P pili were also conjugated to BSA and tested for their ability to co-transport this molecule following oral administration to mice.

When various ratios of BSA/pili were fed to mice, it was found that BSA/pili conjugates prepared at ratios of greater than 1:20 (BSA/pilin subunits; there may be hundreds of subunits per whole pilus molecule) did not generate either anti-BSA or

Table 4 **Antibody response to DNP-modified Lectins[a]**

		Immune response			
		Anti-DNP		Anti-Carrier	
Immunogen	Dose (µg)	Serum IgG	Sec IgA	Serum IgG	Sec IgA
K99	20	<4	<4	875 + 62	3.9 + 5.1
K99	100	<4	<4	1352 + 128	16.7 + 2.3
DNP_6K99	20	21 + 10.5	<4	64 + 7.2	<4
$DNP_{18}K99$	500	1024 + 77	42 + 9.6	128 + 27.4	76 + 12.9
DNP_2K99	500	1176 + 164	28 + 14.4	3565 + 192	88 + 21
987P	20	<4	<4	891 + 76	27.8 + 13.6
987P	100	<4	<4	1024 + 89	88 + 22.4
DNP_7987P	20	24 + 3.1	<4	124 + 12.2	<4
$DNP_{26}987P$	500	1024 + 244	14 + 3.1	111 + 34.1	68 + 19.2
DNP_3987P	500	1351 + 196	7 + 1.4	2048 + 166	128 + 38.4
LTB	20	<4	<4	1351 + 211	12.2 + 4.4
LTB	100	<4	<4	891 + 56	4.0
DNP_2LTB	20	24.3 + 5.6	<4	445 + 35	<4
Con A[b]	20	666 + 84	<4	nd	nd
PW-mitogen	20	641 + 119	<4	nd	nd
L. culinaris	20	954 + 48	<4	nd	nd
H. pomatia	20	591 + 127	<4	nd	nd
P. vulgaris	20	1378 + 110	4.8 + 2.3	nd	nd
G. max	20	1529 + 65	3.1 + 6.9	nd	nd
A. hypogea	20	1276 + 242	<4	nd	nd
U. europaeus	20	1583 + 94	<4	nd	nd

[a] The reciprocal of the antiserum dilution that gave an ELISA reading of 0.5 after 45 min at 37°C. Each value represents the mean of 5 mice + 1 SD.[60]

[b] Each lectin was substituted with 4 DNP groups.[65] 987P pili can not be substituted directly with DNP using DNFB, so it was initially reacted with EDAC plus diaminoethane before reaction with DNFB.

antipili responses, even with a dose of 500 μg.[25,65] However, when ratios of 1:20 or 1:40 were employed, good responses to both BSA and to pili were observed. The magnitude of the immune response was readily varied by altering the dose of complex fed (Table 4). Thus, when LLMs were covalently linked to a hapten, DNP, or a large protein, BSA, and fed to mice, the LLMs acted as carriers for the immunogens and subsequently transported these molecules from the intestine into the circulation (as judged by the appearance of antibody-producing cells in the spleen; results not shown) and thereby stimulated a serum antibody response.

Oral presentation of BSA or other proteins mixed with, but not covalently linked to the lectins, pili, or LTB at no stage resulted in the stimulation of a systemic antibody response to the cofed immunogen (results not shown). This is in contrast to the augmentation of response seen when a number of antigens have been cofed with cholera toxin.[66,31,32,34] These authors found that an augmentation of response to a coadministered antigen could be produced by cofeeding antigen with cholera toxin. This effect is presumably due to the mucosal damage caused by the holotoxin (as evidenced by morphological changes[67]) which allows entry of the accompanying antigen into the submucosal area.

C. ORAL IMMUNIZATION AGAINST INFLUENZA VIRUS USING LTB-INFLUENZA VIRUS CONJUGATES

Following the successful demonstration that pili could be used to orally immunize against BSA conjugated to these molecules, influenza virus particles were conjugated to LTB using a two-step glutaraldehyde procedure. The conjugate preparations were fed to mice and serum IgG and bronchial IgA levels were determined.[68,69]

Oral immunization of mice with influenza virus conjugated to the lectin-like carrier, LTB, greatly enhanced the serum IgG response 20-fold above virus not conjugated to the carrier, while the bronchial IgA response to the virus was enhanced roughly 17-fold above that elicited with the virus alone (Table 6). Enhancement of immunity to the virus in the bronchus is particularly important as this is the site of initial invasion and infection. Thus, for effective protection against this virus, it is critical that high titers of antibody are elicited in bronchial secretions.

Table 5   Oral Immunization against BSA using BSA:pili conjugates

		Immune Response			
	Dose	Anti-BSA		Anticarrier	
Immunogen	(μg)[a]	Serum IgG	Sec IgA	Serum IgG	Sec IgA
K99	20	<4	<4	875 ± 62	4 ± 5
K99	100	<4	<4	1351 ± 94	17 ± 2
BSA-K99$_5$	500	<4	<4	74 ± 11	<4
BSA-K99$_{10}$	500	<4	<4	147 ± 48	<4
BSA-K99$_{20}$	500	222 ± 47	126 ± 30	3807 ± 226	84 ± 16
BSA-K99$_{40}$	500	73 ± 19	46 ± 7	3176 ± 391	64 ± 11
987P	20	<4	<4	891 ± 76	28 ± 13
987P	100	<4	<4	1024 ± 83	84 ± 26
BSA-987P$_5$	500	<4	<4	256 ± 49	<4
BSA-987P$_{10}$	500	30 ± 7	122 ± 48	675 ± 110	<4
BSA-987P$_{20}$	500	306 ± 88	110 ± 38	4263 ± 408	194 ± 39
BSA-987P$_{40}$	500	124 ± 47	<4	<4	<4
BSA	20	<4	<4	nd	nd

[a] Total weight of complex fed. Data are mean of 15 mice ± one SD.[60]

Table 6 **Oral immunization of mice with LTB-Influenza virus particles**

Treatment	Number of mice	Serum IgG	Bronchial IgA
Influenza vaccine 0.25 ml	10	0.8 ± 2.53	2.8 ± 2.08
Influenza vaccine 0.5 ml	10	6.0 ± 12.4	10.25 ± 8.8
LTB-Influenza vaccine 0.25 ml	20	17.4 ± 24.8	41.2 ± 34.4
LTB 0.25 ml	15	0.8 ± 3.1	0.03 ± 0.129
Saline	15	0.27 ± 1.03	0.07 ± 0.176

Note: Influenza particles from a commercial vaccine were glutaraldehyde conjugated to LTB and fed to mice on days 1, 2, 8, 9. Mice were bled and sacrificed and bronchial lavage was performed on day 22. Results shown represent the anti-influenza antibody results ± 1 SD.

Data were generated in collaboration with Drs. K. Bergmann and R. Waldman.[62,63]

IV. HISTOLOGICAL LOCALIZATION OF THE SITE OF UPTAKE OF THE LECTIN-LIKE MOLECULE, LTB

In order to investigate the mechanism whereby oral feeding of lectins leads to the stimulation of serum antibodies rather than to the induction of systemic tolerance, a histological investigation of the site of binding and uptake of fluorescently labeled LTB was performed.[69,70] Mice were starved overnight prior to oral administration of antigens, LTB, LTB-FITC, or LTB-TRITC (50 µg in 500 µl of 0.1 M carbonate/bicarbonate buffer pH 9.5). At various time intervals mice were sacrificed by cervical dislocation, dissected, and tissues prepared for histology.

Examination of sections of intestine obtained from mice 30 min post LTB-FITC feeding revealed intense fluorescence associated with the brush border of villous enterocytes in the duodenum and jejunum (Plate 1a*). Fluorescence was marginally stronger over the epithelial cells overlying lymphoid tissue (small lymphoid follicles or Peyer's patches) (see Plate 1c*). No fluorescence was observed in the ileum at this time. Segments of ileum sectioned 1 h after feeding showed LTB binding only to the brush border of patch-associated epithelial cells (results not shown).

Two hours after feeding, the pattern of fluorescence of the epithelial cells of the villous had changed and much of the fluorescence now appeared to have been internalized within the cells and could be discerned as discrete intracellular patches (Plate 1b*). Material in the lymphoid follicles also seems to have been internalized; however, the fluorescence intensity in this region was much greater than that of the villous epithelial cells (Plate 1d*).

Mice were also fed unlabeled LTB and the pattern of binding to the villous epithelium was visualized using indirect immunofluorescence. In this technique, sections were incubated with rabbit anti-LTB antibody followed by fluorescence enhancement using FITC-conjugated anti-rabbit serum. An identical pattern of binding was observed to that seen when the mice were fed LTB-FITC, thus indicating that the fluorochrome had not altered the pattern of binding of the LTB molecule (results not shown).

Binding of LTB-FITC to epithelium could be shown to be a specific receptor-mediated phenomenon because preincubation of LTB-FITC with GM1-ganglioside completely abolished binding to the intestinal epithelium. Similarly, when tissue sections were overlaid with LTB-FITC:GM1 no binding was apparent (results not shown). Binding was not demonstrable after feeding of similar quantities of BSA-FITC.

The pattern of fluorescence found after feeding fluorescently-labeled LTB suggested that LTB, which enters the circulation following oral administration, does so by binding to the cells of the villous epithelium, followed by internalization within these cells and subsequent transcytosis. It must be noted that at no time was any evidence of mucosal damage seen following the feeding of the LTB-FITC. This is in contrast to the known

---

* Plates 1a-d appear following page 230.

mucosal damage seen following oral administration of the intact holotoxin, or cholera toxin. In contrast to the binding to the villus epithelial cells, the binding and internalization of the LTB into the cells overlying the lymphoid follicles is more reminiscent of the mode of entry postulated for most soluble antigens. It must be noted, however, that at no time was any fluorescence found associated with either the villus epithelial cells or the cells overlying the lymphoid follicles following oral administration of similar doses of FITC-BSA conjugates.

V. ORAL IMMUNIZATION OF PRIMATES

Previous studies investigating the potential for oral immunization with lectins concentrated on work in rodents. It was of some interest to determine whether the same immunity could be evoked by feeding these molecules to primates. Adult squirrel monkeys *(Saimiri sciureus)* were fed twice with LTB. Control animals received either LTB injected IM in saline, or LTB complexed with alhydrogel and injected IM. Negative controls received oral doses of LTB premixed with GM1-ganglioside. As can be seen from Figure 1, oral administration of three 500-µg doses of LTB stimulated a serum antibody response which was greater than that seen by the IM administration of two 200-µg doses of the antigen in saline. Addition of the GM1-ganglioside to the LTB prior to feeding abolished the generation of the antibody response. This suggests the possibility of using the LLMs as carriers not only for use in rodents, but also for use in primates and ultimately humans.

VI. SUMMARY

Lectins and the lectin-like molecules, such as pili, toxin-binding subunits, and viral hemagglutinins share a unique property of being able to bind specifically to the sugar

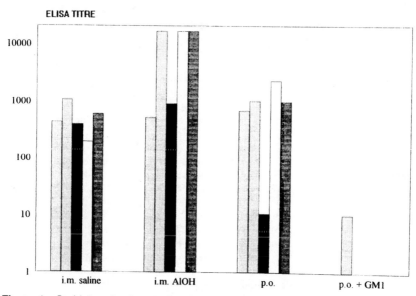

Figure 1 Oral immunization of primates with LTB. Monkeys were immunized with LTB IM in saline (2 doses of 200 µg); IM in Alhydrogel (2 doses of 200 µg); PO in carbonate buffer pH 9.5 (3 doses of 500 µg) or LTB premixed with GM1 ganglioside PO (3 doses of 500 µg LTB + 1 mg ganglioside). Anti-LTB, ELISA titers are shown for individual monkeys.

moieties present on glycolipids and glycoproteins located on the surface of many intestinal epithelial cells. In many instances, the binding of these molecules to these surface glycolipids or glycoproteins results in the internalization and transcellular transport of the molecules from the luminal to the basal side of the villus epithelium. This in turn results in the presentation of these molecules to the immunocompetent cells underlying the villus epithelium or the dome of the Peyer's patches, with a concomitant generation of an immune response. Uptake of these molecules is a specific receptor-mediated phenomenon which can be inhibited by cofeeding molecules with similar structures to the sugar moieties to which the lectins bind. Histological examination of the site of uptake of one of these molecules, LTB, has revealed that the molecule is able to bind not only to the surface of the intestinal lymphoid follicles, but also to epithelial cells overlying the tips and fingers of the villus. Once bound, the LTB is rapidly internalized and can be seen to undergo almost complete transcellular transport across villus epithelial cells within 2 h of feeding. Material which binds to the surface of lymphoid follicles and Peyer's patches appears to be internalized at a much slower rate and can still be found associated with the follicles 6 h after administration. Feeding of haptens or proteins covalently linked to the lectins or lectin-like molecules also results in the cotransportation of the attached molecules across the villus epithelium and subsequent generation of an immune response. Small haptens such as DNP, proteins, and even virus particles have been successfully linked to these molecules and have been shown to elicit serum antibody responses following oral feeding. Studies have been extended to primates, where it has been shown that LTB given orally stimulated a serum antibody response which was comparable to the intramuscular presentation of this antigen. The uptake of the antigen was blocked by coadministration of the GM1 ganglioside to which the LTB binds. Lectins and lectin-like molecules thus represent a unique set of proteins which are able to overcome the almost impermeable barrier which the intestinal epithelium presents to the uptake of large molecular weight molecules. Through a process of RME these molecules are able to cross this mucosal barrier and present themselves, as well as other molecules attached to them, to the underlying immunocompetent cells, thereby eliciting strong immune priming following oral administration.

REFERENCES

1. Rothberg, R. M., Kraft, S. C., and Michalek, S. M., Systemic immunity after local antigenic stimulation of the lymphoid tissue of the gastrointestinal tract, *J. Immunol.*, 111, 1906, 1973.
2. Ngan, J. and Kind, L. S., Suppressor T cells for IgE and IgG in Peyer's patches of mice made tolerant by the oral administration of ovalbumin, *J. Immunol.*, 120, 861, 1978.
3. Richman, L. K., Chiller, J. M., Brown, W. R., Hanson, D. G., and Vaz, N. M., Enterically induced immunological tolerance, *J. Immunol.*, 121, 2429, 1978
4. Hanson, D. G., Vaz, N. M., Maia, L. C. S., and Lynch, J. M., Inhibition of specific immune responses by feeding protein antigens, *J. Immunol.*, 123, 2337, 1979.
5. Tomasi, T. B., Oral tolerance, *Transplantation*, 29, 353, 1980.
6. Mowat, A. McI. and Parrot, D. M. V., Immunological responses to fed protein antigens in mice, *Immunology*, 50, 547, 1983.
7. Mowat, A. McI., The role of antigen recognition and suppressor cells in mice with oral tolerance to ovalbumin, *Immunology*, 56, 253, 1985.
8. Bland. P. W. and Warren L. G., Antigen presentation by epithelial cells of the rat small intestine. I Kinetics, antigen specificity and blocking by anti-Ia antisera, *Immunology*, 58, 1, 1986.
9. Bland, P. W. and Warren L. G., Antigen presentation by epithelial calls of the rat small intestine. II Selective induction of suppressor T cells, *Immunology*, 58, 9, 1986.

10. Richman, L. K., Graeff, A. S., and Strober, W., Antigen presentation by macrophage enriched cells from the mouse Peyer's patch, *Cell Immunol.*, 62, 1100, 1981.
11. Richman, L. K., Graeff, A. S., Yarchoan, R., and Strober, W., Simultaneous induction of antigen-specific IgA helper T cells and IgG suppressor T cells in the murine Peyer's patch after protein feeding, *J. Immunol.*, 126, 2079, 1981.
12. Neutra, M. R., Guerina, N. G., Hall, T. L. and Nicholson, G. L. Transport of membrane bound macromolecules by M cells in rabbit intestine, *Gastroenterology*, 82, 1137, 1982.
13. Bland, P. W. and Britton, D. C., Morphological study of antigen-sampling structures in the rat large intestine, *Infect. Immun.*, 43, 693, 1984.
14. Bass, D. M., Trier, J. S., Dambrauskas, T., and Wolf, J. L., Reovirus type 1 infection of small intestinal epithelium in suckling mice and its effect on M cells, *Lab. Invest.*, 66, 226, 1988.
15. Wolf, J. L., Rubin, D. H., Finberg, R., Kauffman, R. S., Sharpe, A. H., Trier, J. S., and Fields, B. N., Intestinal M cells: a pathway for entry of reovirus into the host, *Science*, 212, 471, 1981.
16. Gonatas, N. K., Kim, S. U., Stieber, A., and Avameas, S., Internalization of lectins in neuronal GERL, *J. Cell. Biol.*, 73, 1, 1977.
17. Helenius, A., Kartenbeck, J., Simons, K., and Fries, E., On entry of Semliki Forest virus into BHK-21 cells, *J. Cell. Biol.*, 84, 404, 1980.
18. Holmgren, J., Svennerholm, L., Elwing, H., Fredman, P. F., and Strannegard, O., Sendai virus receptor: proposed recognition structure based on binding to plastic-adsorbed gangliosides, *Proc. Natl. Acad. Sci.*, 77, 1947, 1980.
19. Carroll, S. M., Higa H. H., and Paulson J. C., Different cell-surface receptor determinants of antigenically similar influenza virus haemagglutinins, *J. Biol. Chem.*, 256, 8357, 1981.
20. Pappenheimer, A. M., Jr., Diptheria toxin, *Annu. Rev. Biochem.*, 46, 69, 1977.
21. Hu, V. W. and Holmes, R. K., Evidence for direct insertion of fragments A and B of diptheria toxin into model membranes, *J. Biol. Chem.*, 259, 12226, 1984.
22. Zalman, L. S. and Wisnieski, B. J., Mechanism of insertion of diptheria toxin: peptide entry and pore size determinations, *Proc. Natl. Acad. Sci. U.S.A.*, 81, 3341, 1984.
23. Leppla, S. H., Dorland, R. B., and Middlebrook, J. L., Inhibition of diptheria toxin degradation and cytotoxic action by chloroquine, *J. Biol. Chem.*, 255, 2247, 1980.
24. Aizpurua, H. J. de and Russell-Jones, G. J., Oral vaccination: identification of classes of protein which provoke an immune response upon oral feeding, *J. Exp. Med.*, 167, 440, 1987.
25. Russell-Jones, G. J. and Aizpurua, H. J. de, Mucosal immunogens, in *Recent Advances in Mucosal Immunology*, Vol. 216B, Mestecky, J., McGhee, J. R., Bienenstock, J., and Ogra, P. L., Eds., Plenum Publishing, New York, 1987, 1791.
26. Gibbons, R. A., Jones, G. W., and Sellwood, R., An attempt to identify the intestinal receptor for the K88 adhesin by means of a haemmagglutination inhibition test using glycoproteins and fractions from sow colostrum, *J. Gen. Microbiol.*, 86, 228, 1975.
27. Svennerholm, A.-M. and Holmgren, J., Identification of *Escherichia coli* heat-labile enterotoxin by means of a ganglioside immunosorbent assay (GM1-ELISA) procedure, *Curr. Microbiol.*, 1, 19, 1978.
28. Holmgren, J., Fredman, P., Lindblad, M., Svennerholm, A.-M., and Svennerholm, L., Rabbit intestinal glycoprotein receptor for *Escherichia coli* heat-labile enterotoxin lacking affinity for cholera toxin, *Infect. Immun.*, 38, 424, 1982.
29. Czerkinsky, C. C. and Svennerholm, A.-M., Ganglioside GM1 enzyme-linked immunospot assay for simple identification of heat-labile enterotoxin-producing *Escherichia coli*, *J. Clin. Microbiol.*, 17, 965, 1983.

30. Gaastra, W. and de Graaf, F. K., Host specific fimbrial adhesion of noninvasive enterotoxigenic *Escherichia coli* strains, *Microbiol. Rev.*, 46, 129, 1982.
31. Elson, C. O. and Ealding, W., Generalized systemic and mucosal immunity in mice after mucosal stimulation with cholera toxin, *J. Immunol.*, 132, 2736, 1984.
32. Elson, C. O. and Ealding, W., Cholera toxin did not induce oral tolerance in mice and abrogated oral tolerance to an unrelated antigen, *J. Immunol.*, 133, 2892, 1984.
33. Fujita, K. and Finkelstein, R. A., Antitoxic immunity in experimental cholera, *J. Infect. Dis.*, 125, 647, 1972.
34. Pierce, N. F. and Koster, F. T., Priming and suppression of the intestinal immune response to cholera toxoid/toxin by parenteral toxoid in rats, *J. Immunol.*, 124, 307, 1980.
35. Holmgren, J., Comparison of the tissue receptors for *Vibrio cholera* and *Escherichia coli* enterotoxins by means of gangliosides and natural cholera toxoid, *Infect. Immun.*, 8, 851, 1973.
36. Holmgren, J., Actions of cholera toxin and the prevention of treatment of cholera, *Nature*, 292, 413, 1981.
37. Hyun, C. S. and Kimmich G. A., Interaction of cholera toxin and *Escherichia coli* enterotoxin with isolated intestinal epithelial cells, *Am. J. Physiol.*, 193, G623, 1984.
38. Pierce, N. F., Cray, W. C., and Sacci, J. B., Oral immunization of dogs with purified cholera toxin, crude toxin, or B subunit: evidence for synergistic protection by antitoxic and antibacterial mechanisms, *Infect. Immun.*, 37, 687, 1982.
39. Ludwig, D. S., Holmes, R. K., and Schoolnik, G. K., Chemical and immunochemical studies on the receptor binding domain of cholera toxin B subunit, *J. Biol. Chem.*, 260, 12528, 1985.
40. Delfini, C., Sargiacomo, M., Amici, C., Oberholtzer, G., and Tomasi, M., Cholera toxin B-subunit protects mammalian cells from ricin and abrin toxicity, *J. Cell. Biochem.*, 20, 359, 1982.
41. Dominguez, P., Barros, F., and Lazo, P. S., The activation of adenylate cyclase from small intestinal epithelium by cholera toxin, *Eur. J. Biochem.*, 146, 533, 1985.
42. Beh, K. J., Antibody containing cell response in lymph of sheep after intra-intestinal of ovalbumin with and without DEAE-dextran, *Immunology*, 37, 279, 1972.
43. Lodinova, R. and Jouja, V., Influence of oral lysozyme administration on serum immunoglobulin and intestinal secretory IgA levels in infants, *Acta Paediatr. Scand.*, 66, 709, 1977.
44. Namba, Y., Hidaka, Y., Taki, K., and Moritomo, T., Effect of oral administration of lysozyme or digested bacterial cell walls on immunostimulation in guinea pigs, *Infect. Immun.*, 31, 580, 1981.
45. Falchuk, K. R., Walker, W. A., Perrotto, J. L., and Isselbacher, K. J., Effect of vitamin A on the systemic and local immune responses to intragastrically administered bovine serum albumin, *Infect. Immun.*, 17, 361, 1977.
46. Dingle, J. T., Studies on the mode of action of excess vitamin A. Release of a bound protease by the action of vitamin A, *Biochem. J.*, 79, 509, 1961.
47. Keele, C. A. and Neil, E., Samson Wright's Applied Physiology Oxford Medical Publications, 10th ed., 1961.
48. Borgstrom, B., Dahlquist, A., Lundh, G., and Sjovall, J., *J. Clin. Invest.*, 26, 1521, 1957.
49. Evans, L., Grasset, E., Heyman, M., Dumontier, A. M., Beau, J. P., and Dejeux, J. F., Congenital selective malabsorption of glucose and galactose, *J. Paediatr. Gastroenterol. Nutr.*, 4, 878, 1985.
50. Dobbins, J. W., Laurenson, J. P., Gorelick, F. S., and Banwell, J. G., Phytohaemagglutinin from red kidney bean *(Phaseolus vulgaris)* inhibits sodium and chloride absorption in the rabbit ileum, *Gastroenterology*, 90, 1907, 1986.

51. Noone, C., Menzies, I. S., Banatvala, J. E., and Scopes, J. W., Intestinal permeability and lactose hydrolysis in human rota viral gastroenteritis assessed simultaneously by noninvasive differential sugar permeation, *Eur. J. Clin. Invest.*, 16, 217, 1986.

52. Davies, S., Maenz, D. D., and Cheeseman, C. I., A novel imino-acid carrier in the enterocyte basolateral membrane, *Biochim. Biophys. Acta*, 896, 247, 1987.

53. Bouhours, J. F. and Glickman, R. M., *Biochim. Biophys. Acta*, 441, 123, 1969.

54. Glickman, R. M. and Bouhours, J. F., Characterization, distribution and biosynthesis of major gangliosides of rat intestinal-mucosa, *Biochim. Biophys. Acta*, 424, 17, 1976.

55. McKibbin, J. M., Fucolipids, *J. Lipid Res.*, 19, 131, 1978.

56. Hakomori, S.-I., Glycosphingolipids in cellular interaction differentiation, and oncogenesis, *Annu. Rev. Biochem.*, 50, 773, 1981.

57. Gill, D. M., Mechanism of action of cholera toxin, *Adv. Cyclic Nucl. Res.*, 8, 85, 1977.

58. Stavric, S., Spiers, J. I., Konowalchuk, J., and Jeffrey, D., Stimulation of cyclic AMP secretion in vero cells by enterotoxins of *Escherichia coli* and *Vibrio cholera*, *Infect. Immun.*, 21, 514, 1978.

59. Joseph, K. C., Stieber, A., and Gonatas, N. K., Endocytosis of cholera toxin in GERL-like structures of murine neuroblastoma cells pretreated with GM1 ganglioside, *J. Cell. Biol.*, 81, 543, 1979.

60. Park, K. and Robinson, J. R., Bioadhesive polymers as platforms for oral-controlled drug delivery: method to study bioadhesion, *Int. J. Pharm.*, 19, 107, 1984.

61. Park, K. and Robinson, J. R., Physico-chemical properties of water insoluble polymers important to mucin/epithelial adhesion, *J. Controlled Rel.*, 2, 47, 1985.

62. Longer, M. A., Ch'hn, H. S., and Robinson, J. R., Bioadhesive polymers as platforms for oral controlled drug delivery. III. Oral delivery of Chlorothiazide using a bioadhesive polymer, *J. Pharm. Sci.*, 74, 406, 1985.

63. Lehr, D.-M., Bouwstra, J. A., Kok, W., Noach, A. B. J., Boer, A. G. de, and Junginger, H. E., Bioadhesion by means of specific binding of tomato lectin, *Pharm. Res.*, 9, 547, 1992.

64. Woodley, J. F. and Naisbett, B., The potential of lectins for delaying the intestinal transit of drugs, *Proc. Int. Symp. Controlled Rel. Bioact. Mater.*, 15, 125, 1988.

65. Russell-Jones, G. J., Lindner, J., and Aizpurua, H. J. de, The use of lectins as carriers for oral delivery, *Proc. Int. Symp. Controlled Rel. Bioact. Mater.*, 19, 40, 1992.

66. Lycke, N. and Holmgren, J., Strong adjuvant properties of cholera toxin on gut mucosal immune responses to orally presented antigens, *Immunology*, 59, 301, 1986.

67. Stavric, S., Speirs, J. I., Konowalchuk, J., and Jefrey, D., Stimulation of cyclic AMP secretion in vero cells by enterotoxins of *Escherichia coli* and *Vibrio cholerae*, *Infect. Immun.*, 21, 514, 1978.

68. Bergmann, K.-C., Waldman, R. H., Bicak, M., and Russell-Jones, G. J., Adjuvant effect of B-subunit of *E. coli* heat-labile toxin on secretory antibody response to oral influenza virus immunization in mice, *Allergologie*, 12, 294, 1989.

69. Bergmann, K.-C., Russell-Jones, G. J., and Waldman, R. H., B subunit of *E. coli* heat-labile enterotoxin enhances secretory IgA antibody response to oral Influenza virus immunization i.m mice, *Schweiz. Med. Wochenschr.*, 121, Suppl. 40/II, 28, 1991.

70. Lindner, J. and Russell-Jones, G. J., Uptake of orally administered LTB by the cells of the Peyer's patch and the mucosal epithelium, *Proc. Aust. Soc. Immunol.*, 168, 1990.

71. Little, J. R. and Eisen, H. N., Preparation of immunogenic 2,4-dinitrophenyl and 2,4,6-trinitrophenyl proteins, in *Methods Immunol. Immunochem.*, 1, 128, 1967.

Chapter 5

Liposomes

Noel K. Childers and Suzanne M. Michalek

TABLE OF CONTENTS

I. INTRODUCTION

Since the discovery by Bangham and co-workers[1,2] that the addition of water to a flask containing a film of naturally occurring phospholipids resulted in the appearance of microscopic closed vesicles, termed liposomes, these vesicles have been studied for their use in targeted delivery of drugs, and more recently, as vaccine delivery systems via the systemic and mucosal routes. This chapter will concentrate on studies using liposomes for delivery of antigen to lymphoid tissues involved in the induction of mucosal immune responses, and on the effectiveness of these responses in protection against infection by mucosal pathogens. Systemic processing of liposomes and methods to target the delivery of liposomes to appropriate systemic or mucosal sites will also be presented.

Liposomes have a number of characteristics which make them acceptable as vaccine delivery systems (Table 1). Liposomes can act as immunoadjuvants and potentiate immune responses to incorporated antigens. Therefore, smaller amounts of antigen are needed to induce an immune response when the antigen is incorporated into liposomes than when given alone. Liposomes can convert nonimmunogenic substances into immunogenic forms, e.g., by rendering soluble substances particulate in nature, making them more effective mucosal vaccines. A variety of substances can be incorporated into liposomes, including multiple antigens, adjuvants, and substances for targeted delivery via cell surface receptors, e.g., cell surface lectins, cytokines, or antibodies to cell surface antigens. Liposomes are taken up by macrophages and by M cells (i.e., specialized epithelial cells covering Peyer's patches[3,4]) for antigen processing and/or presentation to other lymphoid cells for the induction of immune responses. Liposomes are composed of naturally occurring substances (e.g., phospholipids) which make up host cell membranes and, therefore, they represent nontoxic, safe, and efficacious vaccine delivery vehicles for use in animals, including humans. For additional information on liposomes as antigen carriers and immunoadjuvants, the reader is referred to recent reviews by others.[5-16]

0-8493-4866-8/94/$0.00+$.50
© 1994 by CRC Press Inc.

Table 1   Liposomes: a delivery system and immunoadjuvant

1. Small amounts of antigen are effective immunogens when given in liposomes.
2. Substances which are nonimmunogenic in their free or purified forms can be made to be immunogenic by incorporation inside or within the phospholipid membrane of liposomes.
3. Targeting agents and adjuvants can be incorporated into the membrane of liposomes containing antigens to direct their delivery to specific host cells and to potentiate responses to the antigen.
4. Liposomes are taken up by macrophages in tissues and by M cells covering the Peyer's patches for the induction of responses; these vesicles can also substitute for antigen-presenting cells.
5. Liposomes are biodegradable and can be composed of naturally occurring phospholipids which can be safely administered by either the oral or systemic routes for the induction of antibody responses to the incorporated antigen in external secretions or serum, respectively.

II. PROPERTIES OF LIPOSOMES

Liposomes consist of a bilayered (bimolecular sheet) phospholipid membrane (lamella) surrounded by and enclosing an aqueous solution (Figure 1). Vesicles form spontaneously due to the amphipathic nature of the phospholipid molecules used for their preparation. The hydrophilic (water-soluble or polar head) portion of the phospholipids orients towards the aqueous phases, whereas the hydrophobic (water-insoluble) tail points into the bilayer. Thus, in preparing liposome vaccines, water-soluble substances can be incorporated into the enclosed aqueous space, whereas lipid-soluble molecules can be added to the solvent during vesicle formation and incorporated into the lipid bilayer. Water-soluble substances can be covalently linked to lipid-soluble molecules for membrane association which may more effectively direct the delivery of test substances to host cells. The location of the substance inside or on the liposome membrane can alter both the manner in which a liposome vaccine will be recognized and processed by host cells, as well as the antibody isotype of the response induced. Almost any substance can be incorporated into liposomes; however, the solubility, size, shape, or electric charge of a substance affects its location inside or within the membrane or may interfere with vesicle formation. It is also important to ensure that the test substance has not lost its biologic activity once incorporated into liposomes. For example, it has been shown that certain substances such as the B subunit of cholera toxin (CTB) can lose its ability to bind to GM1 ganglioside when incorporated into liposomes (unpublished results of the authors). The loss of binding activity may be due to encapsulation of the CTB or to the procedures used to form the vesicles. In another study, it was shown that by incorporating influenza hemagglutinin into the lipid bilayer of liposomes, the functional and immunogenic activities were largely maintained, while the adjuvant property was enhanced.[17] Despite the current extensive information, studies still need to be done to determine the effectiveness of liposome delivery systems

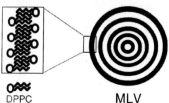

DPPC   MLV

Figure 1 Schematic depiction of the multilamellar vesicle (MLV) characterized by several lipid bilayers composed of dipalmitoyl phosphatidylcholine (DPPC) separated by thin aqueous phases.

for inducing desired host responses based on the nature of the antigen or adjuvant and on their location inside or within the vesicle membrane.

A. COMPOSITION AND SIZE

Depending on conditions used for production, liposomes can vary in size and form. The size of liposomes can range from 0.01 microns[18] to 150 microns.[19] Two standard forms of liposomes can be generated, either multilamellar (Figure 1) or unilamellar vesicles. Multilamellar vesicles (MLV) usually have more than five concentric lipid bilayers (lamellae) separated by thin aqueous phases, whereas unilamellar vesicles (UV) have a single bilayer membrane surrounding an aqueous core and are characterized as being either small (SUV) or large (LUV). Liposomes can vary in their membrane stability, fluidity, and permeability, depending on their lipid content (e.g., ratio of phospholipid to cholesterol). The incorporation of charged amphiphiles renders the liposomal surface positively or negatively charged (e.g., stearylamine or dicetylphosphate, respectively). Each of these properties potentially influences how effective a liposome preparation will be as a delivery system. Therefore, for the use of liposomes as vaccine delivery systems, it is critical to produce well-defined and homogeneous vesicle preparations to ensure reproducibility of results in order to establish the nature of the response induced with the vaccine.

In deciding on the composition of liposomes, it is important to point out that there is a considerable amount of information suggesting that phospholipids, as well as cholesterol, can be immunogenic (reviewed in References 20 and 21). In addition to the presence of naturally occurring antibodies to liposomal phospholipids in normal human or animal serum, both polyclonal and monoclonal antibodies to liposomes have been generated. Antibodies to various liposomal lipids including phosphatidylcholine[22] have been induced, and it has been shown that considerable cross-reactivity of antibodies to one type of phospholipid can be seen with other closely related phospholipids. Under normal conditions, these antibodies do not bind to host cell phospholipids due to the presence of cell surface proteins. It has also been shown that antiliposomal phosphatidylcholine antibodies differ from the antiphosphatidylcholine autoantibodies in lacking the choline-binding properties seen with the latter antibodies.[23] Thus, existing data support the safety of liposomes for use in vaccine development, especially considering the small doses and the oral route by which it would be given.

B. PREPARATION OF LIPOSOMES

Several methods for producing liposomes have been described and reviewed.[11,19,24,25] One commonly used method involves sonication of the aqueous phospholipid suspension. These liposomes are somewhat heterogeneous in size and form. However, to produce liposomes for vaccine delivery, it is necessary to use techniques which reproducibly generate liposome preparations of controlled size and composition and with good encapsulation efficiency and stability. Sonication followed by microemulsification of liposome suspensions is a technique which reproducibly results in homogeneous SUV which have an encapsulation efficiency as high as 74%, depending on the physical characteristics of the substance being incorporated.[26] Microemulsification involves the production of liposomes in a high pressure chamber of an apparatus termed a microemulsifier (Microfluidizer™, Medicontrol Inc., Newton, MA). In the chamber, an aqueous lipid suspension will form high-energy liquid sheets that interact to form small unilamellar liposomes. By controlling the pressure and cycling time, large quantities of liposomes of the desired diameter can be produced.[26,27] This method has been used to generate liposomes containing antigens, especially mutans streptococcal antigens, for use as oral vaccines (see below) and has been recently reviewed.[10,28] Homogeneous liposomes can also be produced by dialysis of detergent from phospholipid-detergent mixtures,[17,29] column chromatography,[30] ultracentrifugation,[31] or membrane extrusion.[32,33] A recently developed method involves the generation of dehydrated-rehydrated vesicles (DRV) (reviewed in Reference 9). This procedure has been shown to result in a reproducible high yield entrapment (~80% of starting material) of various substances, such as tetanus toxoid, influenza virus subunit peptides, recombinant hepatitis B surface antigen, *Leishmania major* antigens, and poliovirus. The liposomes formed are large MLV, which may be too large for cellular uptake and processing. However, it has been shown that microemulsification of these DRV results in homogeneous small (~200 nm) vesicles that retain about 60% of the original starting material,[34] and thus may be of practical use for vaccine delivery. Our group has recently shown the effectiveness of dehydrated liposomes for use as oral vaccines.[35] SUL containing antigen and trehalose (a cryoprotectant)[36,37] are prepared by sonication and microemulsification. These liposomes are then frozen and lyophilized and form SUL once rehydrated. Preliminary experiments indicate a doubling of antigen content following dehydration (our unpublished data). Freeze-drying also adds to the stability (i.e., shelf-life) of liposome preparations by preventing antigen leakage from vesicles as well as preserving membrane lipids and antigens from degradation which occurs with aqueous liposome suspensions.[36] Thus, dehydrated liposomal-antigen-adjuvant preparations should prove to be a practical approach for preparing liposome vaccines for oral use, since dehydrated preparations can be easily packaged into gelatin capsules and stored. Once enteric-coated capsules reach the intestinal tract, they will dissolve, and the liposomes will be released and rehydrated for uptake and induction of immune responses. Although this liposome vaccine may be an effective way to deliver liposomes to the Peyer's patches for the induction of mucosal immune responses, a direct comparison of the various liposome preparations for their ability to induce protective immune responses remains to be tested.

III. PROCESSING OF LIPOSOME VACCINES

A. SYSTEMIC UPTAKE AND PROCESSING

Several explanations have been proposed by which liposomes can be effective vehicles for delivery of antigens and adjuvants for the induction and augmentation of immune responses (reviewed in References 5, 9, 13, 15, and 38). Liposomes, regardless of their composition and size, can adsorb to most mammalian cells. This adsorption will result in the release of associated substances and may be useful for targeted drug delivery. Liposomes are naturally taken up by macrophages and other phagocytic cells in the blood, lymph, and various tissues (e.g., lymph nodes, liver, and spleen), and their intracellular breakdown results in the release and processing of incorporated substances. Liposomes given by the intravenous route are mainly taken up by the liver and spleen, whereas liposomes injected via the subcutaneous or intramuscular route are retained at the site of injection and are taken up by infiltrating macrophages. Evidence has accumulated which suggests that the phagocytosis of liposomes by macrophages is of central importance in their adjuvant effect (reviewed in References 5, 9, and 39). However, it has also been suggested that liposome processing by B cells or dendritic cells results in the presentation of liposomal surface antigens to a T cell subset which differs from the subset involved in macrophage presentation (reviewed in Reference 39). The immunoadjuvant property of liposomes may relate to the ability of antigen-presenting cells to more efficiently take up and process antigens associated with liposomes. The interactions between liposomes and host cells may involve the exchange of lipids or lectins with cell membranes. The adsorption or binding of liposomes to cells can result in their internalization via endocytosis or phagocytosis or their fusion with cell membranes (reviewed in References 5 and 15). However, the mechanism(s) by which liposomes present antigen to host cells for the induction of immune responses and the composition, dose, and method for administration of liposomes for potentiating the optimal desired response require further investigation.

B. MUCOSAL UPTAKE AND PROCESSING

Although the fate of liposomes given orally remains controversial, vesicles composed of cholesterol and certain phospholipids are resistant to damage by bile salts,[40,41] and those resistant to detergents and phospholipases are also resistant to enzymes in the gastrointestinal tract (reviewed in Reference 9). In studies using the rat as an experimental model,[38] we have shown that liposomes, injected into the lumen of ligated segments of the intestine, are taken up by M cells present in the epithelium covering the Peyer's patches. Evidence was obtained, using thin sections for transmission electron microscopy, that liposomes were taken up in endosomes of M cells and appeared to transverse the cell, moving towards the underlying lymphoid cells. Although the mechanism by which liposome-associated antigen is processed and presented to lymphoid cells in Peyer's patches has not been elucidated, the results of this study provided evidence for the induction of a mucosal immune response as manifested by the appearance of IgA antibodies in external secretions (see below). Nevertheless, further studies are required to determine the composition and size of liposomes which are most effective in inducing mucosal responses.

IV. MUCOSAL LIPOSOME VACCINES

The development of liposome applications in vaccine delivery systems has been concurrent with progress in the development of oral immunization strategies. Because of problems encountered in obtaining optimal immune responses following oral immunization, these two areas have converged. The first studies in oral immunization utilizing microbial subunit vaccines were aimed at obtaining protective immune responses to cariogenic bacteria of the mutans streptococci (reviewed in References 24 and 42). Immune responses had been successfully obtained against whole bacteria in an animal model;[43] however, safety concerns that antibodies cross-reactive with human tissues would be induced created an interest in the development of subunit vaccines. To obtain immune responses comparable to whole-cell immunization studies, adjuvant systems with liposomes have been used. As the use of liposomes as a vehicle for oral immunization has evolved, other means of mucosal administration and the use of additional adjuvant strategies are developing. These new approaches will, it is hoped, bring the liposome delivery system closer to large-scale testing of microbial vaccines. This section will summarize the history and current developments in the use of liposomes as adjuvants for potentiating induced immune responses to mucosal pathogens. Several of these studies are listed in Table 2 and are discussed below.

A. VACCINE STUDIES IN ANIMALS AND HUMANS

Liposomes were first used as an antigen carrier for mucosal immunization in a rat caries model in which the immune responses to liposome-incorporated purified cell wall antigens of *Streptococcus sobrinus* were compared to responses obtained using other adjuvant delivery methods.[44] The purpose of the study was to investigate means of obtaining immune responses to purified antigens which afforded as much protection against dental caries as responses obtained with whole-cell preparations. Antigen incorporated into liposomes was found to stimulate as much salivary antibody activity and provide as much protection as antigen administered with other adjuvants such as peptidoglycan, muramyl dipeptide, and water in oil emulsion. The specific antibody responses in groups of animals immunized with purified antigens incorporated into liposomes or given adjuvant were higher than those seen in infected only (control) rats or in rats immunized with whole cells

Table 2 **Immunization studies with liposomal vaccine delivery systems**

Antigen/Adjuvant	Liposome composition	Route of administration	Host	Major findings/References
Cholera toxin/lipoidal amine/lipid A	DPPC, Chol, DP (MLV)	Oral	Rats	Enhanced intestinal IgA response[55,64]
Mutans streptococcal Anti-idiotypic antibodies Carbohydrate Carbohydrate/lipophilic MDP Peptide–CTB Proteins–CTB Proteins Ribosomes	DPPC, Chol, DP (SUV)	Oral	Rats	Adjuvant effect — induction of salivary IgA antibodies; reduced infection by mutans streptococci[28,45-48,58,66]
Mutans streptococcal carbohydrate–protein conjugate		Oral	Rats	Adjuvant effect — induction of serum and salivary antibodies[62,63]
Streptococcus mutans Carbohydrate Glucosyltransferase	DPPC, Chol, DP	Oral	Humans	Adjuvant effect — induction of salivary and serum IgA antibodies[35,61]
Bacteroides gingivalis fimbriae/L18-MDP or GM-53-MDP	DPPC, Chol	Oral or SubQ	Mice	Adjuvant effect — enhanced by GM-53-MDP > L18-MDP (salivary and serum antibodies)[52]

Note: Chol, cholesterol; CTB, choiera toxin B subunit; DMPC, dimyristoyl phosphatidylcholine; DP, dicetyl phosphate; DPPC, dipalmitoyl phosphatidylcholine; MDP, muramyl dipeptide; MLA, monophosphoryl lipid A; MLV, multilamellar vesicles; MTP-PE, muramyl tripeptide phosphatidylethanolamine; PC, phosphatidylcholine; SubQ, subcutaneous; SUV, small unilamellar vesicles.

or antigen only. This study and others[45-48] confirmed the potential usefulness of liposomal antigen delivery systems for use in protecting against mutans streptococci-induced dental caries.

Parasitic and other microbial liposomal-antigen delivery systems for the enhancement of mucosal immunity have been investigated. Rhalem and co-workers[49] found that antigens from *Nippostrongylus brasiliensis* were protective in mice against infection with this helminth when challenged after oral administration, especially when the antigen was given in liposomes. Other studies that have investigated the ability of liposomes to augment the responses (both mucosal and systemic) to oral immunogens have used antigens obtained from pathogens such as *Clostridium tetanus*,[50] *Vibrio cholera*,[51] *Porphyromonas gingivalis*,[52] human immunodeficiency virus,[53] and *Bordetella pertussis*.[54] Because these studies focused on different pathogenic mechanisms than dental caries, the approaches investigated varied somewhat from the original rat caries model. Observing for systemic responses as well as immunization regimens such as oral priming followed by parenteral injection[55] and the use of various liposome components and characteristics are aspects of liposomal immunization which may be important in obtaining optimal immune responses against mucosal pathogens.

Clark and Stokes[56,57] recently published two manuscripts in which mice fed liposomal antigens, in some instances, showed significantly elevated responses in serum but not in intestinal secretions. The authors concluded that liposomes are not a useful adjuvant for oral use. It is likely that certain strong immunogens such as cholera toxin are adversely affected by liposomes by interfering with the recognition and processing of the virgin antigen. Although the authors may be correct in regard to the antigens they were investigating (ovalbumin, keyhole limpet hemocyanin, cholera toxin, and *Escherichia coli* cell wall extract), their results illustrate problems in evaluating mucosal immune responses. As the authors indicated, antibody levels in mucosal responses in their studies were not distributed normally and were characterized by inordinate inter-animal variation. Therefore, their utilization of five to seven animals per group resulted in insufficient statistical power to show a difference in the antibody levels attained. Whether because of problems with sensitivity of assays or an inadequate understanding of the mechanism of protection conferred by mucosal antibodies, it has been our experience[58] (and unpublished results) and the experience of others,[59] that often antibody responses are not significantly different between experimental and control groups; however, differences in protection levels are significant. Therefore, to demonstrate an augmented mucosal antibody response, sufficient numbers of animals/subjects should be tested.

Although the mucosal immune system has been termed "common" because many secretory effector sites are involved in immune responses following mucosal immunization, the magnitude of antibody responses at various sites indicates that compartmentalization does exist. Therefore, oral immunization may be most efficacious for oral and upper gastrointestinal pathogens, but lower intestinal, genitourinary, and pulmonary pathogens may require different approaches for optimal responses. Alternatives to oral immunization using liposomal antigens include nasal, tonsillar, bronchial, vaginal, and rectal routes. Abraham[60] found that intranasal immunization of mice with polysaccharide antigens of pulmonary pathogens in liposomes was more efficient (required less antigen and no additional adjuvants) than oral immunization in preventing mortality when challenged with live organisms.

Oral immunization studies with liposomal antigens in humans are limited to two preliminary studies by our group using the cell wall carbohydrate (CHO)[61] and glucosyltransferase[35] of *S. mutans* (summarized in Table 3). In the first study, a group of four individuals ingested enteric-coated capsules containing liposomal *S. mutans* CHO (500 to 1000 µg/day) for 7 consecutive days. Analysis of salivary anti-CHO IgA antibodies before and after immunization indicated that three subjects responded 4 to 5 weeks

Table 3 **Human salivary IgA immune response after oral immunization with liposomal vaccine**

Oral liposomal *S. mutans* antigen	Subject number	First response	Second response	Third response
Carbohydrate	1	143 (32)[a]	188 (14)	206 (10)
	2	146 (32)	119 (14)	
	3	45 (21)	345 (16)	—
	4	138 (26)	32 (25)	—
Glucosyltransferase	1	39 (28)[b]	—	—
	2	63 (14)	—	—
	3	116 (42)	—	—
	4	31 (28)	—	—
	5	134 (28)	—	—
	6	84 (28)	—	—
	7	238 (21)	—	—

[a] Values = % increase in EU/ml over mean baseline; values in parenthesis = day of peak response.

[b] Values = % increase in specific anti-glucosyltransterase antibody activity per total IgA over baseline; values in parenthesis = day of peak response.

after the oral immunization began. Earlier salivary responses of higher magnitude occurred following second and third immunization of these subjects 6 to 9 months later. In another study, seven individuals ingested capsules containing dehydrated liposomal glucosyltransferase (500 µg; a virulence enzyme of *S. mutans*) for three consecutive days. Analysis of salivary IgA antibody activity to glucosyltransferase showed increases over baseline activity of varying magnitude, with peak responses occurring between 2 and 6 weeks after immunization. Although both studies found strong evidence of salivary immune responses, the numbers of subjects were too small to obtain statistical conclusions. The immune responses were characterized as variable and transient. These findings, in consideration of the animal studies which both support and refute the use of liposomes as effective antigen carriers, illustrate the importance of finding the optimal protocol for induction of long-lasting, and adequate immunity for protection against the disease in question. In the case of liposomal vaccines, factors such as dose, frequency of administration, liposome size, composition and physical characteristics, type of physical association between antigen and liposome, use of other adjunctive compounds (next section), and route(s) of administration are involved in achieving this goal.

As investigators have obtained highly purified microbial antigens, the requirement for immunization strategies to augment the mucosal immune response to orally fed antigens has increased. The cell wall carbohydrate of *S. mutans* has been proposed as a potentially important immunogen for immunization because of the specificity of an immune response which would be obtained. Because the oral cavity is inhabited by many commensal organisms characterized by a balanced ecosystem which, the majority of the time, provides a disease-free environment, it is important that immunization strategies do not adversely alter the microbial balance. Therefore, a carbohydrate-specific immune response against *S. mutans* should not affect colonization with other nonpathogenic streptococci. Although some polysaccharides are strong immunogens (e.g., pneumococcal cell wall carbohydrate), the cell wall carbohydrates of mutans streptococci are weak immunogens. Liposome-incorporation of the carbohydrate of *S. sobrinus*, although found to be immunogenic and protective in the rat caries model, was not as effective as protein antigens.[47] Wachsmann, Bruyere, and co-workers[62,63] found that the carbohydrate of

S. mutans with relatively low immunogenicity was rendered more immunogenic when covalently conjugated to a 74K cell wall protein antigen if given in liposomes.

A novel investigation using liposomal anti-idiotype antibodies to *S. mutans* as an intragastric immunogen was found to induce salivary IgA-specific responses in rats which resulted in significantly lower caries when compared to animals given liposomal nonimmune serum IgG.[58] The results found by these investigators were comparable to protection levels found after injecting anti-idiotypic antibody into salivary glands of the animals.

B. MODIFIED LIPOSOMAL DELIVERY SYSTEMS

In an attempt to obtain long-lasting and protective responses to mucosal immunization using liposomal-antigens, investigators have modified liposomes with various compounds or by altering the liposome/antigen association. In the case of addition of compounds that have inherent adjuvant properties, liposomes, to be useful, should add to these properties by their adjuvancy or other mechanisms, such as protection from inactivation or by promoting uptake by antigen-processing cells of the mucosa.

The rationale for adjuvants chosen for use in mucosal liposome immunization studies has been based on studies with parenteral liposome immunization (reviewed in Reference 9). Analogues of the muramyl peptides (MDP; the minimal component of mycobacterial cell wall with adjuvant qualities) were the first to be investigated as oral liposomal adjuvants. In the original oral liposome/*S. mutans* antigen studies of Michalek and co-workers,[43,44,47] muramyl dipeptides were found to further augment the rat antibody responses as well as caries protection that resulted from liposomal antigens. MDPs have also been found to be useful adjuvants for intragastric immunization of mice with liposomal fimbrial protein from the periodontal pathogen *Bacteroides (Porphyromonas) gingivalis*.[52] Avridine, a lipoidal amine with adjuvant qualities, has also been used with liposomes given orally to rats.[55] This combination of adjuvant and antigen was able to enhance secondary responses to cholera toxin or procholeragenoid, but not the primary response. The importance of immunogen construction was demonstrated by Pierce and co-workers,[64] who showed that lipid A could enhance the development of anti-cholera toxin plasma cells in the lamina propria of intraduodenally immunized animals only when the lipid A was incorporated into liposomes bearing cholera toxin bound to GM1 ganglioside present in the membrane.

The foregoing bacterial and synthetic products are exogenous adjuvants which may be practical for use in animals and humans because of their low toxicity as compared to other effective but toxic adjuvants (e.g., Freund's adjuvant). Another class of potential compounds for use with liposomes is endogenous compounds such as the cytokines IL-2 and IL-4 which were investigated by Abraham and Shah.[65] They found that sIgA titers and specific antibody-secreting cell responses to liposomal bacterial polysaccharides from pulmonary pathogens administered intranasally were greatly augmented when IL-2 was added. In this study, IL-4 did not induce greater responses. Additional studies are needed to identify safe and effective mucosal-specific exogenous and/or endogenous immunopotentiating compounds for co-administration with liposomes. Not only will these adjuvants be useful in vaccine development, but also they will add to the understanding of the mechanism of induction and control of immune responses in the mucosal immune system. Strategies that will promote specific uptake by immune processing cells of the mucosa (e.g., M cell lectins) and selection for sIgA response (e.g., IgA-inducing cytokines) are likely to be one of the keys to useful liposomal vaccine development. In this regard, it is likely that adjuvants identified for mucosal immunization will not be the same as those useful for parenteral immunizations.

V. SUMMARY

During the past 30 years, considerable information has accumulated concerning the use of liposomes for targeted delivery of drugs and/or antigens to host cells via systemic or mucosal routes. Liposomes are microscopic closed vesicles which can be composed of naturally occurring phospholipids for safe use in humans. Types of phospholipids and methods to prepare liposomes have been determined which result in stable, homogeneous vesicles with a good antigen/drug entrapment efficiency. Information has been obtained regarding the composition and charge of the lipid bilayer which would be optimal for incorporating substances into or onto the membrane in order to improve targeting to host cells/tissues, effective antigen presentation, and augmentation of responses. Liposome preparation is simple enough that most laboratories can make them. Convenient procedures are now available to establish the homogeneity of preparations and the biologic and antigenic activity of the incorporated/associated substance(s). These artificial biological membranes have been shown to be taken up by Peyer's patches and result in the induction of mucosal IgA responses in external secretions. Liposomes have been administered intranasally and shown to induce mucosal responses. They have also been safely applied to the eyes and aerosolized into the respiratory tract. The convenience of custom making liposomes that envelope antigen and target proteins for the induction of immune responses makes them ideal for use in vaccine development.

ACKNOWLEDGMENTS

The studies on liposomes from the laboratories of the authors were supported in part by U.S. Public Health Service grants DE 08182, DE 09081, DE 08228, DE 00232, DE 09846, and DE 04217 from the National Institutes of Health. The authors would like to thank Drs. Jenny Katz, Terrance Greenway, Raymond J. Jackson, John S. Schutzbach, and Dawn C. Ward for their critical assessment of this review and Mrs. Vickie Barron for her secretarial support.

REFERENCES

1. Bangham, A.D. and Horne, R.W., Negative staining of phospholipids and their structural modification by surface-active antigens as observed in the electron microscope, *J. Mol. Biol.,* 8, 660, 1964.
2. Bangham, A.D., Standish, M.M., and Watkins, J.C., Diffusion of univalent ions across the lamellae of swollen phospholipids, *J. Mol. Biol.,* 13, 238, 1965.
3. Bockman, D.E. and Cooper, M.D., Pinocytosis by epithelium associated with lymphoid follicles in the bursa of Fabricius, appendix and Peyer's patches. An electron microscopic study, *Am. J. Anat.,* 136, 455, 1973.
4. Owen, R.L. and Jones, A.L., Epithelial cell specialization within human Peyer's patches: An ultrastructural study of intestinal follicles, *Gastroenterology,* 66, 189, 1974.
5. Alving, C.R., Liposomes as carriers of antigens and adjuvants, *J. Immunol. Methods,* 140, 1, 1991.
6. Sato, T. and Sunamoto, J., Recent aspects in the use of liposomes in biotechnology and medicine, *Prog. Lipid Res.,* 31, 345, 1992.
7. Felgner, P.L., Gadek, T.R., Holm, M., Roman, R., Chan, H.W., Wenz, M., Northrop, J.P., Ringold, G.M., and Danielsen, M., Lipofection: a highly efficient, lipid-mediated DNA-transfection procedure, *Proc. Natl. Acad. Sci. U.S.A.,* 84, 7413, 1987.
8. Swenson, C.E., Popescu, M.C., and Ginsberg, R.S., Preparation and use of liposomes in the treatment of microbial infections, *Crit. Rev. Microbiol.,* 15, S1, 1988.

9. Gregoriadis, G., Immunological adjuvants: a role for liposomes, *Immunol. Today*, 11, 89, 1990.

10. Michalek, S.M., Childers, N.K., Katz, J., Denys, F.R., Berry, A.K., Eldridge, J.H., McGhee, J.R., and Curtiss, R., III, Liposomes as oral adjuvants, *Curr. Topics Microbiol. Immunol.*, 146, 51, 1989.

11. New, R.R.C., *Liposomes: A Practical Approach*, Oxford University Press, New York, 1990.

12. Ostro, M.J., Liposomes, *Sci. Am.*, 256, 102, 1987.

13. van Rooijen, N., Liposomes as carrier and immunoadjuvant of vaccine antigens, in *Bacterial Vaccines*, Mizrahi, A., Ed., Alan R. Liss, New York, 1990, 255.

14. Price, C.I. and Horton, J., *Local Liposome Drug Delivery*, R.G. Landes Company, Austin/Georgetown, Texas, 1992, 1.

15. Lasic, D., Liposomes, *Am. Sci.*, 80, 20, 1992.

16. Therien, H.-M., Lair, D., and Shahum, E., Liposomal vaccine: influence of antigen association on the kinetics of the humoral response, *Vaccine*, 8, 558, 1990.

17. Stahn, R.H., Schafer, H., Kunze, M., Malur, J., Ladhoff, A., and Lachman, U., Quantitative reconstitution of isolated influenza haemagglutinin into liposomes by the detergent method and the immunogenicity of haemagglutinin liposomes, *Acta Virol.*, 36, 129, 1992.

18. Cornell, B.A., Fletcher, G.C., Middleburst, J., and Separovic, F., The lower limits to the size of small sonicated vesicles, *Biochim. Biophys. Acta*, 690, 15, 1982.

19. Pagano, R.E. and Weinstein, J.N., Interactions of liposomes with mammalian cells, *Annu. Rev. Biophys. Bioeng.*, 7, 435, 1978.

20. Alving, C.R., Immunologic aspects of liposomes: presentation and processing of liposomal protein and phospholipid antigens, *Biochem. Biophys. Acta*, 1113, 307, 1992.

21. Alving, C.R. and Swartz, G.M., Jr., Antibodies to cholesterol conjugates and liposomes: implications for artherosclerosis and autoimmunity, *Crit. Rev. Immunol.*, 10, 441, 1991.

22. Wassef, N.M., Swartz, G.M., Jr., Alving, C.R., and Kates, M., Antibodies to liposomal phosphatidylcholine and phosphatidylsulfocholine, *Biochem. Cell Biol.*, 68, 54, 1990.

23. Pages, J., Poncet, P., Serban, D., Witz, I., and Bussard, A.E., Relationship between choline derivatives and mouse erythrocyte membrane antigens revealed by mouse monoclonal antibodies. I. Anticholine activity of anti-mouse erythrocyte monoclonal antibodies, *Immunol. Lett.*, 5, 167, 1982.

24. Bangham, A.D., Hill, M.W., and Miller, N.G.A., Preparation and use of liposomes as models of biological membranes, in *Methods in Membrane Biology*, Korn, E.D., Ed., Plenum Press, New York, 1974, 1.

25. Kirby, C.F. and Gregoriadis, G., A simple procedure for preparing liposomes capable of high encapsulation efficiency under mild conditions, in *Liposome Technology*, Vol. 1, Gregoriadis, G., Ed., CRC Press, Boca Raton, FL, 1984, 19.

26. Mayhew, E., Lazo, R., Vail, W.J., King, J., and Green, A.M., Characterization of liposomes prepared using a microemulsifier, *Biochim. Biophys. Acta*, 775, 169, 1984.

27. Childers, N.K., Michalek, S.M., Eldridge, J.H., Denys, F.R., Berry, A.K., and McGhee, J.R., Characterization of liposome suspensions by flow cytometry, *J. Immunol. Methods*, 119, 135, 1989.

28. Michalek, S.M. and Childers, N.K., Development and outlook for a caries vaccine, *Crit. Rev. Oral Biol. Med.*, 1, 37, 1990.

29. Milsmann, M.H., Schwendener, R.A., and Wedner, H.G., The preparation of large single bilayer liposomes by a fast and controlled dialysis, *Biochem. Biophys. Acta*, 512, 147, 1978.

30. Huang, C.H., Studies of phosphatidylcholine vesicles: formation and physical characteristics, *Biochemistry*, 8, 344, 1969.

31. Barenholtz, Y., Gibbes, D., Litman, B.J., Goll, J., Thompson, T.E., and Carlson, F.D., A simple method for the preparation of homogeneous phospholipid vesicles, *Biochemistry*, 16, 2806, 1977.

32. Olson, F., Hunt, C.A., Szoka, F., Jr., Vail, W.J., and Papahadjopoulos, D., Preparation of liposomes of defined size distribution by extrusion through polycarbonate membranes, *Biochem. Biophys. Acta*, 557, 9, 1979.

33. Hope, M.J., Bally, M.B., Webb, G., and Cullis, P.R., Production of large unilamellar vesicles by a rapid extrusion procedure: characterization of size, trapped volume and ability to maintain a membrane potential, *Biochem. Biophys. Acta*, 812, 55, 1985.

34. Gregoriadis, G., daSilva, H., and Florence, A.T., A procedure for the efficient entrapment of drugs in dehydration-rehydration liposomes (DRVs), *Int. J. Pharmaceutic.*, 65, 235, 1990.

35. Childers, N.K., Zhang, S.S., and Michalek, S.M., Oral immunization with dehydrated liposomes containing *Streptococcus mutans* glucosyltransferase (GTF) in humans, in *Recent Advances in Mucosal Immunology*, Jackson, S., Kiyono, H., McGhee, J.R., Mestecky, J., Michalek, S.M., Russell, M.W., Sterzel, J., and Tlaskalova, H., Eds., Plenum Publishing, New York, in press.

36. Harrigan, P.R., Madden, T.D., and Cullins, P.R., Protection of liposomes during dehydration or freezing, *Chem. Phys. Lipids*, 52, 139, 1990.

37. Crowe, L.M. and Crowe, J.H., Stabilization of dry liposomes by carbohydrates, *Develop. Biol. Standard.*, 74, 285, 1991.

38. Childers, N.K., Denys, F.R., McGee, N.F., and Michalek, S.M., Ultrastructural study of liposome uptake by M cells of rat Peyer's patch: an oral vaccine system for delivery of purified antigen, *Regional Immunol.*, 3, 8, 1990.

39. Szoka, Jr., F.C., The macrophage as the principal antigen-presenting cell for liposome-encapsulated antigen, *Res. Immunol.*, 143, 186, 1992.

40. Rowland, R.N. and Woodley, J.F., The stability of liposomes in vitro to pH, bile salts and pancreatic lipase, *Biochim. Biophys. Acta*, 620, 400, 1980.

41. O'Connor, C.J., Wallace, R.G., Iwamoto, K., Taguchi, T., and Sunamoto, J., Bile salt damage of egg phosphatidylcholine liposomes, *Biochim. Biophys. Acta*, 817, 95, 1985.

42. Curtiss, R., III and Michalek, S.M., Vaccines against dental caries due to *Streptococcus mutans*, in *New Generation Vaccines*, Woodrow, G.C. and Levine, M.M., Eds., Marcel Dekker, New York, 1990, 715.

43. Michalek, S.M., McGhee, J.R., Mestecky, J., Arnold, R.R., and Bozzo, L., Ingestion of *Streptococcus mutans* induces secretory immunoglobulin A and caries immunity, *Science*, 192, 1238, 1976.

44. Michalek, S.M., Morisaki, I., Gregory, R.L., Kiyono, H., Hamada, S., and McGhee, J.R., Oral adjuvants enhance IgA responses to *Streptococcus mutans*, *Mol. Immunol.*, 20, 1009, 1983.

45. Gregory, R.L., Michalek, S.M., Richardson, G., Harmon, C., Hilton, T., and McGhee, J.R., Characterization of immune response to oral administration of *Streptococcus sobrinus* ribosomal preparation in liposomes, *Infect. Immun.*, 54, 780, 1986.

46. Wachsmann, D., Klein, J.P., Scholler, M., and Frank, R.M., Local and systemic immune response to orally administered liposome-associated soluble *S. mutans* cell wall antigen, *Immunology*, 54, 189, 1985.

47. Michalek, S.M., Morisaki, I., Gregory, R.L., Kimura, S., Harmon, C.C., Hamada, S., Kotani, S., and McGhee, J.R., Oral adjuvants enhanced salivary IgA responses to purified *Streptococcus mutans* antigens, *Prot. Biol. Fluids*, 32, 47, 1984.

48. Childers, N.K., Michalek, S.M., Denys, F., and McGhee, J.R., Characterization of liposomes for oral vaccines, in *Mucosal Immunology*, Mestecky, J., McGhee, J.R., Bienenstock, J., and Ogra, P.L., Eds., Plenum Press, New York, 1987, 1771.

49. Rhalem, A., Bourdieu, C., Luffau, G., and Pery, P., Vaccination of mice with liposome-entrapped adult antigens of *Nippostrongylus brasiliensis, Ann. Inst. Pasteur/Immunol.,* 139, 157, 1988.

50. Hiraga, C., Ishii, F., and Ichikawa, Y., Oral immunization against tetanus, using liposome-entrapped tetanus toxoid, *Kansenshogaku Zasshi,* 63, 1308, 1989.

51. Chaicumpa, W., Pariaro, J., New, R., Pongponratn, E., Knang Kanaporn, Y., Tapchaiori, P., and Chongsa-Nguan, M., Immunogenicity of liposome-associated oral cholera vaccine prepared from combined *Vibrio cholerae* antigens, *Asian Pac. J. Allergy Immunol.,* 8, 87, 1990.

52. Ogawa, T., Shimauchi, H., and Hamada, S., Mucosal and systemic immune responses in BALB/c mice to *Bacteroides gingivalis* fimbriae administered orally, *Infect. Immun.,* 57, 3466, 1989.

53. Thibodeau, L., Constantineau, L., and Tremblay, C., Oral priming followed by parenteral immunization with HIV-1 immunosomes induces HIV-specific salivary and circulatory IgA in mice and rabbits, *Vaccine Res.,* 1, 233, 1992.

54. Guzman, C.A., Molinari, G., Fountain, M.W., Rohde, M., Timmis, K.N., and Walker, M.J., Antibody responses in the serum and respiratory tract of mice following oral vaccination with liposomes coated with filamentous hemagglutinin and pertussis toxoid, *Infect. Immun.,* 61, 573, 1993.

55. Pierce, N.F. and Sacci, Jr., J.B., Enhanced mucosal priming by cholera toxin and procholeragenoid with a lipoidal amine adjuvant (avridine) delivered in liposomes, *Infect. Immun.,* 44, 469, 1984.

56. Clarke, C. and Stokes, C., The intestinal and serum humoral immune response of mice to systemically and orally administered antigens in liposomes. I. The response to liposome-entrapped soluble proteins, *Vet. Immunol. Immunopathol.,* 32, 125, 1992.

57. Clarke, C. and Stokes, C., The intestinal and serum humoral immune response of mice to orally administered antigens in liposomes. II. The response to liposome-entrapped bacterial proteins, *Vet. Immunol. Immunopathol.,* 32, 139, 1992.

58. Jackson, S., Mestecky, J., Childers, N.K., and Michalek, S.M., Liposomes containing anti-idiotypic antibodies: an oral vaccine to induce protective secretory immune responses specific for pathogens of mucosal surfaces, *Infect. Immun.,* 58, 1932, 1990.

59. Rhodes, M., Baker, P., Christensen, D., and Anderson, G., *Ascaris suum* antigens incorporated into liposomes used to stimulate protection to migrating larvae, *Vet. Parasitol.,* 26, 343, 1988.

60. Abraham, E., Intranasal immunization with bacterial polysaccharide containing liposomes enhances antigen-specific pulmonary secretory antibody response, *Vaccine,* 10, 461, 1992.

61. Childers, N.K., Michalek, S.M., Pritchard, D.G., and McGhee, J.R., Mucosal and systemic responses to an oral liposome-*Streptococcus mutans* carbohydrate vaccine in humans, *Regional Immunol.,* 3, 289, 1991.

62. Wachsmann, D., Klein, J.P., Scholler, M., Ogier, J., Ackerman, F., and Frank, R.M., Serum and salivary antibody responses in rats orally immunized with *Streptococcus mutans* carbohydrate protein conjugate and associated with liposomes, *Infect. Immun.,* 52, 408, 1986.

63. Bruyere, T., Wachsmann, D., Klein, J., Scholler, M., and Frank, R., Local response in rat to liposome-associated *Streptococcus mutans* polysaccharide-protein conjugate, *Vaccine,* 5, 39, 1987.

64. Pierce, N.F., Sacci, J.B., Alving, C.R., and Richardson, E.C., Enhancement of lipid A of mucosal immunogenicity of liposome-associated cholera toxin, *Rev. Infect. Dis.,* 6, 563, 1984.

65. Abraham, E. and Shah, S., Intranasal immunization with liposomes containing IL-2 enhances bacterial polysaccharide antigen-specific pulmonary secretory antibody responses, *J. Immunol.*, 149, 3719, 1992.

66. Michalek, S.M., Childers, N.K., Katz, J., Dertzbaugh, M., Zhang, S., Russell, M.W., Macrina, F.L., Jackson, S., and Mestecky, J., Liposomes and conjugate vaccines for antigen delivery and induction of mucosal immune responses, in *Genetically Engineered Vaccines: Prospects for Oral Disease Prevention*, Ciardi, J., Keith, J., and McGhee, J.R., Eds., Plenum Publishing, New York, 1992, 191.

Index

INDEX